CW00403557

1

MANUAL DE ANALGÉSICOS PARA ENFERMERÍA

AUTORES:
VIRGINIA MARINA GOUTAYER BACHMIAER
MARÍA ISABEL TOMÁS BORREGO

ISBN-13: 978-1984128072
ISBN-10: 1984128078

FECHA DE PUBLICACIÓN:
22 DE ENERO DE 2018

ÍNDICE:

Analgésicos

Los analgésicos son los fármacos empleados para aliviar el dolor. Hay dos grupos:

1) Narcóticos.

Se denominan también opiáceos. El más representativo es la morfina.

Es un alcaloide natural de la Adormidera o Papaver Somniferum. Se usa como patrón para comparar el resto de los fármacos de este grupo.

Se clasifican en dos grupos:

- Opioides menores
Se usan para el dolor moderado
- Codeína.
- Dihidrocodeína.
- Dextropropoxifeno.
- Tramadol.

- Opioides mayores
Se usan para el dolor intenso.

- Buprenorfina.
- Fentanilo. (E)
- Metadona. (E)
- Morfina. (E)
- Petidina. (E)
- Pentazocina.
- Morfina (E)

* (E) Estupefaciente

La morfina es un estupefaciente, actúa sobre los receptores que son estimulados por las endorfinas u opioides de producción endógena.

Estos receptores se localizan en muchos puntos del SNC.

Se distinguen tres tipos:
· m -> "mu"
· d -> "delta"
· k -> "Kappa"

Se caracteriza por tener dos tipos de acciones, unas depresoras y otras estimulantes.

Acciones depresoras:
- Analgesia-> Elimina o disminuye el dolor de gran intensidad, produce

somnolencia y a dosis altas se puede llegar a la hipnosis y coma.

- Acción depresora respiratoria, disminuye la frecuencia respiratoria que puede llegar a producir parada respiratoria a dosis elevadas.

- Deprime el reflejo de la tos.

- Disminuye el peristaltismo intestinal.

- Provoca hipotensión por vasodilatación directa o liberación de histamina y bradicardia.

Acciones estimulantes:

- Miosis.

- Estimula el reflejo del vómito.

- Produce sensación de bienestar y euforia.

- Aumenta el tono intestinal, que junto con la reducción del peristaltismo, produce estreñimiento.

- Aumento del tono de la vejiga por lo que se dificulta la micción.

Se usa en el tratamiento del dolor agudo o crónico de gran intensidad.

En el dolor neuropático (por lesiones de SNC o periférico) es menos eficaz.

Existe una amplia variabilidad entre individuos en el nivel plasmático mínimo necesario para el control del dolor. El rango de concentración en plasma donde se obtiene analgesia con escasos o nulos efectos secundarios es llamada "Terapéutica de los opiáceos", que es específico de cada paciente, por tanto una vez alcanzado el efecto analgésico se debe mantener concentraciones estables del fármaco evitando los picos (que conducen a la presencia de efectos indeseables) y los valles (donde reaparece el dolor)

La administración de morfina en un paciente con dolor crónico, no debe realizarse nunca a demanda del paciente, sino que debe de seguirse un horario fijo que prevenga su aparición.

Ahora se usa mucho una técnica denominada analgésica controlada por el paciente (PCA) que consiste en el automedicamento de analgésico mediante una bomba de infusión que puede ser activada por el paciente, pero cuyos parámetros, en lo referente a dosis e intervalos, están previamente programados para evitar sobredosis.

Se usa generalmente para medicación IV, permitiendo alcanzar concentraciones plasmáticas muy estables dentro de la ventana terapéutica y adaptados a las necesidades de cada individuo.

Esta técnica también puede usarse por vía SC y epidural.

La morfina se puede administrar por distintas vías:

Vías de administración.

- Vía oral; sulfato de morfina.

Existen comercializados de liberación inmediata, para administrar cada 4 horas y de liberación sostenida cada 8 horas.

La dosificación debe ser individualizada, hasta lograr el alivio del dolor.

La dosis inicial 30-60 mg/día.

Solución de Brompton-> jarabe cada 4 horas, las dosis 10ml, variando las concentraciones.

- Vía IV; Cloruro mórfico.

Se puede administrar en perfusión intermitente o continua y es compatible tanto con salino como con glucosado.

Su duración es también de 4 horas.

Esta vía es la más útil en situaciones de urgencia.

La dosis de urgencia es por vía IV lenta a dosis de 0,1 mg/kg.

- Vía IM.

Se usa poco.

La absorción por esta vía va a depender del grado de perfusión tisular.

Una dosis normal es de 10 mg/4 h.

- Vía SC.

Si existe buena perfusión cutánea y no hay edema local, esta vía tiene utilidad en el tratamiento del dolor agudo, pero en el caso contrario la absorción es errática.

La administración crónica en infusión continua e intermitente por vía SC se realiza cada 4 h y se emplea en pacientes en los que la administración oral está contraindicada.

Los niveles obtenidos en plasma son semejantes a los que se obtienen por vía IV.

- Vía espinal, intratecal o epidural.
La morfina actúa selectivamente sobre un segmento de la médula espinal relacionado con la región corporal donde se origina el dolor. Se logra un control efectivo del dolor con una menor dosis y una mayor duración de la analgesia, evitando efectos dependientes de la actuación sistémica del fármaco. La inducción a la tolerancia es muy lenta. También se puede usar cloruro mórfico pero sin conservantes. Si la situación clínica del paciente requiere un cambio de vía oral a la SC, la dosis a de reducirse a la mitad y si es a la IV hay que reducirla 1/3.

Contraindicaciones.
· Pancreatitis.
· Cólico biliar.
· Durante el parto, porque atraviesa la barrera placentaria y produce depresión respiratoria.

- La Codeína.

No es un estupefaciente. Es menos potente que la morfina.

Se usa en el dolor de ligera a moderada intensidad, generalmente asociado a otros analgésicos no narcóticos, como el paracetamol.

Tiene uso como antitusivo en la tos irritativa, apenas produce adicción. No produce adición, pero no se debe abusar de ella.

Efectos secundarios, estreñimiento.

- Metadona.

Si es un estupefaciente.

De potencia y eficacia similar a la morfina, pero su uso a quedado relegado para suprimir el síndrome de abstinencia en pacientes heroinómanos debido a su efecto prolongado.

Debido a este efecto prolongado puede acumularse por lo que hay que tener cuidado.

- La Petidina o mepiridina

Es un estupefaciente. Es un análogo sintético de la morfina, 10 veces menos potente. Desarrolla rápidamente tolerancia y adicción. Produce taquicardia y midriasis por efecto anticolinérgico. No tiene efectos antitusivos y produce poco estreñimiento. Es una alternativa a la morfina cuando existe hiperestimulación vagal. Se emplea en pacientes politraumatizados y en cirugía mayor.

Sustituye a la morfina en el cólico biliar y en el infarto agudo de miocardio cuando hay estimulación vagal (La morfina produce bradicardia y esta se agrava más si hay estimulación vagal).

Sus efectos duran 3-4 horas. Se administra solo por vía parenteral.

- Vía SC.

Produce irritación si se administra repetidamente.

Si vamos a dar dosis múltiples es preferible la vía IM.

- Vía IV.
Puede producir hipotensión.

Efectos adversos
Además de los efectos típicos de los opioides, como la depresión respiratoria, produce efectos neurológicos:
- Convulsiones.
- Temblor.
- Cardiotóxicos; arritmias.

Contraindicaciones
- Pacientes con insuficiencia renal.
Se les acumula un metabolito, "Normeperidina", que es neurotóxico y produce convulsiones que no son antagonizadas por la Noloxona.

- La Buprenorfina.

Ya no se considera estupefaciente, ha pasado a ser un psicotropo.
Lo hay en vía oral y en inyectable. Es un agonista parcial. Si se administra solo, actúa como analgésico, pero si se administra con un agonista puro, antagoniza su efecto,

provocando un moderado síndrome de abstinencia en pacientes previamente tratados con opioides o consumidores de ellos.

Los comprimidos son para administrar sublingualmente, si se tragan, se metabolizan totalmente y no presentan efecto analgésico. Por vía parenteral se prefiere la vía SC a la IV. Es muy potente, de 25 a 30 veces más potente que la morfina y su analgesia es más duradera, de 5 a 8 horas.

Si se administra de forma crónica puede producir tolerancia, pero la dependencia física es menor que otros opioides.

Efectos adversos.
- Nauseas intensas.
- Depresión respiratoria.
- Apenas produce estreñimiento.
- sus efectos cardiovasculares son mínimos.
- Tramadol

Aunque no tiene estructura química de opioide, si actua sobre sus receptores.

Su acción analgésica es moderada, su efecto dura de 6 a 8 horas, se administra 3 veces al día.

Efectos adversos
- Hipotensión ortostática.
- Taquicardia.
- Sequedad de boca.
- Nauseas.
- Vómitos.
- Sedación.
- Cefaleas
- Es raro que produzca sedación respiratoria y estreñimiento.
- Produce de vez en cuando convulsiones y reacciones anafilácticas.

- Fentanilo

· Por vía IV se usa como anestésico.
· Como analgésico; Parches trasdérmicos.
Son útiles en dolor continuo y relativamente constante de origen neoplásico.
En pacientes que están incapacitados o contraindicada la vía oral. Es una

alternativa a la vía parenteral. El efecto persiste horas tras la retirada del parche. Dura 72 horas. Si el paciente presenta dolor se eleva la dosis.

2. Antagonistas de los opiáceos.

- Noloxona

Se utiliza para revertir el efecto de los opiáceos con gran rapidez.
Ampollas de 400 mg.

- Naltrexona

Sólo lo hay por vía oral.
Se emplea en los adictos a opiáceos en las etapas finales de deshabituación para eliminar los efectos residuales.

3) Analgésicos, antitérmicos y antiinflamatorios no esteroideos.

Se denominan también AINE y se determina así para diferenciarlos de los glucocorticoides que son antiinflamatorios con estructura esteroidea. El prototipo de los AINE es el ácido acetil salicílico.

Actualmente hay numerosos fármacos incluidos en este grupo y tienen en común que comparten las acciones analgésicas, antitérmica (antipirética) y la antiinflamatoria.

Con frecuencia se prescriben sin control médico para aliviar dolores de baja intensidad o para bajar la fiebre, pero provocan reacciones adversas algunas bastante graves de las que no son conscientes la mayoría de los consumidores.

El mecanismo de acción de los AINE es inhibir la ciclooxigenasa (enzima que participa en la síntesis de las prostaglandinas, las cuales participan activamente en los mecanismos patógenos de inflamación, dolor y fiebre).

Hay muchos grupos:

+ Salicilatos.
- Acido acetilsalicílico.
- Acetil salicilato de lisina.
- Diflumisol.
+ Paraminofenoles.
- Paracetamol.
+ Pirazolonas.
- Metamizol.
- Fenilbutazona.
+ Acidos propionicos.
- Ibuprofeno.
- Naproxeno.
- Ketoprofeno.
- Flurbiprofeno.
+ Acido acético.
- Indometacina.
- Ketorolaco.
- Diclofenaco.
- Aceclofonaco.
+ Oxicams.
- Piroxicam.
- Meloxicam.
- Fenoxicam.

Son todos analgésicos, antipiréticos y antiinflamatorios, teniendo unos más que otros dependiendo del grupo.

- La Fenilbutazona, Piroxicam y Endometacina, destaca su efecto antiinflamatorio.
- Paracetamol -> Efecto antiinflamatorio irrelevante. Se usa solo como anestésico y antipirético.
No es estrictamente un AINE.

- Todos estos fármacos se administran por vía oral, aunque algunos tienen preparados para inyectar; Metamizol, diclofenaco.
- También los hay en preparados rectales; Endometacina, Naproxeno-
- También los hay de uso tópico, pero sus efectos son cuestionables.
- Piroxicam; se puede administrar por vía sublingual. Es una forma galénica con elevados efectos analgésicos.

Efectos adversos

1) Los más frecuentes son los intestinales. Afectan a la mucosa gástrica y a la duodenal y provocan lesiones que van desde la hiperemia hasta grandes úlceras.

También pueden producir diarreas, estreñimiento, pirosis, esofagitis.

Los pacientes con mayor riesgo son los tratados con altas dosis o con tratamiento muy prolongado.

Hay un gran irritante que es el AAS y también el Piroxicam.

El resto se encuentran en una situación intermedia, siendo los de menor toxicidad, el metamizol y el ibuprofeno administrados a dosis bajas. También el paracetamol.

Para evitarlo hay varias alternativas que se aplican a los grupos de riesgo:

1) Administrar con Misoprostol.

2) Administrar con inhibidores de protones.

3) Administrar con antihistamínicos H2.

2) Efectos hepáticos.

Aumento de las transaminasas, aunque no es muy frecuente y al disminuir las dosis vuelven al los niveles normales.

El Diclofenaco, es el que mayor poder hepatotóxico tiene.

El Paracetamol también. Forma en el hígado un metabolito tóxico que se neutraliza con el glutation.

Si las dosis de paracetamol son muy elevadas, pueden provocar una necrosis aguda en el hígado, por no existir suficiente síntesis de glutation.

No se debe de pasar de 4 g/día de paracetamol (2 comp/6 horas).

3) Efectos hematológicos.
· Anemia aplásica.
· Agranulocitosis.
· Trombocitopenia.
· Hemorragias.

Los producen principalmente; Metamizol, Indometacina, Diclofenaco y Fenilbutazona.

Los pacientes más susceptibles son los que tienen déficit de la enzima glucosa-6-fosfato deshidrogenasa.

4) Efectos neurológicos.

Principalmente la Indometacina.

Se manifiesta en forma de:

· Somnolencia.

· Alucinaciones.

· Confusión.

5) En tratamientos crónicos puede producir hipoacusia permanente y sordera, sobretodo los salicilatos.

También pueden producir pérdidas de sordera transitorias, como son la Indometacina, la Fenilbutazona y el Ibuprofeno.

6) Cutáneos.

· Lesiones vesiculares.

· Eritema.

· Urticaria.

· Fotosensibilidad (más frecuente con Naproxeno y Ketoprofeno)

Aplicaciones terapéuticas

- Tratamiento del dolor leve o moderado, de origen somático o músculo esquelético.

- Dolor postoperatorio, odontológico, cefaleas, dolor visceral (cólicos renales, dismenorrea,...) y en los primeros escalones de la terapia del dolor oncológico.

- Si se usan como antiinflamatorios son a dosis superiores que si se usan como anestésicos.

- Enfermedades reumáticas.

- Gota y tendinitis.

- Como uricosúricos (facilitan la eliminación de ácido úrico) y como antipiréticos; sobre todo el ácido acetilsalicílico y paracetamol.

- El AAS se usa como antiagregante plaquetario para prevenir una trombosis coronaria o cerebral (a dosis bajas).

No se aconseja el uso de dos AINE al mismo tiempo.

Sin embargo aumentan la eficacia si se combinan con un opioide o narcóticos (ej. paracetamol codeína).

Hay que usarlos con precaución en pacientes con úlcera gástrica, cardiopatía, nefropatía, neuropatías y trastornos hematológicos.

El efecto antiinflamatorio no es inmediato, tarda 5-6 días.
· Metamizol -> Si se administra vía IV rápida produce hipotensión.
· Si hay que usar un AINE en el embarazo, se prefiere el paracetamol o el AAS a dosis bajas, y siempre después del primer trimestre.
· El antídoto específico para la intoxicación por Paracetamol es la "N-acetil-cisteína" al 20% en las primeras 8-24 horas, para metabolizar y neutralizar el metabolito tóxico producido por el Paracetamol.
· Los AINES más modernos son:
    - Celocoxib.
    - Rofecoxib.
Actúan muy selectivamente sobre un parte de la encima Cox y presentan menos efectos secundarios y son más potentes, pero son caros.

Antiinflamatorios antigotosus.

La gota es un procedo inflamatorio debido a la retención de ácido úrico.

Se manifiesta con un fuerte dolor en el dedo gordo del pie debido a la formación de uratos no solubles y forman unos cristales llamados tofos.

Si no se trata a tiempo evolucionan a una artritis gotosa o gota crónica. En el ataque agudo de gota el fármaco de elección es la Colchicina.

- Colchicina

Son gránulos que controlan el ataque de 24-48 horas, son de 1 mg y se dan cada 24 h.

No se puede pasar de 15 mg en todo el tratamiento.

Si se sobrepasa aparecen vómitos, diarrea, hemorragia y llegar hasta fracaso renal y shock hipovolémica.

Sino funciona el tratamiento se usan los AINE que son menos eficaces pero también menos tóxicos.

Gota crónica

Si llega a la gota crónica hay dos líneas de actuación en el tratamiento.

1) Fármaco que disminuye la síntesis del ácido úrico. Alopurinol.

- Alopurinol
Es un potente inhibidor de la enzima xantina-oxidasa que es necesaria para la síntesis del ácido úrico.
Se administra por vía oral y se empieza con 100 mg al día que se aumenta progresivamente hasta llegar a los 400 mg. Se administra 1 vez al día y se mantiene una media de 6 meses.
Tiene pocos efectos adversos -> Alguna molestia gástrica.

2) Fármaco que disminuye el ácido úrico al aumentar su eliminación renal. Estos fármacos se llaman Uricosúricos.

Los uricosúricos disminuyen la reabsorción de ácido úrico en los búlbulos renales aumenta su eliminación.

- Probanecid

Es el más clásico.

- Benzbromarona

El que se usa actualmente.

Son comprimidos.

Con estos fármacos se debe beber muchos líquidos para tener una buena diuresis.

Basado en los apuntes de la asignatura de
Farmacología   de la Escuela Universitaria de
Enfermería de "Cabueñes" Plan 97, Segundo Curso.

27092357R00020

Printed in Great Britain
by Amazon

Nicola Thorne is the *author* of a number of best-selling
novels which include *Where the Rivers Meet, Bird of Passage,*
the Rivers Meet, Bird of Passage,*
The Askham Chronicles (*Never Such Innocence,*
Promises, Bright Morning and *A Place in the Sun*). Born in
South Africa, she was educated at the LSE. She lived for
many years in London, but has now made her home in
Dorset.

By the same author

Silk

a novel by
Nicola Thorne

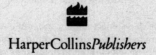

HarperCollins*Publishers*

HarperCollins*Publishers*
77–85 Fulham Palace Road,
Hammersmith, London W6 8JB

This paperback edition 1993
1 3 5 7 9 8 6 4 2

First published in Great Britain by
HarperCollins*Publishers* 1993

Copyright © Nicola Thorne 1993

The Author asserts the moral right to
be identified as the author of this work

ISBN 0 586 21736 3

Set in Meridien

Printed in Great Britain by
HarperCollinsManufacturing Glasgow

All rights reserved. No part of this publication may be
reproduced, stored in a retrieval system, or transmitted,
in any form or by any means, electronic, mechanical,
photocopying, recording or otherwise, without the prior
permission of the publishers.

This book is sold subject to the condition that it shall not,
by way of trade or otherwise, be lent, re-sold, hired out or
otherwise circulated without the publisher's prior consent
in any form of binding or cover other than that in which it
is published and without a similar condition including this
condition being imposed on the subsequent purchaser.

For Sybil and Basil Brooke
with love and many thanks

CONTENTS

PROLOGUE

Worlds to conquer

Under cover of darkness no one saw the youth swing himself aboard the ship using one of the ropes tossed over the side from a cargo hatch on the foredeck.

The port of Alexandria was a busy one with craft of all kinds – the swift feluccas propelled by sail and oar, the slow *dahabeih* used for journeys down the Nile, ocean-going liners, tramp steamers plying their wares among the ports of the Mediterranean and the heavy-duty cargo ships, like this one, which crossed back and forth across the mighty oceans of the world.

It was nightfall, the silhouettes of the ships anchored in the bay visible against the pinky opalescence of the evening sky. Lights from the small craft, busy finding the night's moorings, were reflected in the oily waters of the bay, and the young man stood anxiously on the deck, fearful that his journey might be ended before it had begun.

He saw a movement by the gunwale and ducked behind a hatch while a sailor, casually lighting a cigarette, passed by. Then, keeping to the shadows, the visitor made his way swiftly along the boat and through a door. Here he found himself in a dimly lit corridor with port-holes on to the deck on one side, a number of doors on the other. He tried the handle of one, it was locked. Then another, locked too. Someone from within called out and he hurried along to the end just as he heard the sound of a siren as though the boat were about to weigh anchor and put to sea.

He tugged desperately at a door and it opened. Inside it was pitch dark; there was a stench of polish, of spirits, some sort of cupboard with pails, brushes and brooms. The boat lurched as though it was preparing to leave dock.

He sat on the floor and leaned his head against the wall. Nothing worse could happen to him than had happened already. He was very, very tired.

He didn't know how long it was before the door was thrown open and the shadow of a woman loomed on the threshold. She gasped, put a hand to her mouth, but before she could scream he sprang up.

'Don't,' he whispered grabbing her arm, 'please don't. I won't hurt you. Please . . . I've come a long long way. I desperately need to get away.'

'What have you done?' She took her hand away from her mouth and he could sense her trying to make out his features in the semi-dark.

'I've done nothing to be ashamed of. I promise you. Please help me. I'll make it worth your while. I'll never forget you. Please.'

He was about twenty, she thought, maybe younger. He had several days' growth of stubble on his face, worn jeans, a shirt under a torn jacket and rope-soled shoes. He had very beautiful dark brown eyes and his expression was one of gentility, but also of sadness. His English was poor.

'You know what happens to stowaways,' she said sternly.

'I know. Give me a break,' he repeated. 'Please.'

She appeared to think for a long time before making up her mind.

'If I'm found with a knife in my throat I deserve it; but I'll trust you. This is a cargo boat, but we carry passengers. It so happens one of them hasn't joined the ship and there's a cabin free. You're in luck.'

4

'You'll never regret it,' he said, seizing her hand and bringing it to his lips, a gesture she found incongruous, charming, and also somehow reassuring.

That night they lay together in the single bunk in the cabin and she felt they were like two orphans who had found each other in the storm. She would never know why she'd behaved as she had. A stewardess on the ship registered in Southampton, the captain would sack her without a moment's thought if he found out. The stowaway was much younger than she was; he was vulnerable. He needed a mother more than a mistress. But she was lonely, too. He appeared to have no family and nor did she; they were outcasts, wandering on the face of the earth.

When she fell asleep her companion continued to lie on his back, wide awake: it was hard to believe that he was on his way to the west and prosperity, that he had found shelter and a woman who needed him as much as he needed her.

She was beautiful in a strange sort of way, part Egyptian – part what? He didn't know. They had talked very little, hungry to make love.

It always happened to him just when he thought his luck had run out. He found somewhere: a refuge, a woman, a new way of life. Perhaps now he had reached journey's end. With a deep sigh he put his arm around her, watching the reflection of the bright, garish lights of Alexandria fade through the porthole as the ship sailed out on the high tide towards the open sea, taking him with his aspirations, his hopes of worlds to conquer.

PART I

*A partridge in
a pear tree*

CHAPTER 1

Sitting on a table, swinging her long shapely bare legs, Ginny took stock of Simeon Varga who stood at the end of the room talking to the agency boss, Len Morgan. Arguing might be a more accurate description. The meeting, which had just ended, had been an acrimonious one; tempers were frayed, voices often raised to anger. It was very hot and the men had discarded jackets and loosened ties, or removed them altogether.

Ginny, warned by the weather forecast for the day, had worn the minimum: a cotton dress – although stylish, from Conran – no stockings, low-heeled sandals. The business suit with its accessories had been left in the wardrobe.

Now she perched on a table near the window, wishing that she could open it to admit a refreshing breeze, but at twenty-eight floors up from ground level the windows of the office in Victoria didn't open. The air conditioning was not as effective as it might have been and the atmosphere was hot and oppressive, undoubtedly contributing to the tension.

It certainly hadn't helped that such an important meeting should be held on a rare hot English summer's day.

Ginny had not previously met Simeon Varga, but already he was becoming a legend in the business community: an innovator, an entrepreneur who went after deals; someone with an instinct for success. Yet the man

9

himself was a mystery: reclusive, withdrawn, some said even shy. No one was quite certain where he'd come from and he was secretive about his private life. Len Morgan had said that Simeon Varga was an assumed name. Yet it suited him.

Just then the subject of her speculation turned round and looked straight at her. She raised a hand and smiled, and he quickly said something to Len, who turned away as Varga walked over to Ginny, picking up his jacket on the way and slipping his arms into the sleeves. She noted that it was impeccably cut, lightweight, and more suitable to a hot day than the suits worn by the other men in the room, who had included two of Varga's advisers, his accountant and the media director of the advertising agency, besides herself and Len Morgan, whose executive assistant she was.

'Thank you for the contribution you made to the discussion, Miss Silklander,' Varga said, holding out his hand. 'In fact I think you made more sense than anyone.'

'Kind of you to say so.' Ginny jumped off the table and smoothed down her dress. His steady gaze made her feel awkward, as though she were somehow incorrectly dressed in this room full of men in suits.

'I'd like to take the points you made a little further. Would it be convenient for you to call at my office?'

'Of course.' She felt pleased, flattered but, at the same time, rather nervous of how Len might take this snub.

'Could we meet tomorrow morning at nine?'

'Nine?' She looked at him startled.

'Nine is quite late for me. I'm in the office by seven.'

'Nine it is, then.' Ginny looked straight into his eyes. It would not do to let him know that one was the least afraid or in awe of him.

Then with a curious half-smile he turned his back as the men from his entourage joined him, also shrugging their arms into their jackets, knotting their ties, taking up documents and document cases from the paper-strewn boardroom table.

'Tomorrow at nine, Miss Silklander,' Varga said and turned abruptly to his associates, indicating that they should follow him from the room.

Ginny gazed after them, aware of Len standing beside her, knowing that he was angry. His face was red and his breathing laboured. He was overweight and he smoked too much, but it wasn't just because of that, or the heat.

'What a bugger he is,' Len said crossly. 'He's the most awkward cuss I've ever come across.'

'Oh I don't think so, Len.' Ginny turned to him and smiled. 'It's simply that he's more than your match.'

'Big-headed, over-confident.' Len ignored her. 'What *is* he, for Christ's sake?' He drew out a cigarette from his crumpled packet, lit it, coughed until his face was purple, and then exhaled.

'You should give that up, Len,' Ginny said casually, going over to pour him a glass of water from the jug on the table.

'Now don't you start.'

'I'm sure Mr Varga doesn't smoke.'

'I'm sure he doesn't. He's got everything perfectly under control. Tell me, Ginny,' Len leaned against the door, cigarette in his mouth, 'now if he's so clever why does he need us?'

'He knows what he's doing,' she said. 'He needs our expertise, but he won't be browbeaten. He did, however, like my ideas; enough to ask me to go and see him tomorrow. At nine.'

'Nine.' Len smiled. 'He'll be lucky.'

Just before nine the following morning Ginny drove her Golf GT into the yard of Varga's factory, parked, got out quickly and on the dot of nine was in the reception area, where she was told that Mr Varga was expecting her. 'He always gets in at seven,' the receptionist informed her superciliously.

'Sorry I'm late,' Ginny murmured as she was shown

11

into his presence. 'Two minutes, I think.'

'I like you, Miss Silklander, I really do.' Varga came towards her, reaching for her document case and showing her to a chair. He then sat not at his desk but in the chair facing her and joined his hands under his chin, regarding her gravely. Anyone else and she would have thought they were making a pass.

'It *is* Miss Silklander, isn't it?'

'It is.'

Inwardly she bridled at the chauvinistic question. But this was business, an important, potentially very important, client, whatever Len Morgan said.

Already she was taking papers from her case and spreading them on the coffee table between them. The office was furnished functionally: teak furniture, steel filing cabinets, curtains that had probably come ready made from Marks and Spencer. The wall to wall carpeting was good quality cord. There was a table next to his desk with a battery of VDUs, telephones, and a fax machine; a large castor oil plant wilted in the corner. On the walls hung reproductions of a few well-known paintings, chosen without much discrimination or taste. It was an impersonal ambience which told you very little about the occupant.

Varga was watching every move, his expression carefully guarded as if to ward off the unexpected question. His black hair, brushed straight back from his high forehead, curled slightly at the sides. His smooth olive skin made him look younger than he was: Len had said he was about forty. He had a delicately curved mouth, an aquiline nose and a pair of beautiful brown eyes that somehow seemed to contrast with his perceived personality. The eyes remained watchful, cautious, suspicious. Above all the overwhelming impression they made was one of sadness: deep, impenetrable sadness. She imagined that at some time in his life he had been badly hurt. The eyes were those of a person who had reason to distrust his fellow men.

'I was up most of the night going over my plans,' Ginny said. 'My partner didn't get a wink of sleep.'

'Oh, you've a partner?' Varga smiled briefly as if registering the fact.

'Well, I had until this morning. He looked rather tired at breakfast.'

Varga's smile became expansive.

'You have a dry sense of humour, Miss Silklander.'

'You may as well call me Ginny,' she said offhandedly. 'We tend to use christian names in our business.'

He nodded, but didn't say, 'And you must call me Simeon.' She hadn't expected that he would. She knew he didn't yet quite trust her.

'You see the whole point of employing public relations advisers, Ginny, is that I need to be better known, my products more widely advertised without my spending a fortune. If your company doesn't come up with something positive I shall not hesitate to dispense with its services. I'm no sentimentalist.'

'I think Len Morgan is fully aware of that.' Ginny glanced at the typed pages in front of her, placed her hand on her brow and studied them. The temperature had plummeted several degrees overnight and she wore a lightweight houndstooth business suit over a navy vest with a round neckline. Her thick black hair fell across her face and her eyes were the colour of cornflowers, a deep royal blue: remarkable eyes. Her nose was broad, her mouth rather large and, though she could not strictly be called beautiful, she was arresting. Tall, striking – people always looked at her twice.

Her figure was fashionably thin, small-bosomed, narrow-hipped – long lanky legs and slim hands with tapered fingers, the nails polished as though with an old-fashioned chamois buffer rather than varnished. She seemed the epitome of the young modern successful woman, as ambitious as the male and as capable. At twenty-seven she was, indeed, in her prime: experienced, able, trusted.

She was not the quintessential English rose, but she was the quintessential English woman of a style Varga particularly admired. His admiration was palpable. He felt at ease in her company as he had not felt at ease among her companions in her office the day before.

'Now,' his manner changed and became businesslike. 'Your suggestion yesterday was that to achieve my ambitions it was not enough for Ace to grow. I should buy another company. Why do you think that?'

'Because,' she said slowly, 'I am convinced it will be very hard to give your company the proper image. The products you manufacture are too downmarket. It is very hard to give a higher profile to a brand that sells in cheap stores. I'm sorry to tell you this, and I know it upsets you, but nevertheless it is true.'

She saw that Varga's sallow skin had turned a dull red and his mouth had tightened into a stubborn thin line.

'Country Bouquet has been taken by some of the big multiples; the whole range has been taken by . . .'

'But that's not the image you want to project, is it, Simeon?' She was going to use his christian name anyway. 'You want to be up with Patou, Lanvin or Dior, and that's where all your profits and prestige will come from.'

'You expect *me* to buy a Patou or Lanvin?'

'Oh no,' Ginny sighed and glanced with resignation at her notes. 'What we are looking for, that is if you agree, is a company with a good name that is in difficulties . . . not as easy as you think,' she said quickly, noticing the expression of irritation that flitted over his face. 'But my boyfriend happens to be a merchant banker, which is why he spent most of last night working on this with me. His computer is plugged into the office terminal and he went through as many of the possibilities as he could. So far,' she sighed and brushed the thick hair back from her face again, 'he's come up with nothing; but today he's going to look at the foreign markets, preferably

French. A French perfume would set you up and give you just the image you need.'

Simeon sat back in his chair, appearing suddenly interested and thoughtful. His surprisingly mobile features made his expression more conciliatory, the alert brown eyes unsuspicious at last. Ginny thought that, far from being a business entrepreneur who had taken his pharmaceuticals company from nothing to a full Stock Exchange quotation in ten years, one would have imagined him a savant; an academic, a thinker, rather than a man of action, a tough almost mean negotiator with a lousy temper.

A man of contradictions: Simeon Varga.

Ace Pharmaceuticals had been a small company which tested products for larger companies. Varga had bought it when its shares on the USM were a few pence, not because he knew anything about pharmaceuticals, but because he wanted it as a vehicle for his ambitious ideas. It already manufactured a fragrance called Fleur which was fresh-smelling and inexpensive. Varga had tried to exploit this into a range of cosmetics, renamed Country Bouquet, increase its outlets and make it grow.

Applying his considerable energies Varga had aggressively marketed his product, re-packaged it, but its low cost meant the range was only destined to grace the bathrooms and the dressing tables of people who bought in multiples and counted their pennies, who were undiscriminating about the subtleties of a fragrance and just wanted something to splash about.

Thinking that promotion was what was needed Varga had been recommended to the firm of public relations consultants started and run by the brilliant Len Morgan, a man, Varga thought, very like himself: aggressive, ambitious, anxious as he was to topple the smug products of the British ruling classes who he believed still reigned over the top echelons of industry with their access to money, privilege and the endless ramifications of the 'old boy network' created by the public school system.

Len Morgan was less secretive about his origins than Simeon Varga, who could never be persuaded to talk about himself at all and resolutely declined to give personal interviews. The product must succeed on its own, Varga had insisted: he and his family had nothing to do with it.

Morgan was intrigued by the man more than the product; yet he had tried to lift it from the supermarkets to some of the better stores like Selfridge's and the Fraser Group, but without success. Country Bouquet was linked to the multiples, mail order catalogues, and the stormy meeting the day before at Morgan's skyscraper offices in Victoria had been to tell Varga just that.

It was then that Ginny Silklander had come up with the idea of buying in order to expand. Another company, another product, another image.

That was why she was here.

Ginny Silklander was a classless all-rounder who happened to be a product of an old baronial family. She was a high achiever who had taken a degree, done a secretarial course, worked first on a newspaper, then with an independent television company where she met Len Morgan who had been engaged to promote the network.

There was a handful of public relations companies with the skill to be trusted by large organizations and important men with their secrets and Len Morgan was the latest in the line. He had worked in advertising, PR, television and newspapers. Yet, unlike Ginny, his background was middle class, grammar school, provincial university, which he left without a degree.

Taking Ginny round the factory after their talk Varga proved himself versatile and knowledgeable about all aspects of the business, pausing in the extensive, well-equipped laboratories to show her the latest high-tech gas chromatography and mass spectrometry machines whose purpose was to analyse and measure the

16

components of the ingredients used in the manufacture of cosmetics.

It was amazing how many machines there were, yet how few staff.

'We are fully automated, you see.' Varga proudly indicated a room full of machines run by two white-coated personnel. 'And this is only the lab where we do our testing. We never use animals; I am quite against it. Here,' he led her into another room even larger, equipped with yet more machines, but with more staff peering down microscopes or working on the columns of figures produced by the VDUs on their benches. 'Here we do our testing for the products of other companies. This was the core business when I started it.'

'You actually started it from scratch?' Ginny looked at him admiringly.

'I bought it,' he said with a shrug of his shoulders, 'when the shares were only worth a few pence, penny shares as we call them. I think it was 7p. Now they're worth 376p, and rising. Which is why I came to see Morgan.'

Varga stopped by an empty bench and leaned against it, causing Ginny to stop too. 'I tell you, Ginny, Morgan has not done much for *me* for a fee of fifty thousand a year. I am not exactly satisfied with him.'

'You should see what he charges other companies.' Ginny smiled. 'That's peanuts.'

'To me it is a lot.'

'Your share performance has improved since we came on the scene. However,' Ginny put a hand firmly on the bench and leaned towards him, 'I think now you are wasting your money unless you diversify in order to enlarge. There are certainly a lot of better things you could do with that fifty thousand, unless you change your outlook.'

In silence Varga led her along the corridor towards the entrance where a receptionist looked up uninterestedly from her desk.

'Did you come by taxi?' Varga enquired.

'Car.'

He stood in the reception area frowning, hands in his pockets.

'This boyfriend of yours, the merchant banker. What's his name?'

'Robert Ward.'

Varga took a card out of his breast pocket, scribbled a number and handed it to her.

'If he comes up with any bright ideas over the weekend, this is the number of my private telephone. Call me at any time, night or day.' He then abruptly turned his back on her and disappeared through a half-open door, leaving her to find her own way to her car as though he'd already forgotten her.

Ginny's family and the Wards had known one another for generations. The Ward family was about as old as the Silklanders and Robert's father, the thirteenth baron, had been at school with Gerald Silklander. They were even related, but the degree of kinship was too remote to be significant.

Robert also came from a large, comfortable family and, sharing the same background, friends since childhood, they had always been at ease with each other, but it was only in London that familiarity had blossomed into love.

They had a lot in common: intellectual interests, sporting interests, above all business interests. They were both ambitious. Robert worked for the merchant bank Law, Fairhurst, and again there was a close family connection; the present senior partner, Eliott Law, had been at school with Gerald Silklander.

Robert and Ginny moved in that kind of world where doors were always opening, where privilege and connections were like the links in a chain. They lived in a small house in Kentish Town, north London, and both sets of parents would have preferred it if they had married. Robert would quite have liked it, too, but Ginny thought it would harm her career if she was Mrs Robert Ward, and she wanted to be sure of a partnership in the agency before she took such a step. She thought they might marry when she was about thirty and she would dutifully have a couple of babies while retaining her interest in the business.

Robert was tall and fair-haired, blue-eyed, pink-cheeked, an athlete, a Blue, a member of the Garrick Club, captain of his cricket club and a local Tory councillor. One day he thought he might stand for Parliament. The only thing that he and Ginny disagreed about was politics. She wasn't a true blue Tory like Robert. In fact she was apolitical, the archetypal floating voter. Robert, however, considered himself a progressive Tory and in his ward, where people of all kinds rubbed shoulders, he did a lot to alleviate the plight of those who were less well off. He was a kind and compassionate Tory rather than a greedy, grasping one.

Domestically he was good too. Whoever got in first started the dinner and thus it was almost ready when Ginny arrived home late on the evening of the day she had seen Simeon Varga.

'Sorry, darling,' she said, kissing him. 'I should have rung.'

Robert stoically popped another handful of nuts in his mouth and poured her a glass of white wine.

'No matter. Tomorrow there's a council meeting, so it's your turn. How was Varga?'

Ginny flopped into a chair and sipped her wine, looking thoughtful.

'He's a strange man.'

'Was he interested in the proposal?' Robert sat on the sofa beside her, an apron round his middle, a scotch, the second or third that evening, in his hand.

'I think so. Did you come up with anything?'

Robert rose and, putting his glass on the mantelpiece, reached for a large envelope he had stuck behind the carriage clock in the middle of it. The house was Victorian

19

and had been lovingly furnished with as many pieces of genuine Victoriana as they could find; the carriage clock had been made by Frodsham in England in an age when thousands of the clocks had flooded the market from overseas, particularly France and America. The clock had been a housewarming present from the Silklanders and was always kept ten minutes fast as Ginny was a poor timekeeper, a fault which punctual Robert tolerated.

Robert handed the envelope to Ginny and then, while she read the contents, refilled her glass.

'Oriole,' she murmured, leafing through the pages of the report which he had put together during the day. 'I've heard of it. I think . . .' she looked up at Robert, who nodded vehemently.

'It was as prestigious in its day as Chanel or Lanvin, and dates from about the same time, the twenties. Oriole's L'Esprit du Temps was worn by our grand-mothers, the bright young things. It is badly in need of an injection of cash, and ideas. A new product. L'Esprit du Temps sells nothing like the quantities it used to. I think Varga is just the man if what you say about him is correct . . . and I'm sure it is,' he added loyally.

'How much would they be looking for?'

'About five million francs . . .'

'£500,000, not bad.'

'It's also quoted on the Bourse; that will be useful.'

'Would you be interested in financing Varga?'

'We might.' Robert looked at the clock and checked it with his watch. It was now after nine. 'Let's eat, darling. I haven't had a bite all day since a sandwich and a pint at lunchtime, except for these nuts.'

They ate as usual in the kitchen which looked on to a small yard prettified by a leaning lilac tree with honey-suckle and clematis climbing profusely over the wall.

To start Robert had provided taramasalata from the Greek delicatessen in the high street, and to follow were grilled lamb chops and salad made with feta cheese. Neither of them drank much so they finished off the white, a Chablis. Robert was a connoisseur. A small shed next to the house which had once housed coal had been made into a wine cellar, and Robert kept it well stocked.

They spoke little during the meal. Afterwards they sat drinking coffee, having shared the clearing away and stacked the dishwasher. They sat on the bench in the yard, Robert's arm loosely round Ginny, a prelude to the intimacy they would enjoy at bedtime.

'Hot,' Ginny said, fanning her face. 'Do you think we might move out of town, Robert?'

'Are you serious?' He looked at her.

'How about Brighton? We could commute. Lots of people do.'

'I think you must be getting broody, Ginny.' He tightened his arm around her bare shoulder. She had changed into shorts and a strapless top as soon as she came in.

'Oh no, I'm not thinking of domesticity.' She looked mockingly at him. 'Don't kid yourself. I'm thinking of a better way of life – open spaces, the sight of the sea. Perhaps we could buy a boat?'

'Ginny, if you're serious,' Robert refilled their cups from the percolator, 'sure, let's get a country place. I'm all for it. A little place near the sea would suit me fine. But I think we should remain in London during the week. I've got my political work.'

'Of course.' She bit her lip. Truth to tell the political work was the one thing that got her down. That and having to be nice to the constituents. What would it be like if he got a parliamentary constituency?

As if reading her mind, Robert said: 'There *is*, as a matter of fact, likely to be a vacancy in a constituency near Brighton. The member, a Tory, isn't standing again. If I could get on the short list I think I'd be in with a very good chance.'

'I *thought* politics would come into it,' Ginny said wryly and, with a sigh, she sat up and walked towards the fence. She stood for a moment or two inhaling the subtle

21

fragrance of the pinky-orange Albertine which reminded her of summer holidays and the country cottage she so wished to have.

She felt Robert's hands on her shoulders and turned.

'You *have* said you accepted it, darling.' He looked anxiously into her eyes. 'The prospect of a life in politics.'

'I know and I do.' She reached up and tenderly brushed a lock of hair away from his eyes. 'You too accept my wanting to work. In a relationship there has to be give and take. I think we do pretty well.' She continued to stroke his hair. 'I know you'd like to be married, Robert, and have kids. You'd like that now. I know you're making a sacrifice for me.'

'I'm committed to you, Ginny,' he said, gently drawing her body close to his and kissing her.

Later she lay in bed unable to sleep, aware of his steady breathing beside her, his arm flung loosely around her bare waist. It was hot and there was no sheet on the bed; their moist bodies gleamed in the moonlight that shone through the open window.

She wasn't thinking about Robert but about Simeon Varga, about his brown, velvety eyes, warm, full of life, but also sad; unfathomable, interesting eyes. She recalled his long, brown thin hands, the fine dark hairs on the backs. His nails were round and pared, beautifully kept. He wore a gold signet ring, no wedding ring, but she knew he was married: an Anglo-Italian wife, two children. That was all. He gave nothing away, remained very protective of his privacy.

Despite his uncertainty, his restrained but stylish and expensive clothes, there was an animal magnetism about him: he exuded sex in a strong, powerful way like no other man she'd ever known. It worried and unnerved her that he should be on her mind when she and Robert had just made love; when they were committed to each other for the rest of their lives.

*

The limousine that had collected them from Charles de Gaulle airport on behalf of the Paris arm of Robert's bank came to a stop in front of the unimposing premises in an anonymous suburb on the outskirts of Paris. Looking at the façade Ginny's heart sank. Even the sign ORIOLE was in need of repair. One of the Os had a deep crack in it and the E was lopsided. The building was shabby and badly in need of restoration. She looked at Robert, who shrugged offhandedly, while Varga gazed straight in front of him as if he hadn't noticed.

He'd sat next to Robert on the flight discussing the sales figures for Oriole and the kind of money that would be needed to buy it. The result seemed to have made him pensive and he had said little in the car.

Ginny could tell that Robert was rather taken aback by Varga, whom he'd met for the first time that morning shortly before the plane took off. Apparently other predators were after Oriole and there was little time to lose. Robert, however, maintained the sangfroid of the international merchant banker, giving nothing away; face grave, thoughtful; immaculate in his grey pinstripe suit, blue shirt with the stiff white collar and Garrick Club tie.

As soon as the car stopped the chauffeur left his seat and ran round to open the door. On the steps of the Oriole building stood three grave-faced men, their expressions bleak and unwelcoming. One of them stepped forward and gravely shook hands with Robert who, speaking perfect French, introduced first Varga and then Ginny.

'Gustave Jacquet, the managing director of Oriole,' Robert said, and then turned as M. Jacquet introduced his colleagues: the marketing manager and the finance director. He then stood back and gestured towards the door while, with a deprecating cough, the finance director led the way.

The inside of Oriole was as unimpressive as outside. The entrance hall was dark and musty, badly in need of redecoration, and the office into which M. Jacquet led the party looked as though it had had very little attention since the firm was founded a few years after the First World War.

A secretary emerged from an inner door and M. Jacquet ordered coffee, then he invited his guests to be seated before sitting down at his desk himself, the two directors ranging themselves on either side of him. Ginny noticed that Varga kept his eyes on Jacquet, seemingly impervious to his surroundings.

Jacquet joined his hands neatly in front of him, and avoiding Varga's penetrating gaze, looked straight ahead.

'You know, gentlemen, and Mademoiselle Silklander, that this enquiry is not welcome. We do not regard a hostile bid . . .'

'I assure you there will be no hostility.' Varga also spoke impeccable French. 'If the business suits us we shall invite your co-operation. Without that there is no point in proceeding any further.' He glanced at his watch. 'Not even to drink coffee.'

'Ah!' Jacquet leaned back and glanced nervously at his colleagues. 'This is not what I understood. I thought you wanted to *own* the company? It was founded by my grandfather and has been run with pride by my father and myself since then. My son is poised to take over. The last thing *I* wish is to relinquish control of it.'

'But I understood you needed investment to proceed.' Robert's tone was conciliatory.

'Investment, yes. It is not the same thing as control. But if you only wish a share . . .'

'I wish control,' Varga said firmly, 'but on a friendly basis. We reorganize the finances, restore the building, and you remain in charge to develop new lines and,' he turned to Ginny, 'with the aid of the company represented by Mademoiselle Silklander, promote your greatest asset, L'Esprit du Temps, maybe with new packaging.'

'L'Esprit du Temps came out of the first war,' Jacquet said in a broken voice. 'My grandfather had been a "nose" for Lanvin. He founded the company even though he had been gravely wounded and his sense of smell was almost destroyed by gassing. My father was a young apprentice and had developed the "nose" even before he left school. L'Esprit du Temps owed its success to him, a young man scarcely out of short trousers. My father was a genius: alas, he lacked the killer business instinct.'

'History is all very well,' Varga said drily, 'but now we need to advance towards the millennium. You do agree, Monsieur Jacquet, don't you?'

Jacquet shrugged his shoulders. His jacket didn't fit well. He looked pathetic; his face was that of a tired, worried man who had hung on for as long as he dared rather than see his company go under. Maybe he didn't pay himself enough in his effort to keep going.

At that moment the secretary entered with a tray of coffee cups which she passed round with a face devoid of expression. Somehow it seemed as though she too had lost hope, and Ginny imagined that the whole place was full of tired, hopeless people.

And so it turned out when they were conducted through the laboratories with the old-fashioned equipment, along the winding corridors that led from one part of the building to the next. There was the same dismal atmosphere of defeat, the same forlorn expressions on the faces of the laboratory technicians, the secretarial workers, the clerks in the despatch and invoicing departments.

The tour took about an hour. Jacquet explained everything as though he were in a great hurry. Varga asked a few pertinent questions; Robert and Ginny said very little. Finally, back in the main office, there was silence for a few moments as if Varga was searching the recesses of his mind for the right words.

The finance director, who had not joined them on the tour, had not reappeared and the marketing manager gazed disconsolately in front of him, his expression that of a man who expected very soon to lose his job. Even Varga seemed to have difficulty in voicing his feelings.

'Well!' Jacquet said, nervously. 'As you see, there is a need for investment.'

'There is a need,' Varga said in a low, patient voice, 'for complete restructuring if you are to survive. With the equipment you have, Monsieur Jacquet, it is a wonder to me that you are still in business. Some of it dates from before the Second World War.'

'We have relied very much on L'Esprit du Temps.'

'There is an urgent need for new equipment, new product development. New . . .' Varga stood up, 'thinking and restructuring; a complete change of attitude and outlook on the part of your staff. The whole place smells of decay and defeat. I have to see whether the investment I may make would be worthwhile – for me and for you.' Varga then leaned over and shook Jacquet's hand firmly. 'We will not detain you any longer, Monsieur Jacquet. My advisers will shortly be in touch with you, to give you a decision, one way or another.'

CHAPTER 2

Len Morgan looked at the clean-cut limbs, the alluring expression on the face of the model and nodded with approval. He flicked through the various poses: the outdoor girl, the slinky siren of the night, the pouting *femme fatale*, the girl about town, and wondered, as he often did, how the same person could show so many aspects of herself in one sitting.

'Good,' he said to Ginny, who had brought him the portfolio. 'Has Varga seen them?'

'I thought we should show Varga when we have made up our minds.' Ginny sank back in her chair. 'He is such a perfectionist that if he rejects them we'll have to start all over again.'

A picture in his hand, Len turned and studied her.

'He really is an oddball, isn't he?'

'Very.' Ginny reached up to brush her hair away from her face. 'I don't know if I like him or hate him.'

'As strong as that?'

'Well, not hate. He's cold.' Suddenly she shuddered, as though an icy blast had blown through the room. 'You don't know what he's thinking. I've never known anyone quite like him.'

'Yet he likes you. Admires you. He particularly asked you should be put in charge of his account.'

'Oh I know, and he likes Robert. He says he's straight. Robert is not as sure of his opinion. When we first went to see Oriole, Varga promised they would all remain in their jobs. Now he's considering getting rid of the Jacquet family altogether. Robert says it's not quite straight. He's going back on his word.'

'I suppose it's good business. He found the company worse off than he supposed.'

'He said he paid too much. He's spent weeks combing the books. Besides, Varga thinks the Jacquet family have no real talent in the perfume business. The talent of the grandfather, his "nose", was not passed on. That's why they've developed nothing significant for sixty years. The revival of L'Esprit du Temps is just an attempt to shore up an old image.' She looked through the portfolio of photographs again. 'Without a new product Varga thinks he has bought a pig in a poke.'

'L'Esprit du Temps encore.' Varga leaned across his desk and, for once, he was smiling. 'I like it. I really do.'

'You like the girl, or the idea?'

'I like the whole campaign. Was this your idea or the advertising agency's?'

'The agency.' Ginny flipped through the visuals. 'I am supposed to talk about you in high places. Get you a good image with the press, or rather better than it is already. Robert, meanwhile, is insinuating your name among influential bankers.'

'Robert *has* been enormously helpful.' Varga rose from his desk and began to pace the room. 'Does he do it for you, or what?'

'He does it for business.' Ginny gave him a relaxed smile. 'His bank are making quite a lot of money out of you, Simeon. They don't do it for fun, certainly not for me.'

'Nevertheless I have a feeling there *is* another dimension to all this, a more personal one.'

'Oh certainly there's a personal element. He knows I'm ambitious, and if I handle it well Len might make me a partner. I might then marry him . . .'

28

'Oh! I begin to understand . . .' a smile flickered across Varga's saturnine features. 'It is a complicated way of wooing the lady.'

'I think we should get back to business.' Ginny's manner became brisk and workmanlike. 'I like this model because she's feminine, but not soppy. The new woman for the new image the company wants to put across.' She held up a photograph, staring at it intently.

'Exactly right,' Varga said with approval. 'Not just the company, the group. I am going to buy the remainder of the Oriole shares and merge it with my group. Ace Pharmaceuticals will be renamed AP International. Oriole will be only a part, a not insignificant one, of what will soon be a global company with a global image, and you, Ginny, are an essential part of this. With my experience and your creative flair, together we'll make it.'

He crossed the room and, producing a small wrapped package from one of the drawers in his desk, presented it to her with a slight bow.

'Just to say "Happy Christmas", Ginny, and to thank you for all you've done.'

Situated on a Northumbrian hill and surrounded on three sides by deep coniferous forest, Silklands was a fourteenth-century baronial castle, starkly beautiful from the outside, austere and grand within, with thick walls, stone staircases and huge fireplaces large enough for roasting sheep, as had been done in centuries past. The Silklanders had come over with the Conqueror and had been among the Marcher barons who had swept the country pillaging and looting, decimating the indigenous population on behalf of the Norman king. *Soieterre* became Silkland, the suffix 'er' gradually appearing in legal documents centuries later.

The Silklanders had intermarried with their Scottish brethren across the border, and the mother of Ginny, her three brothers and sister, had been Moira McFee, beautiful in her youth, graceful and dignified in middle age.

The Silklanders had never been wealthy and rather got by with what money there was. They had been able to maintain the ancestral home thanks to the ability of Gerald Silklander, seventeenth baron, who had a little more financial flair than his ancestors, and his son Angus who efficiently ran the farm which embraced thousands of acres of land.

Ginny had had a happy childhood with her brothers Roderick, Lambert and Angus and her only sister Pru. They enjoyed the usual country pastimes of people who lived in castles, whose family went back for centuries and who had all the preconceptions, and to some extent the prejudices, of old nobility.

There was a continuation of these attitudes into adult life. Angus and Pru had married into their own circle and had children who, almost inevitably, grew up like their parents. Lambert, an art dealer, had married a smart, clever woman with the same interests and abilities as himself. Even Ginny – whom the family had always considered a rebel, not quite like a Silklander as though something had been wrong in the genes – was living with a man she had known since childhood.

Thus it was a great family gathering that customarily assembled at the castle year after year to celebrate Christmas. The rituals never varied. Before lunch on Christmas Day the family gathered round the giant fir in the hall where hot punch was served by the helpers, to whom it was as precious a tradition as to the family and who fell on their presents with the same enthusiasm as everyone else. The tree, annually cut from the estate, was almost as high as the ceiling. The lights sparkling amid the tinsel and glitter always took Ginny back to those magical days when, huddled around the enormous fire, they listened to the carol singers especially assembled at the castle.

And nor had this changed. Muffled against the cold

they stood just inside the door, their red, enthusiastic faces as photogenic as a picture postcard. Ginny, sipping her punch, leaned contentedly against Robert's knee and joined in the chorus:

> Star of wonder star of night
> Star with royal beauty bright
> Westward leading
> Still proceeding
> Lead us to that perfect light.

Afterwards the singers, family and helpers mingled, exchanging greetings. There was laughter and reminiscences of past Christmases. Some of the carollers were new members of the choir, grown up perhaps to take the place of an older member who had dropped out for reasons of ill-health, old age or, maybe, death.

This was the best of England, Ginny thought, and wondered how Simeon Varga was celebrating the festivity; a thought she banished as quickly as it had come. She watched her mother slipping in and out of the crowd, first with a tray of punch, then a plate of mince pies. Her father, his back to the fire, had a glass of malt scotch in one hand, a briar pipe in the other. He was tall, rubicund, grey-haired — the epitome of the English country squire whose image seemed, despite the so-called march of progress, to change so little.

Moira Silklander loved nothing better than having her brood under one roof at Christmas time. It was the single occasion in the year when they all assembled, adults and children, and she prepared for it for weeks, if not months beforehand. Angus was responsible for the home-reared beef, the venison, lamb and poultry from the home farm; all the eggs that would be used in pastries and consumed at breakfast. The vegetables were grown in the extensive gardens, the wines came from Roderick, who was a wine merchant in London, the malt from the still private McFee whisky distillery in Aberdeenshire.

31

Dressed in a tartan skirt and polo-necked jersey, with a tartan stole across her shoulders, Lady Silklander moved slowly from one guest to another, most of them old familiars, tenants or estate workers, with an embrace or a hug.

Eventually she came to Ginny and Robert, who had been sitting, statue-like, intent on watching the proceedings. Ginny jumped up to help her mother, who looked at her approvingly before putting out a hand to finger the diamond brooch in the shape of a partridge in a pear tree which was pinned on the suede jacket she wore with a long suede skirt and high boots.

'I don't remember seeing that before, darling. It's pretty. So Christmassy too. It looks very expensive. A present from Robert perhaps?'

Ginny clasped the brooch and wished she'd not worn it. There'd already been one row on account of it.

'It was from a grateful client, Mother.'

'Well he must be very grateful. Surely they're not real diamonds?'

'I think so.' Ginny nervously fingered the brooch, aware that Robert had risen and stood looking at her, a deep frown on his face.

'You know quite well they are, Ginny. Why don't you tell your mother?'

'I am not telling her,' Ginny said angrily. 'Please don't insinuate things, Robert.'

'I'm sorry.' Moira Silklander looked nonplussed. 'I shouldn't have mentioned it. I didn't mean to start a row.'

'It would have been very odd if you hadn't mentioned it.' Robert angrily extracted a cigarette from his case. 'It is a remarkably beautiful and, I should imagine, *extremely* expensive jewel, chosen with great care. Tactful, however, is not a word I'd use to describe a present like that.'

'Oh for *goodness'* sake, Robert.' Ginny stamped her foot. 'You are really making a mountain out of a molehill. You know perfectly well that this was a present from

Simeon Varga because I have done a lot for him. I introduced him to you, and *you* have done a lot for him too. Did he not send you a case of whisky?'

'A case of whisky, though acceptable and certainly most welcome, doesn't have quite the intimacy or significance of a diamond brooch costing about five thousand pounds . . .'

By this time the crowd gathered around the tree had grown quieter as some strained their ears to hear better, while others pretended not to listen. Gerald Silklander, with ill-concealed irritation, walked up to his wife and daughter.

'Is something the matter?'

'It's a silly little tiff between Robert and Ginny.' Moira Silklander kept her voice purposefully low. Then, with a note of urgency: 'Really, Gerald, please get people talking again, and Ginny, Robert,' she took each firmly by the arm, 'please come with me.'

Robert looked as though he was going to refuse, but Lambert Silklander started the conversation going again in a loud, authoritative voice and those present took their cues from him and all started talking at once.

Moira hurried them along the corridor into Gerald's study, where she carefully closed the door as Ginny and Robert obstinately took their places on either side of the fire.

'Now what exactly *is* this between you two?' Moira demanded. 'You're going to spoil our Christmas. I noticed something last night at dinner and so did Pru. Gerald even said to me in bed that he thought you were very quiet, Ginny, not like you at all; and you and Robert hardly danced together afterwards.'

As always on Christmas Eve there had been a family dinner followed by an informal dance, the carpet rolled back in the great drawing-room. It was just before dinner that Ginny had shown Robert Varga's seasonal present and then immediately regretted it. Now she regretted it more than ever.

'Look, Mother,' she put a placatory hand on her mother's arm while with the other she began carefully to unpin the offending ornament, 'Robert is being very silly, very jealous and absurd.'

'I really think I should go, Moira,' Robert began.

Instantly Moira looked alarmed.

'Go? Where? On Christmas Day? Spoil the *whole* party? And what will your parents say?'

'Oh, I shan't go home. I'll go back to London.'

'No you won't, Robert.' Ginny turned savagely to him. 'Because if you do *I* shall move out. I shall pack my things and go and stay with Lambert in Belgravia and that *will* be the end of our relationship.'

'I see.'

Robert now finally lit the cigarette that he had carried in his hand from the hall, fingers shaking slightly. Then he put his lighter carefully back into the breast pocket of his Harris tweed jacket and blew smoke into the air with affected nonchalance.

'If that's what you wish, then of course I'll stay.'

'If you were married you wouldn't behave like this,' Moira Silklander burst out, sitting down in a chair opposite the couple. 'I know I'm old-fashioned but there is *so* much to be said for marriage and its binding ties . . .'

'Mother, it doesn't bind in these days . . .' Ginny said ruefully.

'But there is more of a commitment,' Moira insisted. 'It's a deeper, profounder relationship, sanctified by law, blessed by the church, and this neither of you appear to understand. Why, your father and I would have parted long ago if we hadn't been married . . .'

'Really?' Ginny raised her head in surprise.

'Yes, probably.' Her mother's tone sounded less certain. 'I think you could say that of most married couples, given a long span. The vows of marriage hold us together. It should be a bond. It *is* a bond. Now I think, Ginny darling, that you should return the brooch to whoever gave it to you and announce your engagement to

Robert.' She got up and inspected a calendar on the wall behind her husband's desk. 'An ideal time for the wedding would be late spring or early summer. You've been living together for three years: don't you think that is quite long enough? As you clearly intend to stay together it's time you made it legal and both your family, Ginny, and yours too, Robert, will be very thankful.'

Ginny finally finished unpinning the brooch, but kept it clasped in her hand, turning it over and over in her palm. She had known when Varga gave it to her that it would provoke outrage if she wore it. It was an exquisite piece of workmanship from Van Cleef and Arpels that must have cost a lot of money. But, apart from that, and much more important, was the sentiment behind it which she had seen only too clearly in Simeon Varga's eyes when he had given it to her. Immediately there had been an increase in the tension between them, an enhancement of the physical chemistry, an awkwardness as they'd said goodbye, wished each other a happy Christmas. The betrayal of his feelings that the present expressed, and her acceptance of it, meant that things between them could never be the same again.

She had nearly not shown it to Robert and yet, in a way, she knew she had to. Its very existence was a declaration and a provocation at the same time.

Robert rose and threw his cigarette in the fire that roared up the chimney. Every room in the castle had a fireplace and was kept fuelled, as in the old days, by a man whose sole duty it was. Although staff no longer lived in, the Silklanders had enough tenants to work in the castle, something that eluded the Wards, who had shut off half the family home in Wiltshire because of the lack of staff. But there was no central heating in the castle because of its effect on the old panelling, and even with fires the place was freezing; hence the thick jerseys and skirts worn by most of the women visitors, the sturdy Harris tweed jackets and corduroy trousers of the men.

'You know, Moira, that I agree with you,' Robert said,

his eyes on the crackling flames. 'It is my greatest wish to marry Ginny, and it is *Ginny* who doesn't want to get married. If you can talk to her and persuade her – and perhaps this crisis may have helped to straighten things out between us – I should be only too grateful. Now,' he glanced reprovingly down at Ginny, 'I'd better return to the hall and try and behave normally.'

Ginny stared for a few moments at the closed door after he'd gone, still twisting the jewel in her hands. Her mother went over to the fire and threw a few more logs on to it. Then she sat down on the sofa next to Ginny and tucked her hand in her daughter's.

'Is it serious, darling?'

'Is *what* serious, Mummy?' Ginny's tone was defensive.

'This man . . . the one who gave you the brooch?'

'It is not serious at all,' Ginny said furiously. 'That's what makes me so angry. He is a client, called Simeon Varga. He is a quite brilliant businessman who engaged Len's services and Len put me in charge of his account.'

'What sort of business, dear?' Moira's beautifully modulated voice had just the right note of tact.

'Pharmaceuticals, and he has just bought a French company which makes L'Esprit du Temps. Have you ever heard of that, Mummy?'

'Of course I've heard of it. It was your grandmother's favourite fragrance. I think I even have some of it on my dressing table. It is a *very* famous perfume, a little old-fashioned now, but very well known.'

'Exactly, and one day Simeon Varga is going to be just as well known.'

'And you are in love with him?' her mother asked gently.

'Mummy!' Ginny was on the point of exploding again. 'Why do you *have* to make everything so personal? No I am not in love with Simeon Varga, not one little bit. I agree the brooch was extravagant but he's rich. Rich people often do things like that.'

36

'Has he a wife?'

'Yes he has, and two children. But it's all very well for you, Mummy, in this close-knit community, this far-flung neck of the woods, to forget that London is very cosmopolitan. There friendships between men and women can be based strictly on business.'

'The gift of a brooch of such singular beauty and value was hardly *businesslike*.'

'Yes it was. He wanted to please me. He wanted to please Robert, too, and sent him a case of malt whisky. He couldn't give him a diamond brooch, anyhow.'

'I can quite understand that Robert is upset. Now, darling,' her mother folded her hands in her lap, 'in order to forget this nasty business I *do* hope you're going to be sensible and do as I suggest.'

'I will *not* be blackmailed.'

'It is *not* blackmail, Virginia. It is common sense. Robert is the nicest man you could hope to meet. We all love him.' Her mother only called her by her full name when she was angry.

'He is and I love him too.'

'He would like to be married. I know it. You know it. It would make him happy and us *and* the Wards very happy. More importantly, I think it would make you very happy too, Ginny darling. And no man in his right mind, business or no business, would dare give a diamond brooch to a married woman.'

The Hon Robert John Ward to the Hon Virginia May Silklander.
    The engagement is announced between Robert, eldest son of Lord and Lady Ward of Ockle House, Warminster, Wiltshire, and Virginia, younger daughter of Lord and Lady Silklander of Silklands, Northumbria.

Simeon Varga read the announcement through twice and then, putting *The Times* on his desk, stared thoughtfully out of the window. It was not a very attractive view across the corrugated iron roofs of the sheds housing the laboratories, and beyond that was a six-storey building belonging to a shoe company.

Ace Pharmaceuticals, if it expanded, was soon going to need new premises and his thoughts had turned to the new industrial estates proliferating on the outskirts of many major towns. A move to the country would be rather nice, say Kent or Sussex, somewhere easily accessible.

He began to wade through the documents that had just arrived, delivered by hand from Law, Fairhurst, merchant bankers, yet he was aware of a curious restlessness and, after a few moments, he picked up *The Times* and read the announcement yet again. He then picked up the telephone and asked his secretary to connect him with Len Morgan Associates.

'Miss Silklander, please.'

'Of course, Mr Varga.'

There was a pause and then a few seconds later he heard the soft cultivated tones of Ginny and he knew that his pulse quickened.

'Happy New Year, Ginny,' he said.

'A very happy New Year to you, Simeon.'

'I see it is a particularly happy one for you.'

'Oh . . . yes.' She laughed awkwardly.

'So you decided to take the plunge?'

'*I* didn't decide. My mother threw us into the pool.'

'*Noblesse oblige.*'

'Something like that.'

'You must let me take you both out to dinner to celebrate. I must say, I didn't realize you were so well connected. The "honourable".'

'Well,' she sounded embarrassed, 'it's not so important is it? Unfortunately these wretched announcements have to be so formal.'

'Anyway, congratulations – and to Robert. Now Ginny, I have got the documents from the bank

38

regarding Oriole and I urgently need to talk to you.'

'Me personally?'

'Yes.'

'Sure. When?'

'Can you have dinner?'

'Dinner?'

'I'm tied up until six.' He purposely kept his tone brusque. 'I thought we could discuss it over food.'

'Not a bad idea. Do you need Robert?'

'Not yet. This is not the celebration dinner. I wanted to talk to you first. I hope Robert won't mind.'

'Of course he won't *mind*. Shall I come to your office at about six, then?'

'I shan't be at the office. Can we meet in the foyer at Claridges at seven?'

'Sure. See you then.'

Ginny put down the telephone and sat there thoughtfully for a few minutes. Would Robert mind? Robert wouldn't know. She put through a call to his office and left a message saying that she had to see a client and would not be home for dinner. She spent the rest of the afternoon working on the complex affairs of another client and then drove to Mayfair, parking as close as she could to Claridges. There she took a chair in the foyer and waited, shaking her head at the waiter who offered to bring her a drink.

Shortly after seven Varga arrived, hurrying in through the main entrance, and stood looking round impatiently while the doorman approached him. Watching him, Ginny thought this continual energy of his was one of his most appealing characteristics; he was so alive, his body seemed charged like a dynamo waiting to spring to life even when he was still. He was the antithesis to laid-back Robert who, deceptively, always seemed about to doze off.

Their eyes met. It was most definitely an encounter, a challenge offered and accepted across the foyer. The moment passed almost immediately and, quickly handing his coat to the hall porter, he went over to Ginny and shook her proffered hand. The frisson between them, however, was not yet over and they looked at each other expectantly, excitement lurking in their eyes.

'Congratulations again,' he said. 'You must be very happy.'

'I am.' She smiled at him and her expression was unmistakable: it was about him, not Robert, and then they both looked at the waiter who hovered in front of them.

'Champagne, I think. It *is* a celebration, after all.'

'That would be lovely.'

Varga looked towards the dining-room. 'And I thought we'd eat here. The food's good and it's a cold night. Does that suit you?'

'Perfectly.' Everything suited her. She felt on a high, adrenalin flowing through her body.

'And Robert didn't mind?'

'Not at all. Business is business,' she replied off-handedly.

'Very sensible. You will of course carry on with the business after you're married?'

'Of course.'

'Because I need you.'

'Anyone could do what I am doing; but for the time being you're stuck with me.'

Varga leaned forward and helped himself to nuts.

'I found it strange,' he murmured looking into her eyes, 'because you told me distinctly you would not be getting married for some time. Just before Christmas you said . . .'

'It was Christmas that made the family feel they could put pressure on us,' she said quietly. 'Christmas seems to have that kind of effect. It's not the least bit normal is it? All the holly and tinsel make it so artificial. Anyway, the atmosphere was such that I thought I'd capitulate. Both families wanted it so much.'

'Robert is a very lucky man. Now,' Varga looked up

as the waiter brought glasses of champagne; his brisk manner returned and, undoing his briefcase, he took some documents from it.

'I wanted to tell you specifically, you are the first to know, Ginny, that I intend to buy out the Jacquet family and install my own personnel.'

She felt rather shocked at such a swift development. 'Have you told them?'

'Not yet. I am acquiring more shares through nominees, and when I have seventy per cent I will tell them I want the rest.'

'But what caused this change of mind?' Ginny looked puzzled. 'Robert warned me, but it's exactly the opposite to what you said to them in France.'

'A lot has happened since that day,' he replied, his manner imperturbable. 'I have grown to know them better and not to like what I find. I have made several trips when I wasn't expected. I suspect they have no real knowledge of the perfume business but are cashing in on the name. Oriole will remain separate, but part of my conglomerate AP International, which will become world-wide in its scope. I have huge plans. As Ace Pharmaceuticals I already have a Stock Exchange quotation and you will see that we will grow very soon. Very soon and very big.' He leaned back and, looking like a supremely happy man, raised his glass.

'To you, Ginny.'

'Thank you, Simeon. And to you.' She held hers towards him.

'To you and Robert,' he went on, 'and to us, of course, just you and me.' He paused. 'And, now,' he replaced his glass and drew his chair nearer to hers. 'I am ambitious, you know that. I am going to expand very rapidly. The banks are behind me. I badly need someone I can trust at my right hand. I read of your engagement today, I must say with some dismay, as well as pleasure ... for your happiness, of course.' The end of his sentence was almost a rider.

'Oh?' Ginny looked slightly startled.

'I wanted to offer this post to you.'

'What post?'

'Of my executive assistant, my right hand, with, naturally, a seat on the board, anything in fact that you like, any title you wish.'

'Oh, but, Simeon, I couldn't. I know nothing . . .'

'You know a great deal. You are an accomplished young woman.' Then, with a teasing smile, he added: 'The Honourable Virginia Silklander will look good on my notepaper. You will, of course, remain an honourable even after you're married?' For a moment he looked at her anxiously.

'Of course,' she said laconically. 'Once an honourable always an honourable. Anyway Robert is an honourable too . . . and his father's heir.' She looked at him mischievously. 'I might even be a lady.'

'You would be *Lady Ward*?' Varga was impressed.

'In time, *if* I married Robert, when his father dies. Yes, I will be. I'm surprised it matters to you so much, Simeon.'

'It doesn't matter to me in the least,' Simeon said offhandedly. 'It is the effect on others that is important. But if you came from Brixton I would still want you on my board.' He paused and smiled at her reassuringly. 'But unless I am mistaken you said *if* you marry Robert. It is not certain?'

'Simeon, who can say what is certain in life?' she answered enigmatically.

'Quite right, who can?'

'And Robert is upset about the present you gave me.'

'Ah!' He took a sip of champagne. 'I wondered if you would tell him.'

'I had to. It upset my mother, too. It was *very* kind of you, Simeon,' she drew back the jacket of her black Chanel suit and he saw it gleaming on the lapel of her white silk blouse, 'but there must be no more. In a way it precipitated our engagement.'

42

'Oh, I didn't think it would do *that*.' Varga looked momentarily crestfallen.

'People misunderstand, you see. You and I know it had no ulterior meaning but to people like my mother diamonds are very significant. One thing led to another . . .' She entwined her fingers and smiled. 'As for your offer, I shall have to consult my fiancé.' She shut her mouth primly and he knew she was mocking him, tantalizing him like a witch. His mouth felt strangely dry.

'But you wouldn't let him hold you back?' he enquired tensely.

'I don't expect so,' she replied. 'But I should have to see what it entails. I have to know all your plans.'

'Then let us eat,' Varga said, rising with alacrity, his sense of an excitement that was almost unbearable returning, and beckoning to the waiter. 'There is such a lot to tell you.' He then put his arm gently round her waist and escorted her to the dining-room.

Sometime well after midnight Ginny crept into the bedroom she shared with Robert and, without putting on the light, began to undress. She heard a rustle from the bed; the lamp on Robert's side suddenly illuminated the room and she saw him lying there, fully awake, looking at her.

'You're terribly late,' he said, glancing irritably at the clock. 'I was worried.'

'No need.' She sat on the bed and began to take off her tights, tossing them nonchalantly on the floor. To Robert's despair Ginny was perpetually untidy.

'Who did you see?' His voice strained, he puffed up his pillows and leaned against them, arms folded, staring at her.

'Varga.'

'I knew it.'

'Oh, *Robert*!'

She took off her pants, undid her bra and, nude,

43

walked to the bed and felt under the pillow for her nightdress. As she leaned forward Robert clutched her and dragged her down beside him.

'*Robert!*' she cried furiously, trying to free her arm.

'I could . . .' his face reddened and the veins swelled in his neck as his grip on her arm grew firmer. 'I could . . . oh God, *what* is the matter with me?' He abruptly let go of her arm and put his hands over his face. She could see they were trembling. Robert was in a terrible state.

'I felt I could kill you,' he said quietly, looking at her. 'Just then I had the urge to kill you or rape you. Do something violent. It was awful. Ginny, I'm so jealous.'

His trembling disturbed her and, quickly pulling her nightdress over her head, she went round to his side of the bed and sat beside him. She felt shaken, too, and the ugly red weal round her arm hurt her. Tentatively she put out her hand towards him.

'I simply don't know *what's* got into you, Robert. You have some obsession about Varga and it's *not* like you. I've had other male clients, and you've never reacted this way.'

'That's just the point,' Robert said, still trembling. 'Varga is different. I know it. I don't like him and I don't trust him.'

'But you've done *all* this work for him. Surely you must have *some* trust in him?'

'I'm not talking about work.' His trembling ceased and he angrily scratched his head. 'You must know what I mean.' He gazed into her eyes, so close to his. 'Varga likes you. I know he does. It sticks out a mile; and you like him. There's a chemistry between you. I noticed it the moment I saw you together . . .'

'But *I* don't feel any chemistry . . .'

'Don't lie,' he said roughly. 'You must. It's *there*. Unspoken but *there*. It was even obvious when we went round the Oriole factory in the summer. He would defer to you in subtle ways; he was acutely aware of you, of your presence. I can't explain it, but my jealousy began even then. I was ashamed of it and I still am, but I wish, Ginny, I *wish* you'd give up his bloody account and let someone else handle it.'

'Robert . . .' She rose from the bed and began to walk up and down the room. 'Varga is an important client. He's important to the agency. I believe in him. Len believes in him. He thinks he is going to be big. I know he is. He's already gone terribly far in a very short time.'

'Not *so* short.' Robert's tone was derisive.

'Well, comparatively short. He is single-minded enough to do all he says he wants to do. Tonight he was telling me about all his plans and they're enormously exciting. Ace is going global.'

'To hell with him. You don't need the money, and you don't need the prestige.'

'Robert, darling . . .' she leaned towards him, 'if I give up a client on the basis of misplaced sexual jealousy what do you think Len will say? Varga is not molesting me. He's not importuning me. He treats me as an equal. We had dinner tonight and there was not a single personal nuance all evening. It was all about his plans to take over Oriole completely.'

'Which isn't very honourable, as he gave his word . . .'

'It's not "nice", but it's good business. I can see that.'

'You're getting very hard, Ginny. Hard as he is. He's influencing you. I don't like it.'

'What *you* don't like,' Ginny said, sitting down again, 'is that my attitude to business is the same as yours, as the men you deal with. People like you, Robert, would, in your heart of hearts, like to deal exclusively with men. Women worry you, women in the workplace that is. That's why you want us to get married; so that I belong to you. You want me to have babies so that I will stay at home. You want to tie me down, Robert, and I'm not having it.

'If I told Len to take me off the Varga account my

45

standing in his estimation would sink to zero, and he would never give me another chance again. That way there would be no better alternative for me than to be Mrs Robert Ward and forget all about a career. It would also influence the way he felt about women in employment. Besides,' she looked defiantly at him, 'Varga has lots of good ideas.'

'A gentleman doesn't break his word,' Robert said huffily.

'"Gentlemen",' Ginny replied with heavy sarcasm, 'do it all the time, and you know it. What you don't like, what you can't stomach, is that Varga didn't go to the right school and he doesn't belong to the right clubs. He's not one of you. Not one of the boys.'

'I object to those remarks, Ginny,' Robert said stiffly.

'They are true.' Ginny wagged her finger at him. 'The City is full of shibboleths, full of prejudices, and people like Varga don't fit in. Len Morgan doesn't fit in. But then he's not in the City, thank God.'

'I like Len. Len is different.'

'Len is no threat.'

'Then why is Varga?'

'I don't know,' Ginny said, with an air of defeat that was unusual for her. 'I'm very sorry now that I involved you in the business, that I brought you in. I should keep these compartments in my life completely separate, and that was my mistake. I simply thought it was good for you, good for Varga and fun for me. I saw an exciting hotch-potch of things and I was silly. But you see, Robert, it's because I'm a woman ... another bloke putting you in touch with Varga would have been all right.'

'A "bloke" would not have given you a diamond brooch.'

'There you go again!' She rose angrily and getting up from the bed swept into the bathroom and began vigorously brushing her teeth.

When she went back into the room the light was off

and Robert was either asleep or pretending to be asleep. She slipped into bed beside him and lay there for a long time, stiffly, yet desperate for the comfort of his arm around her; the need to know that everything was all right between them.

But it didn't come, he didn't move, and eventually she drifted off to sleep just as dawn was beginning to break over the city.

CHAPTER 3

Gustave Jacquet and his son Pierre remained motionless after Varga had finished speaking. Although Robert, who accompanied him, knew his plans, he found the situation embarrassing. Ratting on one's word was not, by merchant bank standards and despite what Ginny had said, a gentlemanly thing to do.

It was Jacquet *père* who found his voice first, his son remaining speechless.

'But Monsieur Varga, you *promised*; we would remain to run the company; you would leave us control.'

'I have always said *I* would have control,' Varga said in his gentle, reasonable voice. 'I made that quite clear.'

'But on the rest you have gone back on your word.'

'In view of what I have discovered since I bought control of the company I have no option but to release you from your contract, Monsieur Jacquet.'

'Perhaps you can explain why?'

'The facts.' Varga pointed to the documents in his hand. 'The products, the cash flow. I have to make a considerable investment in Oriole, more than I envisaged. To start with, your machinery is fifty years out of date. *You* lied to me about this. It is useless. It has to be automated, new processes introduced. I would also like to make a change of personnel. The people you have are mostly too old and too set in their ways. I'm sorry, but they will be well compensated for their redundancies.

Therefore I have decided to make a clean sweep.'

'And my son?'

Varga momentarily seemed to lose his composure. 'Alas, I am afraid he too . . .'

'But he has an excellent "nose".'

'Unfortunately untried, as you have introduced no new outstanding perfume for many years. No, I would like the name of Jacquet removed completely from the company's notepaper. Of course there will be a generous settlement, and you have your shares. You still have thirty per cent and I can assure you that one day the dividend will be much higher than it is now, that is unless you care to sell them to me first. I will pay you twenty to thirty per cent above the market price, as is usual.'

'Out of the question.'

'Well then,' fully in control again, Varga nodded to Robert and rose. 'That concludes the business for today. A new managing director will be taking over from Monday. I would be glad if you would give him all assistance necessary; but if not . . .' Varga shrugged, 'it is of no real importance. Meanwhile I have engaged a firm of security guards who will keep an eye on the premises until the new man, whose name is Roger Bennet — he's English, by the way, but speaks excellent French — takes over.'

Suddenly Jacquet rose and, rapidly crossing the room, seized Varga by his lapels before anyone could stop him.

'Does that mean you do not *trust* us, Monsieur Varga? You think I would destroy my own company?'

A look of alarm crossed Varga's face and then vanished just as quickly as Jacquet's grip on his lapel relaxed. At the same time Robert, moving anxiously to his side, gently disengaged the hands of the overwrought man.

Varga fastidiously dusted his lapels and said with equanimity: 'I think you would be most unwise to harm a single piece of equipment of *my* company. And I'm afraid, in the light of this incident I must ask you to leave the premises immediately.'

Jacquet looked despairingly at his son Pierre who,

appearing mesmerized by what had happened, seemed to spring to life and, stretching out his hands, made an impassioned appeal.

'Monsieur Varga. My father is not a well man. His blood pressure is too high. This business has disturbed him deeply. I am sure if you will give me a few minutes to talk to him . . .'

'I'm afraid, Monsieur Jacquet, the expulsion order applies to you too,' Varga replied brusquely. 'You will perhaps now be kind enough to escort your father home, and in view of what you tell me about his health perhaps he should see his doctor. Now, the officials from the security company are already in the building. All locks are in the process of being changed. Once I am satisfied that you and your father have left I shall leave too and be returning to England.'

Jacquet the elder appeared on the verge of making another lunge at Varga but his son grabbed his arm, murmuring sharply into his ear; then, shaking his head as if in a daze, the father let himself be led to the door where, together with his son, he paused for a moment.

'Do not think we will forget this, Monsieur Varga,' Pierre Jacquet said solemnly. 'We shall neither forget nor forgive.'

Varga made an irritable gesture of dismissal and, after the door had closed, sat down heavily in the seat formerly occupied by Gustave Jacquet. He got out his handkerchief and mopped his brow.

'Well,' he paused to glance at Robert, 'not very pleasant, but these things never are.'

'You look as though you're quite experienced in sacking people.'

Robert, shaken too, had taken a cigarette from his case.

'Not in my presence if you don't mind, Robert,' Varga said sharply. 'I do not allow smoking.'

Robert looked as though he was about to ignore him and then, as if recalling the fate of Gustave Jacquet, thought better of it and returned his case to his pocket.

'Thank you,' Varga smiled. 'I am not only doing myself a favour but you too. Now, about the matter you mentioned a moment or two ago, you are quite wrong. I have never done this before. I have sacked people, of course, but never been forced to dismiss the managing director from a company he owned until recently. And, believe me, I did not enjoy doing it. Most emphatically I did not. To be attacked was a totally new experience *and* most unpleasant. One I hope never to repeat. However I'm beginning to realize that such unpleasant actions may be necessary and, if they are, one must approach them from a position of strength. You have seen the figures, Robert. You know . . . you are a businessman yourself. Would *you* have left the Jacquets in charge? Who knows what harm they might have done?'

Robert felt himself in deep waters. He realized he did not, after all, know Varga at all. The many months he had spent working with him had not prepared him for this ruthlessness, the toughness of the stance he had taken with the Jacquets that day.

'I don't think they would have done any actual harm,' he murmured after a while. 'On the contrary. They had a very good knowledge of the business, but they lacked capital. They had let it stagnate; but it was still a good business adequately managed. With encouragement they might have done quite well.'

'You really think so?' Varga said with a sneer. 'Of what use is "adequate"? I want an exceptionally run, well managed business and, I assure you, I would not have got it from the pair we have just sent on their way.' His eyes narrowed. 'I am a little surprised at you, Robert. A little dismayed. I thought you had more mettle?'

'I am sorry to have disappointed you, Simeon.' Robert felt stung by the rebuke. 'I am primarily a banker and not an entrepreneur. I must keep risks to the minimum.'

'Of course you must.' Varga's manner underwent another lightning change. 'And I assure you I appreciate what you have done for me.' Rising, he crossed the room and took hold of his arm in a comradely clasp. 'Together we will do great things, eh?'

'I hope so.' Robert's manner remained reserved. Varga's swift changes of mood unnerved him.

Later, as they drove towards the airport, Varga's hand languidly on the strap as the limousine glided smoothly through the night, he said, 'I intend a big reconstruction of Ace Pharmaceuticals.'

'Oh?'

'With your help, naturally.'

In the lights from the dashboard Robert was aware of Varga's keen scrutiny.

'I want Ace Pharmaceuticals to become AP International – of which Oriole is only a part.'

'I thought you intended to merge with Oriole?' Robert sounded surprised. 'As part of a larger pharmaceuticals group?'

'That was the original intention, but you see, Robert, I have decided not to confine myself to the pharmaceuticals industry, or to its allied fields like perfume and cosmetics. My plans are expanding. I think there is a lot of money to be made much more easily in other spheres.'

'Such as?'

'Electronics, for example. The microchip, computers. These are the really fast-growing, fast-moving industries. AP International will thus be an umbrella and, eventually, the pharmaceuticals and perfume side will form merely a small part of it.' He sat back in his seat and Robert, grateful for the dim light which hid his expression, still could not keep the surprise from his voice.

'Is it wise to rush into things, Simeon? Isn't it better to look before you leap?'

'Oh, I look, I look,' Simeon said impatiently. 'I have looked, don't worry. This isn't a sudden whim. It is part of a plan, years of thought. I have been gradually building up to this step for a long time, ever since I first bought

Ace when the shares were seven pence each. Have I made a wrong move since?'

Robert had to agree that he hadn't.

'Not as far as I can see. But Morgan suggested you enlarge. Didn't that idea come from him?'

'Oh no!' Varga leaned his head back against the soft leather upholstery and laughed. 'By no means. I had this plan years before I met Morgan, or Ginny. I have always wanted to extend my fields of influence. Others do it, why can't I?' Lightly Varga touched the back of Robert's hand. 'And I am a prudent man, Robert. Please don't think I am not. I do look before I leap. I engaged Morgan because I wanted to improve my image. Even by then my company's shares had increased tenfold since I bought them. But I am anxious for the City to have confidence in me. I want to belong. That is why I have moved very slowly in order to build up the image of a prudent financial manager. I take risks, but not too many. I think I have done that very well, don't you?'

'You have.' Robert nodded vigorously.

'To buy Oriole was merely a sideline, an extension. I don't think I paid too much for it. Throw in another million or so to improve it out of all recognition, to bring in proper management, a first-class "nose". Then, hey presto, another small company will be on its way to great things: as part of AP International. Do you understand?'

'I do understand; but it has always been part of my philosophy, Simeon, that the most prudent businesses stick to what they know. You know absolutely nothing about electronics.'

Varga touched the side of his nose and winked.

'I knew nothing about pharmaceuticals to start with. People thought I was a trained pharmacist but I was not. Oh no.' He saw the look of surprise on Robert's face. 'I never pretended, people *thought* it and I didn't contradict them. But I never lied. Did I ever lie to you, Robert?'

'Not as far as I know.'

'Well I can tell you I never did. And I never will. The

main road to success in business is the ability to read a balance sheet — above and below the line — winkle out the hidden assets. If you have as good a nose for business as an expert has for a perfume you can manage anything. Do I make myself perfectly clear, Robert?'

'Perfectly.' Robert swallowed nervously as Varga's hand tightened round his wrist.

'I trust you, Robert. I take you completely into my confidence. You and Ginny . . . my right and my left hand.'

As the car arrived at the airport and stopped before the main terminal, Varga paused before alighting and gazed solemnly at his companion.

'Very soon I shall have my own jet waiting here to pick us up. You just see. It won't be very long.'

Ginny leaned confidentially towards her companion seated across from her at the lunch table.

'AP International are the shares to watch.'

'Really?' The financial journalist, used to being the subject of confidences, tips and attempts, both blatant and subtle, to influence his column in one of the main quality newspapers, wiped his mouth.

He knew it was Ginny's task to influence him and what he wrote, but he respected her and the company she worked for as he respected few others. Len Morgan was an ex-newspaperman, had served many years as an industrial editor himself and was known to be discriminating in his clientele, and almost as truthful as it was possible to be in the shifting sands of the PR world. In this world full of people trying to influence him and tell him stories, Nick Bowyer invariably put in a discreet call to Ginny when he wanted to know what really was going on in half a dozen top companies represented by Morgan Associates. If he could, then he was not averse to returning the favour.

It helped, of course, that he and Ginny had been at university together. They'd been in the same year, though not the same faculty, and had been fellow members of the dramatic society. He had been Vanya to her Sonia.

Nick had also married a mutual friend and had two young children. He was well established in the small hierarchy of financial journalists whom people read and respected.

Nick finished his filet mignon, took a sip of the excellent Rioja that accompanied it and dabbed his lips again with his napkin.

'AP International. I'll remember.'

'Simeon Varga.'

'Varga.' Nick sat back and shook his head. 'Yes, I've vaguely heard of Varga.'

'Now is the time to sit up and take notice.'

Nick got out his notebook, opened it at a clean page and put it on the table in front of him, listening as Ginny talked.

'He bought a pharmaceuticals company about ten years ago,' she continued. 'Its paper shares were worth seven pence each. He worked hard to establish it, invested in new equipment and built up a reputation. He's a finance and ideas man. Also he doesn't believe in borrowing too much money so, for a time, it was a slog.'

'That's refreshing.' Nick made a note. 'Not over-gearing, very refreshing.'

'Recently he bought a small French company at a knock-down price, called Oriole. It makes a fragrance called L'Esprit du Temps.'

Again Nick shook his head.

'Your grandmother would have worn it.' Nick scribbled some more.

'Varga did the same with Oriole that he did with Ace Pharmaceuticals. He kept the gearing low by restructuring his company and calling it AP International. He's bent on further acquisitions. The shares are now 407p and the P/E ratio is ten.'

'Not bad. Varga.' Nick heavily underlined the name,

55

and scribbled some more, flicking over the page.

'He hates personal publicity, by the way.'

'Oh?' Nick looked at her. 'That's good. That's a change. I like discreet businessmen. The trouble is once they get rich it's into the fast cars, the country houses and the bimbos – that's where the money really goes.'

'He wants the attention for his company and its performance, not himself. He is being advised by Law, Fairhurst.'

'Robert's company. Well that's good news, too. What do you want me to do, Ginny?'

'Just a small piece in your paper at the moment. Shares to watch, that kind of thing. You're *so* influential, Nick. A line or two from you can do wonders.'

'And you're a shameless flatterer.' Nick leaned towards her as she picked up the bill. 'When's the wedding by the way?'

Ginny stared at him blankly.

'August, I think.'

'You "think"? It's nearly that already.'

'I haven't really had time to plan weddings. There's so much to do.'

'I suppose your mother will see to all that sort of thing.'

'I suppose she will.'

Ginny got out her American Express card and began calculating the size of the tip, as though she wanted to change the subject.

'Saw Nick Bowyer today,' Ginny said as she creamed her face in front of the mirror. It was a sample of Oriole's new night cream and it smelt good. She rubbed her hands together when she had finished and held them to her nose.

Robert put down the *Financial Times* and looked at her. 'How is Nick?'

'Fine.' Ginny rose from the dressing table and went over to the bed, pulling back the duvet and slipping under it. 'He's going to write a discreet paragraph or two about AP International. He hasn't heard much about Varga.'

'Sometimes I wish none of us had ever heard much about Varga.'

Robert removed his reading glasses and put his arms around her. She was cold and unresponsive, her body stiff, her attitude that of someone lost in thought, too often her manner these days; far too often. He slipped a hand inside her nightdress and began to caress her breast. Ginny sighed impatiently.

'Oh, *Robert*!' Gently she disengaged his hand.

'Ginny!' Robert took his hand away and turned to face her. 'We simply must talk.'

'There is nothing to talk about, for God's sake.' She turned on her side, cradling her head on her hand. Then she reached out and switched off her light. 'It's awfully late, Robert.'

'Ginny, we have not made love for weeks.' She felt his breath on her cheek, his heart pounding against her shoulder. He drew up her nightdress and inserted his hand between her legs.

She turned over to resist him, but his mouth clamped down harshly on hers. She tried to scream and beat him off, but he straddled her without any foreplay and thrust himself violently into her, climaxing almost immediately.

His body on hers was heavy, his breathing harsh, his pulse rate almost alarming. She felt fearful, angry and disgusted; bruised, wounded, possessed by a feeling of deep revulsion for a man so close to her who could treat her like an object.

She pushed him off her and he lay beside her, inert. She thought he was sobbing, but she couldn't feel any pity for him – only sorrow for them both.

'You raped me,' she murmured. 'That was rape.'

'You asked for it,' Robert said between sobs, 'my God, Ginny, you asked for it.'

'That's what they're all supposed to say,' she muttered, rising shakily from the bed. 'And, as they are again all supposed to say — I never thought it would happen to me.' Then she went into the bathroom, and when she had finished washing herself she tottered along to the cold spare room and flung herself down upon the bed.

> The marriage arranged between the Hon Robert
> John Ward and the Hon Virginia May Silklander
> will not now take place.

Simeon Varga put down the paper and sat for a long time tapping his fingers on his desk. He reached for the phone and then changed his mind.

'Let her wait,' he said to himself.

Instead he buzzed for his secretary and asked her to come in with her dictation pad.

Dorothy Richards had been with Simeon Varga since he had bought Ace Pharmaceuticals. She had been secretary to the then managing director, whom Varga had displaced with even less ceremony than he had used with Gustave Jacquet. But in this case most of the staff had not been happy under the previous ownership and welcomed the change. They liked Varga's manner, brisk but fair; they appreciated the way he consulted those who knew more about the business than he did and the fact that he was the first to admit that he knew nothing, eager to learn.

So little had been known about the new owner and little more had been learnt. Mrs Richards had never met his wife; she was never asked to send flowers or remind him of his children's birthdays. He was not the kind of man who had pictures of his family on his desk.

To her he was always 'Mr Varga', though he called her Dorothy despite the fact that she was in her fifties. She had been widowed early, was childless and not only dependent on but devoted to her work. She had mastered all the intricate new advances in computers and word processors, had kept abreast of the times.

She respected Varga. In a way she was devoted to him, yet he gave nothing of himself away; no personal dimension at all. It was all work, work, work. Work was everything.

Varga was ready for her when she came in and greeted her with his customary detached smile. He started to dictate almost before she sat down but she was used to this. There was no chit-chat, no exchange of pleasantries. Indeed he knew as little about her as she knew about him. But whereas she would have liked to know more she felt that Simeon Varga was completely uninterested in her, that if she were run over by a bus and killed he would feel about as much emotion as a total stranger; simply ring an employment agency and ask for a replacement.

'A letter to Mr Twaki Miko of the Yokkaichi Electronics Company, Japan, Dorothy. You have details on file. Mark it extremely personal and confidential.'

'Yes, Mr Varga,' she firmly drew a line.

Dear Mr Miko

Further to my recent visit and our discussions on this matter I have pleasure in confirming my interest in purchasing a majority share in the Yokkaichi Electronics Company at a price per share of 170 UK pence.

The letter was a short one as the details had already been ironed out, and concluded with Varga's best wishes and hopes for a successful partnership.

There were several more letters, a request for a reservation to be made on a flight to Paris in a few days' time.

'Just yourself, Mr Varga?'

'Just myself,' Varga confirmed. He sighed and looked at his watch. 'Get me the details for the Yokkaichi purchase, Dorothy, and confirm my appointment with Mr Burton at Le Gavroche.'

'I did that first thing this morning, sir. The restaurant is apt to be booked up.'

'Thank you, Dorothy.'

A 'thank you' was rare. Varga seldom showed gratitude. Though he was courteous to his employees, they knew it was unwise to expect verbal thanks. Usually a nod was considered sufficient. His employees, after all, were doing a job they were expected to do, so why thank them for doing something for which they were well paid?

'You think of everything,' Varga went on, 'and I hope one day you will be properly rewarded.'

Mrs Richards blushed to the roots of her tinted hair.

'I am well rewarded already, Mr Varga.'

'I'm glad to hear it, Dorothy. Now tell me, if I moved our headquarters to central London, how would you feel about joining me?'

'Well . . .' Mrs Richards appeared nonplussed. 'Whereabouts in central London, Mr Varga?'

'I haven't decided, but probably Mayfair, just round the corner from Le Gavroche, as a matter of fact. There are premises I like in a mews. An international company must have central headquarters. I intend to expand, Dorothy, quite rapidly. I can't expect jet-setting businessmen to come to Croydon.'

Dorothy Richards looked at the floor, her blush deepening. She didn't see why not. Croydon might not have the kudos of Mayfair, but it was where she had been born, married, widowed and lived all her life. In her opinion there was a lot to be said for Croydon.

'I would be quite happy to travel *anywhere* in London, Mr Varga. Mayfair would suit me very well.'

'Excellent, Dorothy.' Varga rose and began to pack documents into his briefcase. 'You can be sure I shall consult you before the new premises are bought or adapted.'

Dorothy was still smiling her gratitude at such solicitousness as he walked out of the room. She then went to the window and watched him get into his car. She wondered how long it would be before the Volvo was replaced by a Jaguar, or maybe a Rolls?

Piers Burton sat studying Varga's face as he expounded the advantages of acquiring an electronics company situated in far-off Japan. One had heard of him, of course. AP International was a rising share on the Stock Market, though one which was still regarded in some quarters with caution. So little was known about him personally though, thanks to his clever management, a lot was known about his company, his ambitions and his management style: subdued, low-key. The City liked that. There were too many high-flyers bent on cultivating their own image. There were too many with life-styles that were too flamboyant: women, horses, yachts and fast cars. No one knew a thing about Varga; but someone like him, with proven business ability yet a dislike of publicity, was much approved of, especially with a bank like Burton, Larosse, which had been founded by Piers' great-grandfather and was known to be steady, reliable and dull, reluctant to take risks, the very qualities in Varga which appealed to the bank.

However, any project that it put itself behind was assured of solid support. It would guarantee an increase in the City's respect, a rapid rise in the price of shares.

Yet Piers asked the same questions as Ginny and Robert had.

'Why electronics, Mr Varga? Surely it's an area you know absolutely nothing about?'

Varga passed a hand over his closely shaved chin.

'I know a lot about business, Mr Burton. You, I can see, know a lot about banking. You don't just invest in companies whose businesses you are familiar with, do you?'

'No, we . . .' Momentarily Piers looked nonplussed.

'Exactly. *You* don't specialize in, say, fruit or meat or oil or . . .'

'No, of course not. We are willing to back any venture we consider viable.'

'And *I* am willing to look at any business I consider viable and, in the long term, profitable. Preferably its shares should be below market value, yet the company itself, due to poor management, must be ripe for development. Unlike many Japanese companies, Yokkaichi seems to fulfil both qualifications. A family-run business, the premature death of the father precipitated into the chairmanship a son who was not quite ready. Under my guidance, however, I think he will do well.'

Varga passed the attentive banker an envelope. 'The figures are all here. Study them, please, and get back to me, by tomorrow morning if you can.'

Piers looked at the bulky envelope doubtfully. There was a visit to Covent Garden planned for the evening, dinner afterwards.

'Well . . .'

'There *are* other banks, Mr Burton, and I think they will be as ready to listen to me as you are.'

'Of course, but may I ask,' Burton's manner became confidential as he leaned forward, 'hasn't Robert Ward been handling your business? Have you been to him?'

'Some of my business,' Varga said guardedly. 'I do not intend to put all my eggs in one basket in the same way that you don't back only one client. And you will not be the last to be approached, I can assure you. I wish to expand very rapidly, but one step at a time. The risks to be shared by various merchant banks. I buy a business, reorganize it and then invest in it. Where possible I keep the same personnel . . . except in France. There I was ready to give them a chance, but they were not up to it and my changes have paid dividends.'

Varga placed another envelope on top of the one he had already given to the banker. 'I think in there you will find all the details of the Oriole concern and I am sure you will agree they are most satisfactory.'

'I'll look at both sets of figures with interest.'

Burton popped a piece of cheese in his mouth, finished his claret and, for the first time, gave his host a friendly smile.

Varga rather liked him. Despite their differences, he was a bit like himself.

After lunch Varga stood on the pavement in Upper Brook Street leaning through the taxi window bidding goodbye to Piers Burton, who was carefully carrying the two envelopes. The banker smiled again; Varga waved and stood watching the taxi drive off towards Grosvenor Square.

He consulted his watch – he was a man governed by time – and then walked into Park Street and towards Oxford Street before turning into a mews at the back of the Grosvenor House Hotel.

Here stood an elegant mansion that had been adapted, probably at the end of the nineteenth century, from what had presumably been the stable blocks. It had only recently been converted into offices and still had at the back a walled garden with a fish-pond and statues redolent of an age long gone.

Having been constructed before the planning regulations became so strict, it was to all extents and purposes totally fake, Adam in style outside and modern within. Varga's heart had warmed to the place and he imagined that it was because it answered some call deep inside him for gracious living; for a need to forget about his past, dig up and discard his roots.

There was still a FOR SALE notice prominent outside the house, but it would not be there for very long. Varga produced a key from his pocket, unlocked the solid oak door with its brass furnishings, and walked into the cool gleaming reception hall with a marble floor, pillars rising to a glass atrium which gave it more light as well as height.

In the middle a solid but obviously fake marble statue of a Greek discus thrower dominated the hall, and behind it a large floor to ceiling mirror made the reception area seem twice its size.

Varga stood there for a few minutes gazing at himself reflected in the glass: a sober, staid man of business in a dark coat over a dark suit, a hat in his hand. Varga always wore a dark trilby, usually pulled well over his brow. Behind him, the open door looked out on to the Mayfair pavement and the red brick wall of the garden of the house opposite, which was hidden from view by trees.

He went to the door and closed it. He switched on the lights and inhaled the smell of new paint, freshly varnished wood, as though it had been a fragrance of great allure such as he hoped Oriole would one day come up with. Then he removed his coat, put it with his hat on the bottom of the stairs, and walked up to the first floor and along the corridor to the large back room overlooking the garden, which would be his office.

It had double windows leading on to a balcony and throwing them open he stood for some time gazing at the backs of the houses, all of which had been converted into offices. Inside he could see people moving about, girls at their VDU screens, someone watching a television set. Maybe it was an advertising or PR company like Ginny's; he felt happy.

Varga went back through the french windows, closed them behind him and wandered out of the office into the reception area next door, where Dorothy would sit with her screens, through that to an outer office where the other secretaries would gather with theirs. Up another flight to the second floor where his expanded staff would sit: his finance manager, Tony Liddle, his marketing manager, a projects director yet to be appointed, and so on.

He inspected the lavatories, the facilities, the small but well equipped kitchen, the stores where the paper and office accessories, the computer supplies and so on would be kept.

Then he walked back along the corridor and paused

at the head of the stairs, looking up at the opaque glass surrounding the dome. Despite the fact that it was a dull, brooding day which promised rain, he imagined that, through it, he could see the sun.

A few hours after leaving his future office in Mayfair, Simeon Varga rang the doorbell of a house in Mill Hill on the outskirts of London. After a few seconds the door was opened by a pretty woman, possibly in her mid- or late thirties, who looked at him unsmilingly before standing back as though reluctant to admit him.

'I thought you were coming yesterday,' she said accusingly.

'I'm sorry, I couldn't make it.' Varga took off his hat and, aware of the same familiar feelings of dread with which he always approached the house, entered it.

For eleven years it had been his marital home. He had taken his bride there, carried her over the threshold as in story books, and his two children had been conceived there and born in Edgware General Hospital a few miles away.

It was a detached house with a nice stretch of garden back and front and four good-sized bedrooms. It had been a gift to the bride from her father and, despite the snub, to Varga it had been the pinnacle of the dreams of a formerly stateless man, with no history of a happy family home or a prosperous future. Eleven years was a very long time.

Simeon Varga had always been ambitious, but ambitious in a different way from what he was now. Then he had been ambitious to have a house half as nice as the one in Mill Hill, a pretty wife like Claudia and two happy children like Andrea and Mark, now seven and eight respectively and at a private school. All seemed to be going well and then something changed; something very deep that affected not only his private life and his dreams, but his life as a whole.

His ambition, once to be the chairman of a medium-sized company like Ace Pharmaceuticals which would give him and his family a decent living, to be a happy family man taking his wife and children on holidays, playing with the kids in the garden, maybe a dog and a cat as well, had changed. As his company had grown his expectations had grown. He found that making money was easy and he knew he had a gift that could make him one day into a very rich man, a millionaire, maybe, many times over.

Claudia had seen that ambition change direction in the years they had lived together; had seen passion turn to lust, and then to indifference, and a happy family life into routine.

Her once contented husband became like a man possessed, keeping all hours, leaving home early and arriving back late. They seldom had an evening out, and games in the garden with the children and holidays abroad were things of the past.

His family hardly ever saw him and then, one day, he didn't come home at all.

It had been very hard for Claudia Varga, a chic and attractive woman by any standards, to realize that her husband no longer wanted her; harder still that he no longer wanted the home or the children, though his dutiful weekly visits were routine. Dutiful, weekly and awful. She dreaded them. Mark and Andrea dreaded them too and did their best to be out when their father called. And if they were at home they both usually cried as soon as he left and made life hell for her.

No wonder she turned sour, especially when he said there was no one else and this breakdown of his family life was solely on account of his business. He had fallen in love with one style of life and out with another.

But it was more complicated than that. Had the seeds in fact been there before they were married, before Claudia had even been carried over the threshold on their wedding day?

Claudia came from a close-knit and very conventional Italian family dominated by her mother Fortunata who, now a widow, lived with her eldest son in a large house in Highgate. The Berninis prided themselves on the family name, though it had no known connection with the great seventeenth-century sculptor and artist Giovanni Bernini, architect of St Peter's in Rome. The modern Berninis had come as silversmiths from Naples at the end of the nineteenth century and established themselves in the east end of London. Within a generation a fortune had been made, and there was a showroom in Albemarle Street and one in the Via Veneto in Rome. In the rarefied world of the expensive jeweller theirs was an honoured and respected name, on a par with Cartier and Tiffany.

The close-knit Berninis would have liked the only girl to have married one of their own kind and not a man without fortune or background with whom she had fallen in love. The patriarch Antonio had distrusted Varga, but maybe he was over-possessive of his attractive daughter, who, by then in her mid-twenties, was clearly anxious for a husband.

There was little love between the Berninis and Varga even when he showed an aptitude for business they should have suspected from the beginning. He was proud, he knew they had snubbed him and in his way he was just as stubborn as the expatriate Italians who merely tolerated him as a son- and brother-in-law.

When Antonio Bernini died Claudia's brothers and her mother continued what was almost a vendetta against her husband, which grew fiercer as his indifference to Claudia became apparent and husband and wife drifted further and further apart. They eventually occupied separate bed-rooms and one day Simeon left home altogether.

If anything governed the Bernini family it was a resolve, headed by the vindictive matriarch, to pay back Varga in kind for the insult he had administered to the daughter of the house of Bernini.

Varga put his hat down in the hall and looked around him.

'Where are the children?' he asked, removing his coat and hanging it on a peg. Then, slowly, he went into the sitting-room which looked as it always did, perfect, not a thing out of place, impersonal, anonymous, never a home. Unlike most Italian home-makers, Claudia hadn't the gift.

'Today they are at a children's party,' Claudia replied sulkily.

'They are always somewhere when I call.' Varga looked severely at her. 'Sometimes I think it is deliberate. You are trying to alienate them from me, Claudia.'

Claudia reached for a cigarette and put it in her mouth, disregarding the look Varga gave her. It was some time now since she had tried to please him or cared what he said. Her canny Italian father had made her too independent when she married Simeon; she was spoilt and rich enough to do as she liked. She rudely blew smoke into his face and he recoiled angrily, turning to look through the french windows at the neat well-cut lawn, the tiny flower beds maintained by a weekly gardener. It was almost autumn and a layer of leaves from the trees surrounding it lay on the path. He thought of the bright, light building in Mayfair he had just left, full of promise, and contrasted it with this house full of lost hopes. This was the end; that was the beginning.

It was like leaving the dead and, except for his children, he wished he could bury it for good. The children though were Berninis in looks as well as spirit. They were pious, obedient, docile, mother's children. Even he could see how little character they had. They sided with their mother, reproaching him with their accusatory expressions, their sullenness when he was with them.

He wondered why he cared, but a father had to care. His father had never cared about him.

Claudia sat down and crossed one elegant leg over the

other. She was short and always wore very high heels. She dressed immaculately, carefully. Nothing was ever allowed to slip. She used too much make-up. She would age quickly, yet since Simeon had left her her face had become more mask-like, sometimes even the cracks showed when she smiled. When he was not around she smiled a great deal and had started to drink perhaps more than she should.

'The children were here yesterday when you *said* you'd come,' she went on in the same accusing, nagging manner.

'I couldn't come. I said I'm sorry.'

'You could at least have telephoned.'

'Yes, I should have telephoned.' He put a hand to his head which was already beginning to buzz as it always did when he came back to this depressing place. 'I should have rung and I didn't. I'm very sorry. Claudia, I've been putting together a very important deal. I was at the office all night. I completely forgot . . .'

Claudia got up and with an oath ground her cigarette out in the heavy cut-glass ashtray.

'I don't fucking care *where* you were or *what* you did,' she stormed, making him wince because he hated obscenity in women almost as much as he hated cigarette smoke. Now she indulged in both to excess. She had become so distasteful to him as a woman that he wondered how he could ever have loved her, desired her, made love to her. In his mind he compared the tall, elegant aristocratic Virginia Silklander to this granddaughter of an Italian immigrant and found her wanting.

Claudia ranted on regardless. 'When you *say* you are coming I *expect* you to come or, if not, to *telephone*. I expect that, do you hear? The kids expect it. Christ knows, as a father you do little enough for the poor bastards. Once a week . . .'

He tried once more to be patient. 'I *always* come when I say I will. If I can . . . my business is expanding.'

69

'Is it?' Claudia threw back her head and her laugh was shrill and artificial. 'Right, if it is I'll have some more money. I need a new car. I wouldn't mind a new house. You see, Simeon Varga,' she lifted her finger and wagged it viciously at him, 'I want to take you for everything you've got and I *intend* to. You won't find my family forgiving or tolerant . . .'

'As ever,' Varga murmured.

'As ever.' She thrust her face close to his. 'They never liked you. My God, they were right. We'll take you to the cleaners, Simeon. Believe me.'

'I believe you, Claudia.' Simeon passed his hand over his face again and his fingers remained tensely on his forehead which was throbbing. Then he lowered them and stared at her.

'I must tell you I want a divorce. This farce of a marriage must end. Then I *will* see the children in my own time, alone and at my own place. I . . .'

'No divorce,' Claudia screamed, thrusting out both hands. 'Never, over my dead body. I am a Catholic, my children are Catholics. We got married in a Catholic church. You made vows, Simeon. Never, never. No divorce. Never. My father, were he alive poor man, would kill you. The shock will kill my mother. You know the laws of the church have always controlled our family.'

Simeon sat down again, his heart beating quickly.

'Only when they suited you. Your brothers are among the greediest men I know. They pay lip service to Catholicism, and so do you. I doubt if any of you other than your mother even believe in a deity. I am talking of practical matters, not of an imaginary heaven. The fact is, we have lived apart for two years. If you will not agree to divorce me, in time the law permits it. There is no question about it, but it will happen.' He pressed his hand to his forehead again. 'The only thing, Claudia, is that if you make it easy for me, civilized, I will be extremely generous to you. If you don't I will fight you for everything you want and,' he looked at her, his eyes flashing dangerously, 'make no mistake about it but I shall win. From now on I intend to get everything in life that I want. No holds barred.'

CHAPTER 4

Ginny stood by the french windows in Varga's office gazing down into the small courtyard. Jets from the fountain cascaded over the basin into the pond below, scattering the fish which played hide and seek among the lilies floating lazily upon the surface of the water. The movement seemed to mesmerize her, but eventually she raised her eyes to the windows of the houses opposite, clearly converted into offices, for this was part of the commercial centre of the metropolis.

Once upon a time Mayfair had been the chosen domicile of wealthy people; great houses had grown up there whose families had given their names to many of the streets and squares: Albemarle, Grafton, Devonshire, Cavendish. Among them had been Silklanders, whose town house, long demolished to make way for an office block, had been a few streets away from here.

Eventually she turned round and found Varga gazing at her.

'Well?' he asked.

'Lovely. It's a beautiful house.'

'It's Georgian in style, but really quite modern.'

'I guessed that.' She pointed towards the house behind them. 'This would have been the mews for the houses over there. Still, they've done this awfully well.' She looked down at the floor. 'I love the carpet. Very good taste, Simeon. Tell me . . .' she paused; 'was it your wife?'

'My *wife*?' He looked at her with surprise.

'I thought –' she hesitated, reluctant to appear sexist. 'I thought perhaps your wife would have helped with the furnishing.'

'My wife has absolutely nothing to do with my business,' he said coldly.

'You never in fact mention her.'

There was no furniture in the room, and Varga leaned casually against the wall, his arms folded.

'My wife and I haven't lived together for over two years. We are divorcing.'

'Oh, I'm sorry.'

'Don't be sorry. We have grown apart.'

'And your children?'

'Will be well taken care of. When the divorce is through I will have them to stay with me. Ginny, your remark about the furnishing is pertinent because my reason for bringing you here was to hope that it was something which might appeal to you.'

'To me?' She looked astonished.

'To a woman of your taste and sophistication. I'm sure you know the ins and outs of the salerooms. And I'm not being sexist,' he concluded with a smile.

'My brother's the person you want.' Ginny ignored his remark. 'He's an art dealer. You couldn't do better than get Lambert to buy for you, and his wife Maggie, who has the most exquisite taste, also does interior decorating.'

'Why didn't I know of them before?'

'Because you never asked me.'

He looked at her and envied her cool self-confidence. Of course she would know all the right people, and they would know the right people, and this would continue to bind them all together in a tight little cocoon, a self-perpetuating, all-enveloping world of the privileged, the noble, the very wealthy, the people who went to the same school and whose families had known one another for generations.

Elegant, beautiful Ginny, perfect in her Dior suit, silk shirt, large white buttons. Her hair parted at the side had the sleekness and vitality, the sheen of a well-bred horse, endlessly groomed, brushed and combed. Her perfume was subtle, fragrant, her accessories fine kid, soft leather, her watch twenty-two carat, her pearl and diamond brooch perfect, unflawed, undoubtedly a family heirloom.

Her black hair, her dark blue eyes, sparkling, mischievous, her parted lips, white even teeth, gave her the sensual allure of an unattainable woman: he wanted her so badly.

He wondered if she knew, could even guess, what a spur she was to his ambition.

She put her head on one side, as if questioning him, breaking the spell, as he hurried on.

'I want this to be like a gracious residence,' he waved a hand about, 'rather than an office. It must be full of antiques; old, valuable. It must provide an ambience of luxury and ease; but it must also be businesslike. You understand, I hope, Ginny?'

'Oh, I understand perfectly,' she assured him.

'Lunch?' Simeon looked at his watch.

'Why not?'

Casually he took her arm as they walked down the stairs, across the cool hall and into the summer sunshine. It was only a short walk away to a favourite restaurant where there was nearly always a table, even if he hadn't booked.

'I think champagne,' Simeon smiled as the *maître d'hôtel* showed them to their seats. 'Could we drink a bottle?'

'I think a glass is enough for me,' Ginny murmured. 'Work, you know.'

'Half a bottle.' Simeon nodded his approval. 'I scarcely ever drink at lunchtime. Have you half a bottle, Giorgio?'

'Certainly, Mr Varga. Half a bottle of the house champagne.' And he hurried away.

'You don't have many vices really, do you, Simeon?'

'You're laughing at me.' He glanced at her as the *maître d'* appeared with the menus.

'I'm not.' She leaned one arm on the table and casually rested her chin in the palm of her hand. 'You don't smoke, you drink very little, you don't like getting into debt and borrowing, you don't court publicity, in fact you hate it. Even then,' she broke a roll which had been placed on her side plate, 'don't you think you're moving a little too fast?'

'No.'

'It's only a year since you bought Oriole. Then Yokkaichi. Now the house . . .'

'I've moved very slowly compared to some people. I have very good cash balances in all my companies. The leverage is exactly right to the P/E ratio per share. I have added a new bank, by the way.'

'Oh?'

'Burton, Larosse.'

'Mm,' she nodded. 'Did you deal with Piers?'

'You know him?'

'Only vaguely, but he's good.'

Of course she would know him; there would be some family connection, some link with the old school tie.

'I haven't of course *left* Robert,' Varga said carefully. 'Hopefully they will handle other deals for me. One must spread the risk.'

Ginny seemed intent on buttering her roll, her eyes on her task.

'You know that Robert and I are no longer engaged?' She raised her eyes and her grave expression made his blood run faster.

'I saw it in the paper.' He spoke as casually as he could. 'I nearly rang you, but thought it was not quite the right thing to do. I'm sorry to hear it.'

'There's nothing to be sorry about.' She brought the roll to her mouth, to the point of taking a bite, and smiled at him. 'Just as well we found out now, before it was too late. Mother rushed us into the engagement and she was rushing us into the wedding.'

'Was there anything . . .' he wanted to appear discreet. 'I hope it had nothing to do with me?'

She looked at him and at that moment she knew. They both knew. They felt happy, expectant, but it would never do to betray the change that had subtly, suddenly come about. Varga wanted to reach out to her and take her hand but he dared not. One mistake, one false move, and he would lose her.

Naturally she didn't give him a straight answer. 'Rather like you and your wife – what's her name, by the way?'

'Claudia.'

'Rather like you and Claudia, Robert and I simply grew apart. The trouble was we had known each other for ever. We played together as children, grew up together. The Wards had a country house near ours – as well as their main home in Wiltshire. His mother is Scots and there were always Wards in our house and Silklanders in theirs. Maybe we drifted together, and now we've drifted apart. That's all there is to it.'

'I gather you broke it?'

'Why do you "gather" that?'

'It's a feeling I have – sorry if I was mistaken.'

At that moment the champagne arrived and they stopped talking as the wine waiter went into the elaborate ritual of pouring, halting as the mousse frothed halfway down the flute, only to evaporate in a surge of tiny bubbles which rose to the surface of the pale golden liquid. Then he began all over again until the glass was nearly full, the ceremony complete. Varga thanked the waiter, took his glass and held it towards her.

'Anyway, let us forget the past and its unhappy memories. To you, Ginny.'

'To the success of AP International and its entrepreneurial chairman.'

'Ginny,' Varga put down his glass and a note of urgency entered his voice, 'I asked you once to come and work for me. I renew the invitation. I knew that, maybe, you were formerly held back by Robert's obvious hostility to me ... oh yes, it was very obvious.' He glanced at her before hurrying on. 'I can't blame him.'

'There was no need for any hostility,' Ginny said in a voice that was very detached. '*I* was quite capable of separating business from anything else. Robert obviously wasn't. In my judgement he lacked maturity.'

'He *was* jealous?'

'It was absurd.' Once again Ginny avoided answering the question directly. 'His stupid jealousy was his undoing; that was the reason for our break-up.'

'Then it *was* to do with me?' Varga experienced a thrill of pleasure at her admission.

'Only indirectly.' She sounded offhand. 'It was a matter of principle. Robert's suspicions were, as you know quite well, unfounded. There has never been anything between you and me.'

'Quite,' Varga gravely concurred.

'Besides, you were married, or so I thought, and it has always been my policy to keep my hands off other women's men.'

'*Very* laudable in this day and age.' Varga sipped his drink, feeling pleased. 'Anyway I shall soon be free . . .'

The *maître d'* arrived to take their orders. Ginny didn't feel hungry, and it seemed that Varga didn't either. Their attitude disappointed the *maître d'*, who made a fruitless attempt to tempt them with the *plat du jour*. They both decided on smoked salmon as a main course and a salad of endives.

The *maître d'* bravely hid his failure and, with a regretful smile, departed. Well as he knew the rich, he found them hard to understand. Why should anyone come to a restaurant of this calibre for something that could be purchased at a delicatessen? No wonder the chef was temperamental.

Varga leaned urgently towards her. 'I need your strength, your expertise. Naturally you will be a director . . .'

'And what would be my title?' A smile seemed to hover on her lips.

'Director of Public Relations, whatever you like. You name it, you will be it. I will pay you whatever salary you require and there will be shares in a fast-growing company which you, Ginny, can help to promote.'

'But I can do that from where I am. As it is I work constantly on your account.'

'Come to Yokkaichi with me next week and see round the Japanese plant. I'd like you to get some idea of what is involved. I'm going to sign the deal and I'd like you to be there.'

'No.' Ginny took another sip of champagne and vigorously shook her head. 'It would be the wrong move at the wrong time. Let's leave it on the slow burner, Simeon.' Then she said in a completely different tone of voice, 'Look, before I forget I'll give you my brother's telephone number. You don't have to use him, but I don't think you'd regret it. Frankly, I think you'll like each other.'

Maggie Silklander was an interior decorator of renown, an expert particularly in the field of Georgian furniture, though with her innate good taste she could have accomplished with ease the decor of an ultramodern apartment in New York.

Lambert's speciality as an art connoisseur was the Renaissance, though like his wife he was knowledgeable and eclectic. Growing up in beautiful surroundings he had been interested in art all his life, and after taking a degree in art history at the Courtauld Institute was employed by Sotheby's.

There he had met Maggie, also a trainee, and they

married when they were both twenty-one. In many ways it was a marriage of ideals as well as an ideal marriage based on common interests.

Maggie was petite, smart, artificially blond. Her looks contrasted well with Lambert's thick black hair and blue eyes which made him as handsome as the same combination made Ginny beautiful. Maggie, though, was as industrious as a bee; Lambert liked to dream. His favourite pastime was spending hours in some old country house where he felt at home valuing pictures. Frequently Maggie came along too to value the furniture. It fitted in with their life-style that they had no children, though no one knew whether this was by accident or design. They certainly never seemed to pine for them or miss having them.

Now they had inspected the new office premises, bare except for the golden brown carpet, which Maggie had eyed rather critically.

'It must not necessarily be *all* Georgian,' Simeon said. 'After all it's quite a modern house.'

'How about abstract?' Lambert looked at him.

'Abstract?'

'Abstract paintings. I have some very good young painters on my books. Maggie's a wizard at abstract too.'

'I don't just want straight lines and blobs,' Varga replied, looking dubious. 'I think I'd rather collect well-known painters, though they can be modern.'

'Oh they can be abstract and well-known,' Lambert said gaily. 'Leave it to me.'

'I could have done without this carpet,' Maggie said reproachfully. 'However it's here and it would be criminal to take it all up. I'll do you a scheme – tell you how much it will cost.'

'And how long it will take to do,' Simeon said. 'I am an impatient man, you know. I want to move in here very quickly. It's an important stage in the development of my plans. By the way I like Japanese.'

'Japanese?'

'Japanese art.' He shrugged. 'Japanese things. After all a lot of my business will be with Japan and it's nice to please one's clients.'

'Japanese?' Lambert looked doubtfully at Maggie. 'We're rather keen on Japanese ourselves. We'll certainly see what we can do.'

'A man without much humour, I think,' was Maggie's comment over drinks later that day at Ginny's. There was a rather deserted air about the house and empty spaces where Robert had taken things that belonged to him: furniture, pictures from the walls. The elaborate hi-fi equipment had been his. There was a big gap there. Maggie thought Ginny looked tired.

'You're talking about Varga?' Ginny turned from the drinks tray and held a glass out to Lambert who stood by her side.

'Yes. Where exactly does he come from?'

'I've no idea.'

'You've no *idea*?' Maggie sounded disbelieving.

'None at all.' Ginny sank on to the sofa beside her.

'Haven't you asked?'

'No. Why should I? Our relationship is strictly business. I don't care where he came from and if he wants to be secretive about it that's his affair.'

'But doesn't it matter where he comes from?'

'Not from my point of view, certainly not from a business point of view. His wife is Anglo-Italian. Maybe he came from Italy.'

'But how can you do his PR if you know nothing about him?'

'He eschews personal publicity. He really doesn't like it. He refuses personal interviews, won't be photographed or appear on the TV. There are quite a lot of moguls who are like that. I am meant to be his front, his mouthpiece. But he makes darn sure I know everything about his company. There is stacks of information on that. He's very meticulous, very careful. He plans

80

everything thoroughly, though that doesn't prevent him moving fast when necessary. He's very hot on deals. He gets wind of something and he's off. He's acquisitive. He's doubled the share price in a year and the City's impressed.'

Lambert sat opposite his wife and sister. 'I don't really know if I like him or not.'

Ginny smiled. 'That's the secret of his charm. He's enigmatic.'

'I wouldn't call him exactly charming.' Maggie shook her head doubtfully. 'He's cold. He scared me a little.'

'Oh, that's nonsense!' Ginny sounded as though Maggie had made a personal affront. 'He's shy, not cold. He really is terribly shy. Frankly I find it appealing.'

'He's sexy,' Maggie said after a pause.

'Do *you* find him sexy, Ginny?' Lambert had a mocking light in his eyes.

Ginny was giving nothing away. 'My relationship with him is strictly one of business. I couldn't work for him otherwise.'

'And what about his wife?' Maggie reached for a nut from a bowl on the table.

'Divorced, or divorcing. That much I know.'

'Children?' Despite what she'd said Maggie was clearly intrigued by Varga.

'Two. I think quite young. And that's all I *do* know. Now,' she put down her glass firmly and stood up, 'I can give you a fry-up or take you round to the local Greek.'

'We've got to get home,' Lambert said. 'We've people coming to dinner. In fact we should have been there at six.' He stood up, rapidly draining his glass. Then as he put it down he said casually: 'Strange here without Robert.'

'Yes, it is in a way.' Ginny bit her lip.

'Any regrets?'

'Only that it is sad to lose a friend.'

'But surely Robert will stay a friend?' Maggie protested. 'You've known him all your life, Ginny.'

'I suppose in time it will come round to that again.' She walked slowly with them to the door. 'Just now we don't communicate.'

'I suppose it had nothing to do with Varga?' Lambert paused and gave her a sly look.

For answer Ginny opened the door and gestured towards the street.

'Off you go,' she said, 'or your guests will be breaking down the door.'

The Silklander family was a close one and those who married into it immediately became drawn into its affairs. Maggie was no exception. She felt closer to the Silklanders than she did to the family into which she had been born. Silklanders had a way of involving everyone in their fortunes.

It was because of this that she worried more about Ginny than Lambert, and after their guests had gone later that night and they were tidying up she said: 'Shouldn't you be worried about Ginny?'

Lambert looked up from the drinks table where he was pouring them each a nightcap.

'Do you think she has a relationship with that man?' Maggie went on.

'Are you referring to Varga?' Lambert smiled. '"That man", as you call him, is our latest and most valuable client. I intend to persuade him to spend a small fortune or, rather, to allow us to spend one on his behalf.'

'You don't really *like* him though, do you?' Maggie frowned and sat on the sofa, beckoning to him to join her. 'I can tell.'

'I don't *dislike* him. In fact I suspect I quite like him. He knows absolutely nothing about art and even less about antique furniture. But that's to our advantage. Not that I want to con him, but that's what we're here for. I think he's pretty straight. Of course he's not one of us.'

'Hideous snob,' Maggie said with a grin. 'Oh, the business side is fine.'

The home of the Lambert Silklanders was an example of a complementary elegance that went with the life they lived in the higher echelons of London society. There they moved easily among the rich, the titled and the celebrated in one form or another, or those who were simply famous for being famous.

Robert Ward had fitted very well into this ambience and he and Ginny had been frequent guests in Cadogan Square. The three-storey town house was the very epitome of gracious living: a large drawing-room was furnished with pieces by William Vile and John Cobb, Matthew Boulton and Hepplewhite, with a Bonnard, a Seurat and a little-known Toulouse-Lautrec, one of his circus drawings, on the walls among others by less well-known masters.

The master bedroom was on the first floor above the drawing-room which had balconies front and back on to the square on one side and the rear garden on the other. On the second floor were guest bedrooms and Lambert and Maggie shared a large, light open-plan office at the top of the house. They were the sort of people, moneyed, aristocratic, who might be expected to have live-in staff, a housekeeper or some such, but they only had a daily woman who also helped out at important dinner parties. The *chef d'oeuvre* in the dining-room on the ground floor was a japanned table by Hepplewhite, but even more priceless was a rare example of a Japanese *karabitsu*, a chest of the Fujiwara period, elaborately decorated with *maki-e*: spray painting with gold dust. This almost priceless piece of furniture had been a wedding present from Maggie's father, an eminent surgeon at a leading London hospital. The dining-room walls were hung with one-leaf *tsuitate* and several-leaved *byobu*: painted screens showing ornamental scenes, sometimes exotic, of exquisite beauty, and the parquet floor was scattered with *tatami* mats.

They certainly knew a lot about Japanese art, but they did not necessarily want to share what to them was a personal addiction with Varga.

'I do think he's keen on Ginny. I can tell about these things. For instance, that break-up with Robert was very sudden.'

Maggie rose and wandered to the window which opened on to the back balcony. It was too dark to see it now, but it was festooned with clematis and roses, the purple buds of *montana* and the yellow flowers of Gloire de Dijon which had crept across the lower part of the house to cover it over the years.

'You don't mean you think that *Varga* is behind all that?'

'Your mother certainly thinks so.' Maggie turned and gazed at him.

'But Mother has never met him. Has she?'

'No, but she says she has an instinct. Ginny talks of him constantly. Well, he's asked her to work for him.'

'My God.' Lambert leaned against the back of the sofa. 'She never mentioned it to *us*.'

'She was close to it, I thought. She told your mother she's not going to, but Moira seems to think she will. He's offered her a directorship. Douglas says his shares are climbing so rapidly that he will soon be a multi-millionaire.' Douglas was Lambert's brother-in-law.

'The sly puss. Maybe we should ask Ginny to dinner and have a good talk.' Lambert rose and refilled his glass.

'Ginny is twenty-eight years old,' Maggie said severely. 'You honestly don't expect her to take any notice of what *we* say. Besides we can hardly criticize him if we're working for him. We don't want to kill the golden goose.'

'True.' Sitting down again, Lambert stretched his legs and gazed in front of him. The Silklanders were not a wealthy family and although Archibald Wickham had money it was mostly thanks to his lucrative practice as a plastic surgeon. He was already on a third, much younger wife, so it was doubtful whether Maggie would ever see any of his money. Their antiques and decoration business was good, thanks not only to their skill but their connections. However one could not afford to lose a free-spending client like Simeon Varga.

Accordingly over the next few weeks they devoted themselves almost exclusively to touring the galleries and auction rooms of London and beyond for pieces which would be suitable for the mansion in Mayfair, the new headquarters of AP International.

The name AP International on the brass plate looked simple but elegant and Ginny stopped to admire it before she entered the main door now guarded by a uniformed commissionaire. The receptionist sitting at the Weisweiler work table (1780) looked up with a professional smile which turned into one of welcome when she saw who it was.

'Miss Silklander, Mr Varga is expecting you. Your brother and sister-in-law have already arrived.'

Ginny turned to give her keys to the commissionaire who would park her car in one of the nearby underground car parks and then ran her fingers along the diamond-shaped veneer.

'Very nice.'

'I believe it cost £25,000,' the receptionist said in awed tones, and she didn't look like a woman who would be surprised by many things.

'Mustn't spill any ink on it, then.' Ginny winked at her and ran lightly up the stairs even before the receptionist had got her finger on the intercom buzzer to announce her.

Ginny paused for a moment by the head of the stairs and looked down into the reception area. As well as the beautiful piece of furniture by the German-born *ébéniste* Weisweiler, who had worked for the Queen of France as well as the Prince Regent of England, there were two Louis XVI armchairs upholstered in heavy brocade, and a low mahogany table, probably by Adam or Hepplewhite, on which were copies of *The Times*, the *Financial Times* and *Harpers and Queen*. Overlooking them all, with an expression of superiority which went well with that of the receptionist, and replacing the fake discus thrower, was a bust of a Roman emperor, probably Augustus and undoubtedly authentic, mounted on a classical plinth.

The whole of the reception area was bathed in natural light from the cupola which had been an inspired idea of the architect, who had converted the building to its present use, to expel the gloom from the mews.

Hearing a movement behind her Ginny turned to see Varga standing there, a hand extended.

'Well, what do you think?'

'Quite breathtaking,' Ginny said enthusiastically. 'Wonderfully good taste, the whole thing.'

'Wait until you see my office.' Varga drew her to the open door and from the threshold she could see a huge bureau-plat that seemed to cover half the room, a duchesse chaise-longue alongside the window and, opposite the desk, two comfortable marquise chairs with cabriole legs. Suspended from the ceiling was a magnificent eighteenth-century chandelier of rock crystal.

The walls of the room were hung with a heavy layered cream paper which set off to perfection the small but impressive collection of paintings, the open spaces an indication that there were more to come.

There was a tiny pastel by Fragonard, an early and relatively unknown work which had still cost, Ginny knew, nearly half a million pounds, because Lambert had rung her after he'd bought it at auction. There were also a Dutch scene by David Teniers the Younger, which had been around £100,000 and had come from a gallery; the head of a girl by Marie Laurencin; a Stubbs and, behind the desk, a collection of miniatures by the eighteenth-century artist Nathaniel Hone, who was one of the founder members of the Royal Academy.

'Super!' Ginny exclaimed. 'The whole thing is super.'

Maggie and Lambert smirked like proud parents.

'I told you,' Varga said proudly, 'I told you over the telephone. How they got this together in such a short time is beyond me.'

'It's the secret of knowing where to look.' Lambert walked over to the beautiful *vernis* Martin lacquer table on which there was a silver bucket containing a bottle of Piper-Heidsieck Rare Champagne and poured a little of the beautiful vintage amber liquid into four tall crystal flutes.

'And having the wherewithal to pay.' Maggie, dressed in a tailored navy dress, raised her glass towards Simeon.

'Don't let's talk about money,' he replied, also raising his glass. 'But first I want to toast Ginny who, in many ways, is responsible for this. Not just the luxury, the house, which is very dear to my heart, and the furnishings, but for making it all possible.'

'I made *none* of it possible!' Ginny protested.

'But you did. Had we left it to Len, as much as I like him, I doubt I would have got so far. It is Ginny who, with single-minded energy, has promoted my company spectacularly in the past year. She introduced me to the best bankers, the best advertising agency. She talked about me to the most influential journalists and media personalities. Finally,' he turned and bowed in the direction of Maggie and Lambert, 'to the finest interior decorator and antique specialist in the business, the finest art connoisseur. Do you know,' he looked first at the Fragonard and then at Ginny, 'my paintings alone are worth over a million pounds.'

'And increasing every day.' Lambert helped himself to a canapé. 'The market is going far and you,' he raised his glass towards Varga, 'are going with it, Simeon. You are on the crest of a wave and I can only see an ocean of endless promise and success ahead of you.'

Varga sat down on the chaise-longue and drew Ginny down beside him. Then he addressed himself to her brother.

'Lambert, I want you to persuade your sister to join me.' He indicated the interconnecting room. 'It only awaits her instructions as to furniture. I have left it bare because it is for her.'

Ginny laid a hand on his arm. 'I told you, Simeon, it is not the right thing, *or* the right time . . .'

'But I think it is.' Lambert, sounding excited, crossed to refill first Simeon's glass and then top up Ginny's. 'Maggie and I have had a chance really to get to know Simeon over the last few weeks. We are very impressed, aren't we, darling?'

'Oh very.' Maggie nodded vigorously.

'You see, Simeon,' Lambert continued, 'Ginny is very precious to us.'

'Of course, and to me too,' Simeon said quietly.

'We want the best for her,' Lambert continued, as though he hadn't heard.

'I'm not a *child*,' Ginny began as if embarrassed by the display of sentimentality.

'Darling, let Lambert speak.' Maggie's glance promptly silenced her. She knew what an important client Varga was for them.

'You're certainly not a child, Ginny,' Lambert continued, 'but you are my sister. I'm proud of you. The whole family is proud of you. You've broken the mould. You and Maggie represent the modern woman: clever, attractive, feminine. You've had a great career. You were the first woman in our family to go to university. You've got a very good job with Morgan; but you are number two, or three or four, I'm not sure. He has any amount of good people all at your level. Here you will be number one, immediately after Simeon.'

'He offered to make me director of publicity,' Ginny said. 'That's not number one. Finance and marketing are more important.'

'I now offer you also a directorship of my company,' Varga cut in. 'A seat on the board. Liddle is important, but you will be important too.'

'What have I done to deserve all this?' Ginny's eyes levelled with his.

'You have the talent, the ability,' he replied. 'I can sense it, feel it. Lambert agrees with me.'

'What does Liddle say?' Tony Liddle was the all-important financial controller who had been with Varga from the beginning.

'Tony agrees you're outstanding. There is no jealousy there, I can assure you.'

'No strings either?' She gave him a sideways look.

'None at all.'

'Then, subject to contract, I accept,' Ginny said, holding up her glass. 'You can blame it on the champagne.'

Lambert and Maggie drove Ginny home after a celebration dinner at the Dorchester round the corner. Ginny sat in the back of the car, feeling tired, a little bewildered, still not convinced she'd done the right thing. Had she been swept along by the glamour, the money, the champagne, the fact that Varga's feeling for her clearly went beyond mere business? In front of her Maggie and Lambert chatted animatedly.

'Varga wants me to make those offices at the back of the house into a *pied à terre* for him.'

'Oh!' Ginny stared straight ahead as they sped along Park Street and, crossing Oxford Street, drove round Portman Square and into Wigmore Street. It was right out of Lambert's way but he'd insisted. They were all on a kind of 'high' that night that had very little actually to do with champagne.

'I don't know if he'll get planning permission,' Maggie went on. 'At present he's in a rented flat in Shepherd Market.'

'I know,' she ventured.

'Have you seen it, Ginny?'

'No.' As Maggie glanced disbelievingly over her shoulder Ginny leaned forward. 'I *know* what you're thinking, but it's not true. If there were anything personal between

89

Varga and me I wouldn't have accepted. In fact I'm still not sure I *will* accept.'

'Oh, but you must . . .' Maggie turned right round. 'You promised.'

'I *said* "subject to contract". I'll have my lawyers go through every word, every syllable. You see, I'm not worth the money. I haven't got the experience *or* the knowhow, whatever Varga says.'

'He's clearly carrying a torch for you. Isn't he, Lambert?'

Lambert didn't reply immediately.

'I hate involving business and personal feelings. I'm all against it.' Ginny flopped back in her seat.

'Clearly he thinks you're very, very capable.'

'I did a good job for him, that's true.'

'That's it.' Lambert thumped the wheel. 'Varga trusts you. He also knows you know people who can be helpful to him. That's what he needs most of all now. Contacts.'

'He has his own contacts. I had nothing to do with Yokkaichi Electronics. In fact I think that was a bad move and I opposed it.'

'He knows you're an independent voice. You'll *criticize*.' Maggie was obviously keen for her to do the job.

'He wants to prove me wrong. He enjoys it. He loves an argument.'

'Why are you against Yokkaichi Electronics?' Lambert was curious.

'It's way outside his experience. He knows pharmaceuticals.'

'Look,' Lambert's tone was laconic. 'Varga is a businessman, pure and simple. Profit and loss, balance sheets. They're all that matter. He says he has his eyes on a newspaper, a range of broadcasting and TV stations in the States, and an oil company.'

'You'll have your work cut out.' Maggie gave her a broad grin. 'It's not a chance you should turn down, Ginny.'

Ginny wondered if, much as she loved her brother and sister-in-law, they had their own interests at heart as much as hers.

Len Morgan frowned, gazed at his desk, thumbed through some papers as if preoccupied. Then he raised his eyes level with Ginny's.

'You know I feel you're making a profound mistake.'

'It's too good an opportunity to miss. I talked it over with my brother.'

'You might have talked it over with *me*.' Len sounded hurt. Ginny gazed at the floor.

'You've really accepted?'

'I told him this morning. Then I came straight over to see you.'

'It would have been better the other way round. You're making a mistake.'

'I can't see *why* you're so set against it, Len. I've been with you for ages. It's time to move on.'

'Yes, but not *that*. I can't explain why.' Len focused his eyes on the ceiling. 'Hell, he's our client,' he said, lowering them. He got up and walked moodily to the window where he stood gazing over that unique view of London, then he turned his gaze to her.

'Let's face it.' Ginny perched on his desk, swinging her legs, in the familiar pose in which he would always remember her. Perhaps he was a little in love with her, too. 'You don't *like* him, do you?' she said.

'I don't know the guy.' Len went back to his desk and sat down, still gazing at her, provocative witch with the long, shapely legs. 'And nor do you. No one does, anyway. He's the most secretive man I've ever known.'

'That doesn't mean you can't *work* with him. He's given me a tremendous chance, Len. I'm to be a director. It's one of the fastest-growing companies.'

'I don't want to lose you, Ginny, but also I don't think this is a good move for you. It's not in your interests.'

'It's not in *your* interests, Len. I think that's the truth.'

Ginny slipped off the desk and straightened her skirt. 'Maybe you're being a bit selfish. Maggie didn't take much to Varga at the beginning. But now they like him . . .'

'He pays the piper, doesn't he?'

'Don't be unkind. They're not all that badly off.'

'I always thought Lambert a greedy bastard, even if he is your brother.'

'Thank you for that compliment.' She narrowed her eyes.

'Ginny, I didn't mean . . .'

'Maybe I don't know you so well either, Len. Lambert is a good, hard-working dealer. Since when was making as much money as you can "greedy"? You do it yourself.'

'Of course. Forgive me.' He crossed his arms, angry at his display of bad humour.

'Look,' Ginny leaned over the desk towards him, 'this conversation is silly.'

'Varga's in love with you.'

'Varga is still married.'

'I don't care. But that's his motive. First you'll be the mistress, then the wife. Is that what you really want?'

A surge of blood seemed to rush to Ginny's head and she felt like hitting him. Instead she said abruptly:

'Do you want me to work out my notice?'

Len grimaced and wrote something on a pad in front of him.

'If I can't influence you I shan't attempt to keep you, Ginny. Mark Foster can take over from you straight away.' He held out his hand and gave her a rueful grin. 'Naturally, I wish you all the luck in the world, but never ever tell me I didn't warn you.'

CHAPTER 5

Giuseppe Bernini, the great-grandfather of Claudia Varga and her brothers, Carlo, Matteo and Paolo, had left the family silversmith business in Naples to set up one in London. It quickly flourished thanks to the skills and money – not much, but enough – at his command. Despite their assimilation into England and the English way of life, the family remained in many ways Italian, with Italian names, Italian customs and, most decidedly, a taste for Italian food. They had also remained strong adherents of the Roman Catholic faith.

The old man would have been proud of his descendants. They had husbanded their original investment, made it grow and continued the tradition of hard work that had been a mark of the Berninis for generations. The house of Bernini was synonymous with fine jewels and craftsmanship. The showroom in Albemarle Street had the elegance of the many art galleries which surrounded it. It was the epitome of good taste: simply the name BERNINI engraved on the stone portico above the door.

Great-grandfather Giuseppe would also have been gratified by the fact that the family remained close to its Italian roots and that his great-grandchildren looked after their widowed mother, the matriarchal Fortunata, who dressed in black and ruled her family partly by excessive affection, partly by terror.

The Bernini home was still where Giuseppe had established it in Highgate overlooking green fields, as it had nearly a hundred years before.

Carlo, the eldest, was unmarried and lived with his mother. She would gladly have parted with him because he was almost forty and she felt a dishonourable stigma attached itself to his single state. She was passionately attached to him, however, as she was to the rest. Some people said Carlo had never found a woman to love as much as he loved his mother. She treated him like a child and he was afraid of her, even though he was the head of the business, a prominent member of the Anglo-Italian community, a patron of charitable causes and a popular man. Many a girl from the same background as Carlo Bernini would have given a great deal to be his wife, and not just for his money. He was a fleshy but handsome man and dressed with impeccable taste and care. Of his two brothers who worked with him in the business, Matteo was married with three children and Paolo, also with three children, ran the Roman side of the House of Bernini.

Claudia, the second eldest, had of course married Simeon Varga. The family had not been pleased about the marriage and had opposed it. Varga was not one of them; without background or fortune, a strange man, secretive about himself and his origins, even to his wife.

The only thing they liked about Varga was his obvious ambition, his intention to make money. He wasn't a scrounger, not after Claudia for her money. He had told them that he was on the verge of buying his own business and he had kept his word. From the shadows of running an export-import business with a letterbox address, he bought a small pharmaceuticals company off the peg and made it grow rapidly.

They also approved of the fact that, although Varga appeared to have no family of his own, he had not asked his father-in-law for money and had protested about the gift of a house. He was proud and they approved of pride;

but they had so wished his origins had been Italian.

Despite the family's foreboding the marriage at first appeared happy. The Vargas dutifully visited the Berninis once a week and for family gatherings: Christmas, Easter and the many birthdays. There were soon two children to join the growing ranks of Bernini cousins and they all got on very well.

They approved of the way that Varga's business grew, expanded and, hard workers themselves, they told Claudia not to complain about the fact that she saw so little of her husband. Bernini women expected to see little of their men. No one made money without hard work.

But when the blow fell the family was appalled. The Vargas stopped sharing a bed. Claudia was in tears, but he refused to move back. Eventually, amid much recrimination, he left her. It was a wonder he dared, because he had seemed as frightened of Fortunata as the rest of them.

It was Fortunata who swore to avenge the dishonour done to her daughter; an abandoned woman who, because of her religious faith, would never be free to marry again unless Simeon died.

The curse of the Bernini descended on Varga, but he cared little about it. He was obsessed with his work, the necessity to do well. Besides, he had another interest.

Matteo Bernini had married into a wealthy branch of the Anglo-Italian community to a girl who had the full blessing of his mother. Diana Bernini spent her time mostly divided between beauty salons, Harrods and working for various charities which would gain her public recognition.

Diana was a rather discontented woman, bored with marriage and eager to make her mark in the world, to be something other than wife and mother, money spender, an adornment. She was good-looking and would have liked to model Bernini jewellery, but that was unheard of. Matteo would have felt it demeaned him as a man to have a wife who worked. People in the community would think less of him.

A sister was another matter, however. Since her desertion it was agreed that Claudia needed an outlet in order to forget. She had expressed an interest in the business and she was encouraged to start as a vendeuse on the shop floor. She was good-looking, too, with the inherited Bernini flair, a knowledge of jewellery and an eager desire to make money, more than she needed; but they all made more, far more than they needed. It was a built-in desire to accumulate excessive wealth.

Claudia had been tremendously successful in the months she had worked in Albemarle Street. She was elegant, seductive, yet the women who came to buy jewellery for themselves, or have others buy it for them, liked her. The brothers, who shared a deep animosity towards Varga, were pleased with her, and with the fact that, despite her conventional background, she had struck out as an independent woman.

Matteo, the designer, had a room at the back of the building where he experimented on his creations rather as a couturier puts together a new collection for the season. It had a skylight to give him the maximum amount of light, fine grinders and microscopic instruments to enable him to assemble his precious stones into harmonious works of art. He spent part of the year travelling, seeking different sources for the various jewels and precious metals he used for his work. He dressed informally in Armani jackets and trousers, Gucci ties and shoes. At work he wore a white overall and, invariably, had a glass in his eye. He could concentrate for hours. His fingers were very long and beautiful, almost like those of a woman, his touch subtle and delicate.

Carlo was the opposite. He dressed formally, his suits made in nearby Savile Row, shirts from Turnbull and Asser across the road in Jermyn Street, shoes handmade by Lobb's of St James's. His hair, unlike his brother's, was fair; their grandmother had been a fair-skinned, fair-haired girl from the Swiss-Italian border. He could have passed any day for an English gentleman and, like his brothers, had been educated at a Roman Catholic public school. Carlo enjoyed the life-style of a member of the wealthy upper middle class. Although he went home to mother every night he enjoyed a number of pastimes, many of which she would never have approved of. He liked eating, drinking, gambling, fast cars, certain forms of vice, and the company of women.

But by temperament he was Italian; he had a dark, brooding Latin nature. He had vowed to his mother never to forgive the man who had cast aside his sister, and promised to avenge her.

Carlo was sitting in his office sipping black coffee and reading the *Financial Times* when there was a knock on the door and his brother came in. Carlo looked up in greeting and indicated a chair but Matteo went round to Carlo's side and placed a newspaper in front of him, indicating a paragraph at the end of the page.

'Did you see this?'

Carlo looked past his brother's finger and his face darkened as he leaned forward and read:

WOMAN TO BE A DIRECTOR OF AP INTERNATIONAL

The first woman has been appointed to the board of the AP International conglomerate which, in the years since it was bought off the shelf by Simeon Varga, has seen its share price increase by 150%. Recently Mr Varga has bought into the Japanese electronics business to add to his expanding empire which includes the French perfumery Oriole. In the twenties L'Esprit du Temps by Oriole was one of the most fashionable perfumes of its day.

Yesterday it was announced that the Honourable Virginia Silklander is to leave Morgan Associates where she has been an executive for the past five years to join Mr Varga as head of Public Relations with a seat on the board. Miss Silklander (pictured left), 28, the younger daughter of Lord and Lady Silklander, recently broke off her engagement to the Hon Robert Ward whom she had known since childhood. Miss Silklander firmly denies rumours of a romance with Mr Varga. He is believed to be separated from his wife, by whom he has two children.

Mr Varga, despite his success in the City, jealously guards his private life and little is known about him. He eschews publicity and refuses all interviews. This trend seems likely to continue as Miss Silklander also refused to discuss any personal questions concerning Mr Varga and said her job was to promote AP International and its products as successfully as she could.

'Well, well . . .' Carlo said, gazing up at his brother, one hand reaching for the phone. 'Well, well, well.'

Morgan's secretary buzzed him through the intercom:

'Call for you, Len. Mr Bernini.'

Len Morgan paused, frowned, searched through his memory which was like a computer, and lifted the phone.

'Mr Bernini?' he said politely.

'Is that Mr Morgan?'

'It is. Which Mr Bernini do I have the pleasure of speaking to?'

'Oh, you know us then?' Carlo sounded gratified.

'If it is *the* Bernini of Albemarle Street, who has not heard of you? Unfortunately, although I've heard of you I've never been able to afford your products.'

'Well, we may be able to do something about that,'

Bernini said affably. 'You find something you like and I think we can give you a decent discount. I'm ringing now because I think we have need of your services.'

'Oh?' Morgan sounded surprised.

'We have a lot of competition in the jewellery market and not only Cartier and Tiffany. A new *Dutch* firm is opening a branch in Bond Street.' Bernini sounded most indignant at the idea of another interloper.

'Well I'd be extremely pleased if we could be of help, Mr Bernini.'

'Maybe you'd like to come and see us?'

'Very much.' Len reached for his diary. 'When . . .'

'Or maybe Miss Silklander? I have heard very good things about her.'

There was a palpable silence.

'Unfortunately Miss Silklander is no longer with us.'

'Oh?' Carlo sounded surprised. 'What a pity. Where has she gone – or I suppose you would prefer not to tell me?'

'You can read about it in today's papers,' Len said, his mind ticking over. Bernini, Varga . . . there was a connection.

'Oh? I'll do that.' Carlo sounded deflated. 'May I presume, then, that you personally would be handling our account if we could come to some arrangement? I know your fees are very high.'

'I think you could assume that,' Len said guardedly. 'But maybe we could do a deal? An eye for an eye, you know.'

The beautiful bureau plat in the corner was the work of Martin Carlin, and there was a high chest of drawers by Charles Cressent, cabinet-maker to Philippe d'Orléans. There were two bergère chairs which were part of the set in the hall, and an elegant sofa whose flamboyant carving and brilliant upholstery marked it as probably Russian. Maggie said she had picked it up for next to nothing in a house sale.

The walls were the colour of primroses and Maggie had chosen etchings by George Chinnery, an early nineteenth-century English painter who had settled in the east. The drapes at the window were of pale blue silk held back by tie-backs of the same material. The whole effect was light and airy, like some elegant drawing-room rather than an office.

Varga stood in the doorway, the excited expression on his face resembling a child's who enjoyed receiving presents. And, in fact, Ginny's pleasure was his pleasure.

'Now, anything else?' Maggie was gratified by Ginny's thrilled reaction, running her hands along the veneer of the desk, gasping with admiration at the chest of drawers, sinking with a satisfied sigh into one of the chairs. 'Anything else at *all* – Simeon says you have only to ask.'

'It really *is* magnificent.' Ginny looked over at Simeon who walked slowly into the room with the measured pace of a cat, or perhaps a leopard. 'I don't know *how* I can be expected to do any work here. It's like a museum.'

'Oh, I shall expect you to work.' Simeon sank on to the chair next to her. 'You can work in a museum, you know.' He looked doubtfully at the pictures. 'I wasn't *sure* about those etchings . . . they . . .'

'They can always go somewhere else if you don't like them,' Maggie said eagerly.

'Oh, but I love them.' Ginny held up a hand in protest. 'One of our ancestors was a merchant in Madras in the eighteen-twenties and Chinnery painted his portrait. Maybe you knew that, Maggie?'

Maggie frowned.

'I can't remember a Chinnery; but isn't that a coincidence!'

'Daddy will be *delighted*,' Ginny said.

'What a good omen.' Varga crossed one leg over the other and neatly joined his hands together. 'I very much hope your parents, indeed all your family, will come and visit you here, Ginny. As well as you, I owe *so* much to Maggie and Lambert.'

'We owe so much to you,' Maggie said wryly, aware that, together, they had spent close on half a million pounds furnishing Ginny's office. On the other hand to be practical, as Lambert said, it was also an investment. 'Now,' she took up her handbag and gloves from the desk, 'I must fly.'

'Don't forget the flat.' Varga rose and held out his arms to her as though to embrace her.

'But have you got permission?'

'Not yet,' Varga smiled. 'But I don't think it will take very long.'

'Oh it will take *ages*. You don't know what these planning people on the council can be like.'

'I think a little something helps to oil the wheels of bureaucracy,' Varga said smoothly. 'You can leave that all to me, or Tony. Personally I don't think it will take very long at all.'

He bent and kissed Maggie on the cheek and then he saw her to the door while Ginny went over to her desk, her expression thoughtful. When Varga came back she was gingerly opening one of the drawers and peering inside. They smelled of old wood.

'It's *ridiculous* to use this for an office,' she said straightening up as he came towards her.

'My dear young woman,' he pretended to chide her, 'you have to learn a whole new style of working.'

'I'll say.'

'You see,' Varga flung open the door of a small adjoining room which was furnished just as a normal office would be with teak desk, tubular metal chairs and the usual array of telephones, fax machines and VDUs, 'here is your secretary's office tucked away out of sight, no antiques for her. Yet slowly you will begin to respond to the ambience of your office,' he raised a hand languidly in the air, 'and you will discover for yourself how inspirational it will be. Now, for your secretary . . .'

'Simeon there *is* something I must ask you,' Ginny interrupted, folding her arms and leaning against the desk. 'When you talk of "oiling the wheels of bureaucracy" what exactly do you mean?'

'My dear,' he raised his eyebrows, 'what do you *think* I mean?'

'I hope you don't mean a *bribe* . . .'

'Really, Ginny,' Varga's expression suddenly changed. 'What a *disgusting* thing to accuse me of.'

'I'm sorry . . .'

'I'm *amazed* you should even think it . . .' Suddenly his face – his expression always so mobile – broke into a smile and she realized he was teasing her. How little, indeed, one knew this man. 'A small gift is all it needs to encourage the wheels to move more quickly. That's all. It was quite certain I should have got permission anyway, as this was once residential.'

'What sort of gift?' she persisted.

'Ginny!' Varga sat down again and crossed his legs, his air that of someone calling on reserves of patience. 'Please, *don't* let us get across each other on our very first day together. I want it to be a special day, a happy day. My dear, in dealing with bureaucrats there is a special technique, a set of rules. You can be sure it is *nothing* dishonest. Now,' he rose and walked towards the door with a positive spring in his step before turning round, 'we must be very clear about our boundaries, Ginny. I will not interfere in yours, and I expect you not to interfere in mine. We must keep our parameters. You do agree, don't you?'

'Of course.' As he vanished through the door Ginny turned again towards the desk and sat down in her exquisite antique chair. Apart from the furniture the office was empty, not a piece of paper or a file in sight. Although there was a point for a telephone there was no telephone. The windows were open and outside the sun shone, but she felt a little chilled and got up to close them. She stood there for some time gazing out of the window at the fountain playing in the garden, then her eyes wandered up to the functional offices on the other side of the wall. No antiques there. Although she was disturbed by her slight contretemps with Varga, in a way she was pleased. It introduced an air of reality into their relationship which in the last few weeks, while details were settled and contracts drawn up, had been too honeyed for words. She was used to the cut and thrust of office life, and here it was rearing its ugly head again.

When, a little while later, she was ready to go, she somehow expected he would be there, offering the usual courtesies, the polite exchanges, the suggestion of a drink, perhaps. But he had left; gone without telling her.

He was setting the parameters of their relationship, showing who was the boss.

The house nestled in a mews behind one of the large London hotels, not far from the offices of AP International. On one side was Piccadilly and Green Park, on the other the cramped yet elegant streets of Mayfair, many of which looked pretty much as they did in its heyday: the eighteenth century.

The mews houses were very desirable, much sought after, and fetched enormous sums on the property market. Instinct, as always, made Simeon Varga look to right and left then behind him, before he inserted his key in the door and slipped inside.

Sometimes there was a person, or people, in the hall, sometimes it was empty. Its opulent decor and furnishings, its air of furtiveness and secrecy, left few people in any doubt as to what kind of establishment it was.

On this occasion the hall was empty and Varga stood for a few moments, his ear cocked, listening. All the rooms were soundproofed but occasionally there was a whisper on the stairs, cautious footfalls, occasionally, very occasionally, a discreet laugh.

But now there was nothing and, looking into the reception room on the ground floor and seeing that too was empty, he gazed quickly up at the screen which kept watch over the outside of the house and then climbed swiftly up the expensively carpeted staircase to the first floor. Then he listened again and, still hearing nothing, he crept along the corridor, put a key into the lock of another door and let himself in.

The room was sumptuously furnished and there was a heady, cloying smell of sandalwood and spice. A large double bed had a satin cover, turned back, and there were heavy satin drapes of a similar material with matching tie-backs at the windows, which were also barred. The walls were hung with richly textured paper, and there were original cartoons depicting exotic scenes of couplings involving men, women and animals in a variety of erotic and unusual positions.

Otherwise the room was sparsely furnished. There was only a richly brocaded chair by the window and a lacquered oriental chest at the foot of the bed, which had at its head two small tables of a similar style and design, and two lamps with pink silk shades.

On one side wall was a built-in wardrobe, and after he had locked the door behind him, Varga opened the wardrobe and, taking from it a heavy silk oriental robe, began carefully to undress. He hung his clothes in the wardrobe, put his undergarments on the chair, and went into the bathroom which was adjacent to the bedroom. There he washed his face and hands, parts of his body, under his arms and between his legs, and brushed his teeth. He inspected his gleaming molars carefully in the mirror and then he combed his hair, patted some skin freshener on his face, re-entered the bedroom, stepped out of his robe and climbed into bed.

Under the influence of the soporific atmosphere he had practically dropped off to sleep when there was a click as the door was unlocked from the outside and the handle gently turned. He opened his eyes and smiled; the woman who came through the door with a tray in her hand, on which there was a bottle of champagne and two glasses, bowed her head in greeting, saying nothing.

She put the tray on the table nearest to him, bent to

104

kiss his brow and then, going to the window, undid the heavy silk ties and tugged the curtains across with a cord.

In the low lamplight Varga watched her as she removed the dress she was wearing, her bra, panties and tights and, naked, went into the bathroom as he had done. He heard running water, the flush of the lavatory, and then she re-entered the room, gently closing the bathroom door behind her.

She had put some sort of oil on her body in the bathroom and as she stood gazing down at him she gently massaged it into her breasts, along her stomach, on her thighs. She was of Eurasian appearance and the sheen on her dark skin inflamed him, as it always did; he held out his arms to her.

'Melissa,' he murmured, hungrily crushing his mouth on hers. Like a cobra uncoiling she stretched voluptuously alongside him, her body seeming to sway in time to the sex act, even though it had not yet begun.

Then, as suddenly, she straightened up and, reaching for the bottle of champagne, which was already uncorked, poured a little of the amber liquid into two tall glasses, waiting as it frothed, watching the bubbles rise to the top.

Still with one hand on her waist, Varga took the glass with the other and, holding it up, said:

'To you.'

'To you.' She raised her glass and toasted him. Then, drinking deeply from it as though she was very thirsty, she replaced it on the table and stretched out beside him again, this time with her arms behind her head.

'How's everything?' Varga enquired, putting his empty glass on the table beside him.

'Everything's fine. And with you?'

'Everything's fine too.' Deeply relaxed, he also clasped his hands behind his head.

'The office?'

'It's all ready. You must come and see it one day.'

'The girl?'

There was a pause.

'The girl is fine, too. She's clever, maybe a little too inquisitive, critical, but we'll see.' He smiled at her, blowing her a kiss. 'As you know I like intelligent women.'

'I hope you didn't take too big a chance on her.'

Varga leaned over and poured some more champagne first into his glass and then into hers.

'I need her. She's extremely well connected. She's the sort of person who will give my organization the class and respectability I want. She knows everyone and everything; but I shall have to be careful with her.'

The woman sank her head deep into the pillow and her body began to rise and fall tantalizingly again. Putting out a hand she tweaked his nose, with the air and expertise of the familiar.

'Take care you don't fall in love,' she said in a low, strange kind of voice that was a cross between an incantation and a croon. 'Take care, Varga. Take care.'

PART II

Noblesse oblige

CHAPTER 6

Ginny looked around at the journalists gathered for the press conference and smiled at the ones who were special friends, those all-important contacts who were needed to put in the right word at the right time; the men and, more often these days, women whose words, columns, articles in the financial pages of the quality papers carried so much weight.

There were not more than a dozen people present and she thought she could count most of them as friends. On Sunday and throughout the following week a series of articles would appear in which AP International would, with any luck, be puffed to the skies. But one false move, one ill-considered word and the results would be the opposite to those intended; the stock, instead of rising, would fall several points on the Footsie scale.

There were one or two special favourites: Denzil van Wyke of the *Daily Financial News*, Martin Hartshorne of the influential *Investment Weekly* and Gloria Keane of the money pages of an important daily.

Ginny was giving them a private briefing in her office over coffee poured from a silver pot, drunk at leisure from porcelain cups; home-made petits fours accompanied it. This rather upmarket image Ginny knew was being imitated, not altogether successfully, by aspiring women executives in situations with the potential of hers. They had tended to go for the very expensive expense account lunch, but increasingly it was coffee and biscuits in the office to indicate seriousness; the pressure of work in the market place.

It was a year since Ginny had started to work for Varga and the progress of his company had been enormous. The shares had advanced 115 per cent in that time, and there seemed no end to the steady and successful climb.

There were, however, a few of the important analysts who worked for banks and financial institutions who remained suspicious of Varga and dubious about his long-term staying power. He was still too secretive, refused to give interviews, avoided photographs, all the things guaranteed ironically to make him a subject of more than unusual interest. He was the grey man of the City; few people even knew what he looked like. The City abhorred flash entrepreneurs who drew attention to themselves. However when a man was too secretive, there were those who wanted to know why. Ginny's job was to put things right, to balance the scales. Ginny had been most of her working life in PR, and with her air of breeding, her good manners and her charm, struck just the right note with the hound-dogs of the City.

Next to her sat Varga's financial director, Anthony Liddle, and discreetly at the rear Dorothy sat operating a tape recorder which she would later transcribe after Varga had listened to the playback.

'Good morning, ladies and gentlemen,' Ginny said.

She was wearing an Yves St Laurent suit specially flown over from Paris the night before. Such was her schedule that it was almost impossible to find time for a fitting but, with great difficulty, she had managed it the previous weekend, an acolyte of the great man coming into the salon especially for her. Her tailored look was now familiar to those who followed the fortunes of AP International and speculated about its growth and the manner of the man who ran it. Ginny was the voice of the company to the world, and the burden was a heavy one.

She knew that in his office Varga would be watching the progress of the press conference relayed to him by a hidden television camera. So far so good, all was going well. A maid dressed in black with a white apron circulated with the coffee pot.

'So,' Ginny shook her head to the offer of more coffee, 'to sum up: this has been a year of unparalleled progress in the fortunes of the company. There has been an increase in our share price of 115 per cent and our P/E ratio is now a healthy twelve.' She looked around with a smile. 'We can confidently predict a similar growth in the year ahead. Anthony Liddle will break down the figures and report on our expansion plans when I have finished talking.'

She glanced at a paper on her lap.

'This year saw our entry into the US market with our acquisition of Mondo Pharmaceuticals which will increase the overall share of the group in the drugs market. In particular we are investigating a new drug to beat the spread of the AIDS virus and Mr Varga has allowed for £100 million in the accounts for research and development. The managing director, Dr Hugo Fahr, is on the board of the group.'

Someone raised a hand in the audience and Ginny smiled.

'Yes, Max?'

'I have heard it reported, Ginny, that Varga has in fact cut the R & D budget in *half* for Mondo.'

'He's trimmed it,' Ginny said brusquely, 'making payroll economies by reducing personnel, closing down one of the laboratories entirely. But the overall investment in pure science remains the same.'

'According to the *Wall Street Journal* the Mondo executives are not happy about it.'

'I'm afraid,' Ginny said with her practised smile, 'that even *friendly* takeovers are sometimes unpopular until the dust has settled. Inevitably a few people find their jobs have changed or, occasionally, disappeared. We

111

regret this, but it is the price of progress as I'm sure you'll agree, Max.'

Max Nagel of the *Overseas Investor* was about to ask a supplementary question, but Ginny held up a hand.

'Do you think you can save further questions to the end, Max? I'm sure either Anthony or I will be able to deal with anything you bring up. Now, Mr Varga has expanded his press group into Canada and also acquired some Italian titles, especially the influential fashion magazine *Ciaou Ciaou*. Here he proposes again to leave the editorial board in full control. He is, in addition, looking at the acquisition of the entire Pronto group so that he will be the third largest publisher of newspapers and magazines in Italy. Next he is looking at tin mines in Brazil and beef in the Argentine, where he has already large interests in canning. We hope that by this time next year we shall be able to give you a fuller update on all of these projects, and some more still in the pipeline.'

It never did to go on too long so she tucked away her notes and turned to the man beside her. 'Anthony . . .'

Anthony Liddle, who had been with Varga from small beginnings, backed her statement with a plethora of figures, statistics and flow charts with which he plotted the rise of the share price. 'There might be a dip when the final tranche for the payment of the Pronto newspaper and magazine group is due but, from then on, we anticipate steady growth all the way.'

Anthony concluded his statement and took a sip of water. Then he carefully sat back, folding his arms with the air of a man confident of his position.

Even this audience, experienced in the wiles of financial directors, looked impressed and for a while sat studying the mass of material they had been expected to assimilate in a very short time. Finally Denzil van Wyke, an elegant, clever man who favoured tweeds, raised his voice:

'Well, that's a very ambitious programme, Ginny, and

112

it's difficult to assimilate all the information you have given us.'

'There's a press release.' Ginny waved a document at him.

'Oh I'm *sure* of that, Ginny.' Denzil gave her a lazy smile. 'But what rather worries me is the diversification of Varga's interests. Why so many different products in so many different countries? Pharmaceuticals here and in the US, newspapers in Canada and Italy, perfume in France, electronics in Germany and Japan, precious metals in India. Isn't Mr Varga overextending himself a little? After all we know so little about him personally.'

'Mr Varga doesn't think there is over-extension.' Anthony took his cue. 'He is careful never to make a move that isn't backed up by sound financial calculation.'

'It would be nice to see him from time to time,' Gloria Keane butted in.

'That's because you're a woman,' Ginny replied and there was laughter.

'Seriously.'

'Seriously, Gloria, you know he always appears at the AGM. He has his shareholders to answer to.'

'Very happily at the moment, I might add,' Anthony cut in. 'I may say that I approve and, in fact, produce all the background figures. I visit all the concerns subject to takeover, go over their books, and discuss them with the auditors. We try to keep friendly; Mr Varga dislikes hostile bids.'

'But are you not too heavily geared as a company? Too much money borrowed from the banks?'

'That has been calculated to leave us with a comfortable ratio of income to borrowings, only twenty-five per cent. If anything we are *under* rather than over borrowed.'

'Well . . .' Denzil shook his head. Ginny felt a spasm of alarm. If Denzil, one of the most important writers, cast a doubt the share price would fall immediately.

Denzil, however, chose not to continue and Gloria

Keane cut in. 'What I can't understand,' she said, 'and I ask again, is why Mr Varga is never here to produce these figures himself. We would very much like to see him and question him more than once a year, when, quite rightly, he always gives preference to questions from shareholders.'

'Mr Varga would like nothing better,' Ginny said reassuringly. 'Except that he is out of the country for so much of the year. Unavoidably. Today, he is in New York.'

'Mr Varga likes being on the spot.' Anthony's quiet note of confidence echoed Ginny's own. 'I do the preliminary reconnoitre. He always follows up. I can assure you every move is soundly based.'

'Perhaps, however,' Gloria persisted with the determination of the experienced woman hack, 'it would be very nice if Mr Varga could be persuaded to call a press conference once in a while to reassure us that he still exists.'

'Oh, he exists all right,' Ginny said with a rueful grin. 'He woke me at four this morning to brief me for this conference. Now, do we have a final question, please?'

As Ginny walked into his office Varga got to his feet, turned off the television and came towards her, his hands extended.

'You were superb, Ginny,' he raised her hand and kissed it. 'You handled them beautifully. You and Tony are a wonderful team.'

Ginny stood gazing at him, that man who was, indeed, infinitely mysterious and who had such a strong power of attraction for her. Maybe that was why. He took her hand and led her to the chaise-longue which faced the blank TV screen. She sat down wearily and kicked off her shoes.

'It's back-aching work,' she said. 'Mind-bending too. Simeon,' she paused and, turning her head, gazed at him, 'why do you have to be so secretive? It's doing you no good.'

'I hate having to dissemble. It goes right against the

114

grain. Incidentally, you're very good at it,' he said approvingly. 'Four AM? That was a very nice touch.'

'Supposing they found it was untrue?'

'Well,' he shrugged, 'how can they? Seeing that I always travel incognito, no one knows anything. And soon I shall have my own plane.'

Simeon sat back, folding his arms, a smile of self-satisfaction on his face. Then he put a hand lightly on her knee and patted it.

'But excellent as you are at PR, dear Ginny, that is the only thing in which you are wrong. It's just the fact that I *am* mysterious, that I *am* unattainable and do not chatter to the press, that makes me interesting, like a woman you know.' He looked at her darkly again. 'A woman can be mysterious, too, and that makes *her* more desirable. Look at all these so-called entrepreneurs, every detail of whose lives are an open book: their wives, their friends, their mistresses, their holidays. Pah! I have *nothing* but contempt for them. Believe me,' he touched the side of his nose and winked, 'I have a very sound instinct, and I know what I am doing is right. Getting you was right; that was a very sound instinct.'

Ginny sighed again.

'Well we'll get a good article from Gloria. She promised it.'

'Splendid. You know I *like* Gloria.'

'Then why don't you meet her?' Ginny looked at him suggestively.

'Because I don't need to.' He allowed his hand to rest lightly on her knee again and she left it there. 'I have you to represent me to the world, and none does it better. I believe I can operate much more effectively if I am anonymous. Believe me. I know.'

She did believe him. It was very difficult not to. He was so right in everything he did, uncanny in his accuracy in predicting events, the movement of the markets. She had never met a person with such intuitive financial instinct.

He never consulted her beforehand but announced that such and such a deal was on, although he had usually sent Tony to make the preliminary investigations. Tony, who was almost as mysterious as Varga, seemed to know everything; the perfect shadow of his boss, trustworthy, discreet. Many of the projects that were examined he rejected and Varga always agreed with him. But the ones they decided to go ahead with almost immediately became money spinners. Parts of the companies that didn't work were sold off, the rest incorporated into the group with the group management principles. The parts disposed of usually covered the original costs of acquisition. The core that remained almost immediately went into profit, thus making the overall balance sheet stronger than ever.

Ginny was aware of his hand on her knee, the well manicured nails, the fine dark hairs on the backs of his fingers. They had never been intimate, never kissed, never touched, yet they were close; so close that she knew that everyone else in the business thought they were lovers.

But they weren't; not yet. She felt like the prey within the sights of an expert hunter. Only she was not afraid, content to bide her time and wait for him to strike.

'Now.' He finally removed his hand and, rising, went over to his desk. Leaning forward he examined the screen of the VDU. 'My next objective is a couple of TV stations in America. I'm flying out tomorrow.' He opened a drawer in his desk and produced a file which he handed to her. 'I want you to examine these and tell me what you think. I'm taking Tony with me.'

'I'm honoured to be consulted,' Ginny said.

'Well I trust you,' he replied. 'I only just found out there were difficulties . . .'

'Simeon . . .'

'Yes?' He looked up at her.

'I know you may think I'm speaking out of turn, that it isn't my business, but . . .'

'*Yes*?' His tone was gentle.

'I don't want you to overdo it.'

'How do you mean, "overdo it"?'

'Our acquisitions at the moment are about one a month. You heard what was said at the meeting. The goodwill shown to you by the financial journalists could easily turn sour.'

'It's your business to see it doesn't.' His tone was suddenly abrupt, almost unfriendly.

'I'm doing all I can, but you saw there was an air of hostility at the meeting today, particularly from Denzil, and he has always been a good friend to us.'

'Yes, I noticed that.' Varga frowned. He then came over and sat next to her again. 'Tell me, is he married?'

'I know nothing about his private life. Why?'

'I thought his attitude to you was, shall we say, slightly amorous. Maybe you could invite him for a drink?'

'Simeon, what *are* you saying?' Ginny exclaimed indignantly.

'I'm only *suggesting*,' he said gently, 'that you should be nice to him.'

'Well for that,' Ginny got to her feet and turned sharply towards him, 'I could resign.'

'*Ginny*!' His voice was pained and he rose too.

'That was a *terrible* thing to say,' she went on. 'Crude.'

'I know. It was a silly thing to say.' He lowered his voice. 'And how angry I would be if you did.' As he looked at her his eyes seemed to melt. 'You must *know*, Ginny, how I feel about you. But I've held back and you have not encouraged me. I know you wanted our relationship to be businesslike, and I respected that.'

'I don't want anything to change,' she said swiftly.

'People think we are lovers already. Tony thinks we are.'

'I know.' She held out a hand and he took it. 'But I think it would change everything. Besides . . .'

'Besides what?'

'I don't *know* you, Simeon. I don't really know you any better than those grumbling journalists.'

'Then get to know me better.' His smile was tantalizing.

She shook her head nervously. 'No, not like that. It would be a very serious step for me.'

'For me too, Ginny. I held back so long because it would be a *very* serious step and not one I would take lightly.'

'Simeon . . .' Then her hand was in his and he stood in front of her. She could feel his breath warm upon her cheek and, as his lips approached hers she closed her eyes, in anticipation of one of the most exquisite, most exciting moments in her life.

They lay in the dark touching each other's bodies. She could imagine she saw his profile silhouetted against the window, but it was very dark indeed. There had been several knocks on the door while they were making love but they ignored them. Twice the telephone had rung and they ignored that too. God only knows what Dorothy thought, but they didn't care. Their lovemaking was a frenzied coupling of two people who seemed to have been starved of sex for too long.

She thought that when the light went on all the magic would go and, as she felt him rise, said 'Don't.' He sat down beside her again and her arm encircled his waist. Their clothes lay around them, discarded on the carpet like the aftermath of an accident.

The shadows of the desk, the chairs, became more apparent as her eyes grew accustomed to the gloom.

He bent his head and kissed her again and she shivered a little with apprehension.

'Cold?' he asked.

'Frightened,' she said, and for the first time in her life she felt she knew the real meaning of possession: something that, once held, could never be let go.

*

The woman entered the lobby of the hotel and was greeted by smiles. All the staff knew her and liked her because she was friendly, gracious and gave good tips. The commissionaire would spring to open the door for her, or close it behind her. The porters saluted her, the waiters hurried to her table if she ate in the restaurant, the barman always knew what she drank.

The lift door opened for her; she entered and it closed behind her. She raised her head watching the buttons as it rose swiftly to the thirty-sixth floor. She suffered a little from vertigo.

She drew a deep breath – part relief, part apprehension – as it stopped at the penthouse suite and she clasped the gun in her pocket as the doors glided open. One never knew.

She had never met the man at the other side before and he came forward to greet her with evident pleasure; shook her hand politely and drew her into the lounge with its staggering view over London.

'Would you like a drink?' he asked, as if to break the ice.

'Champagne, please.'

'Of course.'

He went to the bar and, producing a full bottle of champagne, broke the foil and expertly eased the cork from the bottle, feeling it to be sure that it was properly chilled. He then took a perspex cooler and two glasses from the cabinet and set them on a low table that ran the length of the sofa where she was sitting.

'Won't you take your coat off?' he asked.

'Not yet.' She still had her hand firmly over the handle of the pistol. He laughed, showing two rows of even teeth. In a way he was attractive, except that he had too much flesh on him and she didn't like the expression in his eyes.

'You must trust me, you know.' As the liquid frothed towards the rim of the glass he passed it to her. 'You have the product?'

'I have.'

'Good.' He raised his glass to his lips and toasted her. 'And I have the money. We will have a drink and the transaction is completed.'

She nodded and they drank in silence, warily looking at each other. When she had finished her drink she opened her purse, producing a packet which she handed to him. He sat down beside her grasping it eagerly. Then he gently opened it and took out a polythene pack, opened this and, putting his finger into the soft powdery contents, withdrew it, licking it thoughtfully.

'Good,' he said. 'Excellent.'

'It's top quality.'

He reached in the pocket of his jacket and produced a wad of notes which he handed to her.

'You can get more of this?'

'As much as you like.'

'The price is high.'

'It's the best quality, as I said.' She stood up, pulling her coat closely around her.

'By the way,' he leaned back watching her, 'I wonder if you can get me a woman? You seem to know the ropes. London is such a lonely place for a man on his own.'

Melissa sat down again beside him, a faint smile on her lips. 'This comes extra,' she said, opening her coat, and he saw that she was naked except for a pair of high-heeled shoes and thigh-length stockings.

He drew in his breath and she threw off her coat, the gun in her pocket forgotten.

One could always tell.

CHAPTER 7

'How do you do?'

'How do you do?'

'So nice to see you.'

'And you too, Lady Silklander.'

'We've heard so much about you.'

'And I you.' He had an attractive, engaging smile, warm, melting brown eyes.

'It's nice to meet you at long last.'

Yet Moira seemed unnerved by his presence, as if she didn't know what further to say. She turned for support to Gerald, who stood at her shoulder gazing at the visitor.

'This is my husband. Gerald, Mr Varga.'

'How do you do?' Firm shake of the hand.

'How do you do, Lord Silklander?'

Ginny put a hand to her mouth. She found the situation comical, to say the least. The contrast between this urbane man of the world and her woolly, countrified parents could hardly have been more pronounced. Her father always looked as though he'd just finished mucking out the cowsheds, and frequently this was the case. He was not a man who ever stood on ceremony and he seldom visited London. He only occasionally spoke in the Lords and then on matters of specialized interest to farmers. Father did, however, have a best suit, because there were occasions such as Christmas when he had to wear it, or when he sat on the bench or visited the Lords.

He had evening dress, for his rare appearances at the local balls, which had belonged to his grandfather and which fitted him perfectly. Lady Silklander liked tweed mixtures – heather was a favourite – and she sometimes wore long knitted dresses about the chilly castle that made her look vaguely Pre-Raphaelite. She never wore make-up and her hair was a mess.

The fact was, her parents were typical representatives of the upper classes, to whom appearances mattered little. Ginny loved them for it. It was the way she too had been brought up, but her life in the big city had changed all that.

'Ginny,' her mother said reprovingly, a light in her eyes.

'Sorry, Mummy.'

'Do bring your friend into the drawing-room,' she continued with the same air of gracious condescension. 'Did someone bring in your cases, Mr Varga?'

'I believe so, Lady Silklander.'

Her mother looked past them to the Jaguar, with its boot open and Hamish the gardener collecting the two small bags inside. She frowned.

'You haven't *brought* very much, Ginny?'

'It's only a weekend, Mother. Simeon has a suit hanging in the back of the car.'

'Oh, there was no need.' She clasped Ginny's arm as they walked into the drawing-room followed by the men. 'We're very simple and informal people, Mr Varga. Ginny will have told you. Take us as you find us.'

'I assure you I do, Lady Silklander. And you must take me as you find me.'

They were now in the middle of the room by the drinks table, and Moira Silklander gave him a second going over with her forthright stare.

'*Do* sit down, Mr Varga.' She beckoned to her husband, who was chatting to his daughter. 'Gerald, give Mr Varga a drink.'

'Yes, of course.' Gerald Silklander went obediently to

122

the table. 'Whisky, Mr Varga? It's malt, from the family firm.'

'Excellent.' Varga rubbed his hands together and, apparently completely at ease, smiled at Ginny and patted the place beside him. 'What distillery is that, Lord Silklander?'

'Don't tell him, Daddy, for heaven's sake,' Ginny burst out. 'He'll want to buy it.'

Everyone laughed. The company, now settled round the fire, seemed to grow more relaxed. Simeon felt that he'd passed the test with ease, despite his hostess's penetrating glances.

They each had another drink, then Moira Silklander stood up. 'I'll show you to your room, Mr Varga.'

'Oh, I'll do that, Mummy.' Ginny sprang to her feet.

'*I'll* do it, dear,' her mother insisted. 'You stay and chat to Daddy. It's ages since we saw you.'

Ginny acquiesced gracefully, but managed to wink at Varga and shake her head. Perplexed, he followed her mother out of the room, across the enormous hall and up the stairs to the first floor.

'I'm afraid you'll find it a little cold here,' she said. 'We can't have central heating because of the panelling.'

'Of course.' Behind her Simeon shivered. He was already freezing, but he'd been warned by Ginny. Anyway, there was the cheering thought that in bed at night he would have her body to keep him warm.

'There's a fire in your room *and* an electric heater,' Moira Silklander said, flinging open the door. 'Plenty of extra blankets on the bed.'

Simeon walked over the threshold behind his hostess and then stopped with a sharp intake of breath.

'Something the matter?' Moira murmured, glancing behind her.

'It's magnificent. It's *huge*.'

'Oh, all the rooms here are like this,' Moira Silklander replied offhandedly, throwing a couple of logs on the already blazing fire. 'It's the biggest castle in England.

The biggest *old* castle, if you know what I mean. Parts of it are twelfth century. It is *not* a stately home like Beaulieu or Longleat. It's a castle. An ancient fortification,' she added for clarification.

'Ginny told me,' Varga murmured, noticing that his case had already been unpacked and his night things lay on the bed. 'She is very proud of her family.'

'It's an ancient line. Mine too. The McFees are as old as the Silklanders, warriors before the Bruce.'

'Quite.' Varga's knowledge of English history was scant and of Scottish non-existent.

'And yours, Mr Varga?' Moira Silklander looked questioningly at him.

'Mine, Lady Silklander?' He looked puzzled.

'Your family?'

'Oh, not as old as yours,' he said quickly. 'Now, do you think I might take a bath before dinner?'

'The bathroom's along the hall.' Moira Silklander turned towards the door. 'I'm afraid you'll find it rather cold. No heating. Dinner at eight. Sharp,' she added, looking sideways at him, but she didn't really think it was necessary.

Mr Varga looked to her like a man who would always be on time.

The church was half a mile from the castle, still well within Silklands' grounds. Sunday service was always attended by the family and the villagers, mostly tenants, many of whom worked for the family and lived in tied cottages on the estate.

The rich man in his castle the poor man at his gate no longer applied to this particular section of society where, since the war, a kind of community atmosphere prevailed, more a gathering now of equals than master and servant. There was a little metaphorical forelock touching but nothing more.

Of course respect was still shown to the baron, his lady and family, and they occupied the raised pew at the back of the church that their forebears had occupied for centuries. Lord Silklander was expected to contribute more to the collection than anyone else, and after the service he led the exit from the church and stood chatting with his wife, children and guests to their fellow worshippers.

To Simeon Varga it was quaint, strange but enormously appealing. It was part of that sturdy fabric of English society to which he had always been drawn; which he craved. He yearned for ancestors, a country home, a place in the establishment. There were some things that, as a stranger, he couldn't have, but others for which he would strive.

He sang the hymns with gusto, repeated the prayers, even closing his eyes for the repetition of the Our Father, but most of the time he observed; his beautiful, rather wistful eyes roamed around, missing nothing. No mannerism, no nuance escaped him. He sat between Ginny and Betty, her sister-in-law; he listened to Angus Silklander reading the lesson, saw him acting as sidesman. It was obvious to him that the Silklanders were a vital part of a centuries-old tradition: England at its best, and he loved it.

Not only did he love it but he could be part of it. As Ginny's husband he would be part of this family, and the Silklander blood would flow through the veins of their children.

Finally, after a long, long, long voyage he would be accepted. And to the Silklander family he would be able to bring something which he had and they lacked: money. It did not take a nose as keen as his to sniff out the fact that the family were, if not on its beam ends, short of ready cash.

Old name, no money. It was a familiar condition in the British aristocracy who had lived on position and not husbanded or tried to increase its wealth.

He followed Ginny, her father, mother, brother and sister-in-law into the sunshine where he stood a little apart, the object of interested, kindly glances from the

125

rest of the congregation. He was dressed in tweeds, a checked shirt and a woollen tie, but he was not English. He was not even Scottish. Not only his looks but his air, even the shy, hesitant smile on his face, were foreign. The vicar eventually went over to him, peered myopically at him, and said in an exaggeratedly slow voice: 'And how are you enjoying your visit here, Mr . . . ?'

'Varga,' Simeon said, shaking hands.

'What an interesting name. Where is it from?'

'England,' Simeon said with a smile, pleased with the vicar's evident discomfiture.

Parish chit-chat followed: the dates for the next meeting of the church council were noted in diaries; the ladies' flower-arranging rota; the cleaning of the church.

Needless to say it was the ladies who always cleaned the church, who in fact did almost everything. But the important decisions concerning the parish were still left to the men. There was not a single woman on the parish council, nor was there likely to be. Women wielded power, but it was a concealed power, the sort of power they had learned how to exercise for centuries past: by influencing the men while appearing to obey them.

The group began to disperse. Gerald Silklander, who had been in deep conversation with the vicar, looked round for his brood and then with a wave, his son beside him, set off at a brisk pace across the fields towards the castle which, still half-hidden by the morning mist, looked mysterious and beguiling.

Betty Silklander waited for Varga to catch up with her and, some paces behind, Ginny and her mother followed arm-in-arm.

'It's lovely to be home, Mummy.' Ginny excitedly squeezed her mother's arm.

'It's been too long, darling,' her mother responded with a hug. 'I wish you'd come more often.'

'I've been so terribly busy. Simeon's expanding so fast it is hard to keep up with his ideas.'

'He certainly *seems* very clever.' Her mother's tone was polite, yet cautious.

'He's brilliant, a genius. He doubles his share price practically with each new acquisition.'

Moira didn't quite know what that meant. 'I *wish* some of it would rub off on your father and Angus.'

'But I thought things were going quite well, Mummy?' Ginny glanced at her anxiously.

'Oh they are. I mean *comparatively* well. But it's hard being a farmer, darling, with all these European Community regulations. Your father sits up half the night filling in forms. It's tiring and repetitive. I suppose Simeon has a lot of forms to fill in, too?' She looked enquiringly at her daughter, noting the glow in her eyes, feeling the spring in her step, the quivering body, like some thoroughbred about to take off. She had never seen Ginny so happy, even when she was engaged to Robert – especially, perhaps, when she was engaged to Robert. But the girls who married family friends could never be expected to fall head-over-heels in love. One married a chum, as she had Gerald. She knew with Ginny it was different.

Ginny, her head flung back, burst out laughing. '*Simeon* doesn't fill in forms, Mummy. He has people to do that for him.'

Her mother's eyes swivelled sideways at her.

'You like him very much, don't you, Ginny?'

'I do. Very much.'

'Where does he *come* from exactly, darling?'

'I don't really know.' Ginny studied the ground as she walked, her expression reflective.

'What do you mean, you don't really know?' Moira slackened pace and pulled Ginny back, searching her eyes. Ginny's answering expression was no longer serene.

'Well I don't. I know so little about him.'

'How can you go to bed with a man you know so little about?' Her mother had lowered her voice almost to a whisper, as though she was afraid that the people striding out in front would be able to hear.

'Did *you* know so much about Daddy?' Ginny's reply was rhetorical.

'Yes I did. I knew *everything* about Daddy, as you did about Robert. I certainly knew where he was born!'

'Well I don't.' Ginny raised her chin defensively. 'Simeon is very secretive. I respect it. His past obviously pains him and he doesn't like to talk about it.'

'Maybe he has something to hide?'

Disliking her mother's suggestive tone, Ginny removed her arm.

'That's a horrible suggestion, Mummy. I can respect someone who is reluctant to talk about the past, even if you can't.'

'He gave you that brooch, didn't he?' Her mother's tone was persistent, intrusive. 'He really was the cause of your break-up with Robert?'

'No he wasn't,' Ginny replied defensively. 'He *did* give me the brooch but then it meant nothing. It was only later . . .'

'Of *course* it meant something,' Moira said with asperity. 'A man doesn't give diamonds to a woman without expecting consequences . . . at least Robert realized that, if neither of you did.'

'My relationship with Robert was on the rocks anyway . . .'

'I *never* approved of you living together. It's all you can expect.'

'Mother!' Ginny paused and gave a tired sigh as though the subject exhausted her. 'Mummy, I knew Robert from the age of *two*. *You* knew his parents. My grandparents knew his grandparents. That doesn't make Robert any *better* than Simeon, or any worse. In fact since I have known Simeon I think the way we families marry into one another is rather incestuous. It's horrible. No wonder so many of the progeny are shuttled off into mental homes.'

'None of our family have ever been in mental homes!' Moira expostulated.

'No, but we know a lot of people who have, and look at Robert's great-aunt Evelyn. *Everyone* said she was quite bonkers. It might have been inherited,' she added with a sly look.

'There was certainly something eccentric about Evelyn,' her mother said stiffly. 'But to call her "quite bonkers" is going too far. Lots of families have eccentric members. Some people think your father's a bit eccentric. It's not the same thing as being certifiable; besides, if you know nothing about Mr Varga . . .'

'Oh Mummy, *do* call him Simeon. You were "Mr Vargaing" him all the time at dinner last night. I think he finds it hurtful. He wants so much to be accepted; he's sensitive, you know. He's doing everything he can to fit in and be pleasant.'

'But he's different, darling, isn't he? No matter how hard these people try they can never be *quite* like us. Do you know what I mean?'

Ginny gave a snort of anger and ran to catch up with Simeon and her sister-in-law who were chatting animatedly.

'Everything okay?' Ginny asked, standing between them and linking arms.

'Fine,' Betty replied. 'I was telling Mr Varga about our problems with beef production. Do you know he has come up with a very good idea?'

'Simeon.' Varga looked apologetic. 'Please call me Simeon.'

'Simeon's ideas are quite brilliant,' Betty went on without pausing.

'Simeon is full of brilliant ideas.' Ginny squeezed his arm. 'Why don't you talk to Angus and Betty after lunch?'

'Or come and see the farm?' Betty was enthusiastic.

'Nothing I'd like better.' Varga glanced at Ginny and there was something about his expression, the way he looked at her, that made her able to time the moment at which, without any doubt, she became absolutely and irrevocably in love.

By now they were approaching the drive of the castle and from the gates they could see a car in front of the main door which had not been there when they left for the walk to church.

It was an ancient Bentley, certainly pre-war, and in front of it stood a man and two women talking.

'Oh, Pru!' Ginny exclaimed, clutching Simeon's hand. 'It's Pru, my sister. Oh, how *lovely*.'

She began to quicken her pace, but her mother had already caught up with her and tugged at her arm to slow her down. 'Ginny . . .'

'Mummy, it's Pru and Douglas. Who's the girl with them . . .'

'Ginny,' Moira persisted. 'I'm awfully *sorry*. It was a horrible thing to say . . . about Simeon.'

'Oh, *Mummy*!' Ginny clasped her hand and leaned forward to hug her. 'That's all right. You're just an old-fashioned fuddy-duddy.'

'I know.' Moira bowed her head. 'I deplore it and it's horrible. Why on earth should everyone be like me? I could have bitten off my tongue as soon as I spoke.'

'It's sheer prejudice, Mummy,' Ginny whispered in her ear. 'When Simeon is ready, when he trusts me absolutely, he'll tell me everything I want to know. All I know *now* is that he's been very badly wounded, emotionally I mean. His personal life is so sad, and he loves being here. He likes you and Daddy, and I can see how well he gets on with Betty. Oh, *Mummy*!' Ginny, her eyes still on the car ahead, put her hand to her mouth. 'Robert's there too.'

'Robert?' Moira screwed up her eyes. 'Oh, so it is. Pru and Duggie must have brought him over with his fiancée.'

'Fiancée!' Ginny gasped.

'Surely you know, darling? It was in *The Times* about a month ago.'

'I hardly have time to read *The Times* for the announcements.'

'Well I imagined *someone* would have mentioned it. It never occurred . . .'

'Never mind, it's all right.' Ginny patted her mother's cheek. 'I don't mind in the least. I'm very glad for Robert. Who is she?'

'Well, we don't know her,' her mother's tone was ironic. 'You see, he's actually *marrying* someone we don't know.'

By this time Gerald and Angus Silklander had reached the car and were shaking hands with Robert and the young woman who stood next to him. She was in her mid-twenties, nice-looking rather than attractive, and she wore spectacles. As Ginny approached him Robert, who had been watching her, held out his hand.

'Ginny!' he called and as she clasped it, he leaned forward and kissed her on the cheek.

'What a lovely surprise,' she said warmly, returning his peck. 'I've only just heard of your engagement, Robert.' She then turned to the young woman who gave her a friendly smile.

'I've heard a lot about you,' she said. 'I'm Wendy.'

'How do you do, Wendy? Well,' Ginny looked around again, 'this *is* nice. You see who we have here with us, Robert?'

'Yes indeed,' Robert said with a perfunctory smile as Varga stopped a few paces away from him. 'This *is* a surprise. How are you, Simeon?'

'Very well, very well, Robert. And you?'

'Fine. Wendy, may I introduce Simeon Varga? My fiancée, Wendy Pinctus.'

'Pinctus,' Varga said with a meaningful smile. 'What an interesting name. Is it foreign?'

Ginny started to giggle and she saw a slight blush stain

131

her mother's cheeks as Wendy replied: 'It's Irish, sort of.'

'Don't you work at the bank?' Ginny said suddenly. 'I'm sure we've spoken on the phone?'

'We have spoken on the phone,' Wendy said in a pleasant voice, with a trace of Irish. 'I was Mr Law's secretary.'

'Of *course*.'

'She's now dealing,' Robert said proudly. 'A high-flyer.'

'Not quite in *your* league,' Wendy laughed as she shook Varga's hand. 'We've all watched your progress with admiration, Mr Varga.'

'It's thanks to Robert who helped me to take off.' Simeon clapped a hand on Robert's shoulder. 'Take off *and* sometimes keep me flying.'

'Oh, I don't think I do that any more.' Robert placed a proprietorial arm around Wendy.

'Why don't we all go in and have a drink?' Gerald Silklander pointed to the steps, stroking one of the beautiful labradors which had rushed down in a frenzy to greet him. 'We've a lot to celebrate. You must all stay to luncheon.'

Lunch, like dinner the night before, was a family gathering in the kitchen where, beside the large scrubbed table, there was a black range on which were a number of bubbling pots.

The dining-room, huge and unheated, was used only at Christmas when all the family were present, and fires were lit in it for days beforehand to try to warm it up.

Moira and Gerald Silklander had been born in the days when every big house had a huge complement of servants, yet she had been a teenager during the war and had not been presented at court. When court functions were resumed in 1947 she was twenty and had been working for two years as a landgirl on her own father's Border estates.

Thus, although she had grown up with servants, she

had had her life and, to a certain extent, her expectations changed by the war in many ways which she thought, even at the time, were for the better. She knew that she and Gerald still had attitudes that seemed to her children old-fashioned; but at least by the time she was married she had learned the rudiments of cooking and house-keeping and knew how to fend for herself, skills and attitudes she instilled in all her children. Boys as well as girls were expected to be self-sufficient, make their beds and keep their rooms tidy, help with the washing-up after meals. It was only in recent times they had acquired the luxury of a dishwasher.

Even more recent was a washing machine for clothes which previously had been washed in a tub by one of the dailies and hung out to dry.

Their self-sufficiency had stood the Silklanders in good stead when it was brought home to them that they were by no means as wealthy as their fathers had been, although the McFees owned thousands of profitable acres by the Tweed and lived in a style slightly more elevated than the present-day Silklanders. Moira's brother, who had inherited the property, had three indoor servants including a butler and his wife, and wouldn't have known how to boil an egg.

The Silklanders, however, were still rich in assets. There was some priceless plate and silver, beautiful linen, but they were mostly kept in chests or behind locked doors. The really good pieces of silver were in the bank and would probably never again see the light in Gerald's lifetime.

The kitchen was now the regular eating place for the family, who had no qualms about who they entertained there; the high as well as the most humble. Tenants were frequently entertained to dinner by the lord and lady of the castle, with minor royalty staying the weekend for the shooting.

Simeon Varga had expected quite a different style of life and was surprised when, the night before, he had been ushered into the kitchen and invited to sit down at a table laid with a checked cloth and plain cutlery and the kind of basic wine-glasses that usually went with petrol coupons.

Now, for lunch, there was a succulent joint, best Aberdeen Angus beef from the McFee herd across the border, home-grown vegetables, bread-and-butter pudding and litres of cheap red wine bought from the nearest off-licence.

Simeon was fascinated by the spectacle of the English upper class at table; their manners, habits, the way they ate. Nothing would change, ever. Wherever they were they felt comfortable.

He listened and he watched, absorbing everything.

Nothing escaped his attention about the behaviour and the attitudes of the elite of an imperious nation which had not so long ago claimed to rule half the world.

That tiny island: England.

Angus Silklander was a man very like his father. He was tall, dark-haired and strong: he looked like his father and behaved like him. He had never in his life been very far from home. All the boys had gone to boarding-school in Scotland, and when he left school with not very good A-level results Angus decided that he wanted to learn how to farm and manage the family estates. He had a natural affinity with animals and the land.

When he was twenty-one he married Betty Lewis, whose family were, like his, Anglo-Scots. He met her at a dance in Edinburgh and they were engaged after only six weeks. It had been, and was, a very happy marriage; had produced three children. Betty was extrovert, intelligent, life-giving, just like Angus.

After lunch Angus and Simeon gravitated with their coffee cups to the window of the sitting-room, which overlooked miles of undulating hills. Angus was explaining the topography of the countryside and the problems of reforestation.

'You've heard all about the rain forests? You see, if you cut too many trees without replanting you denude vast areas of the land and that affects animals, crops, even the weather.'

'So your main business is timber?' Varga looked at him with interest. He was like Ginny. They shared the same openness, the same classic good looks.

'Well, not exactly.' Angus thoughtfully stirred his coffee. 'We have beef cattle, sheep, a large dairy farm.'

'Yet Ginny told me things were difficult?' Varga sounded puzzled.

Angus put down his cup on a nearby table and sighed. He wore grey flannels and a tweed sweater, a check shirt with a knitted tie. He looked at home, supremely at ease; a man sure of himself and his place in the universe. His wife had come up and was listening to the conversation.

'It's the EC common agricultural policy,' she exclaimed with a note of exasperation in her voice. 'We are always being told to do this, do that.'

'They change their minds the whole time.' Angus took up the cue. 'And the government is so supine. We farmers want to get on doing what we do best, with the minimum of interference . . .'

'There are ways of circumventing government interference,' Simeon said with a smile.

'Oh?' Angus and Betty exchanged glances. 'How?'

'Oh, there are ways. There must be.' He smiled at them. 'There are ways in my business, so there must be with yours.'

'We have things called quotas . . .' Angus began.

'Ignore them.' Varga too put down his cup and restlessly looked round for Ginny. He spied her in a corner talking to Robert, and his expression of bonhomie suddenly left him.

'Why don't you come over and have a look round our place?' Angus said with enthusiasm. 'I hear you're a wizard at business. Maybe you can give us some tips?'

'I'd like that.' But Simeon's attention was only half on

135

them, his eyes on Ginny and her erstwhile fiancé.

'This afternoon?' Betty was trying to take his attention away from Ginny and Robert. 'Or tomorrow?'

'We fly back tomorrow, alas,' Varga sighed. 'And in the afternoon I am going to Mexico.'

'Golly!' Betty sounded impressed. 'But why not this afternoon?'

'Yes,' he said suddenly. 'Maybe Ginny would like to come too? I'll go and tell her.' It was obviously a relief to him to interrupt the conversation between Robert and Ginny.

While Angus, Simeon and Betty were engrossed in the subject of farming, Robert and Ginny had seemed to gravitate naturally together after lunch, and sat drinking their coffee on a sofa in the corner of the room. Pru and her husband Douglas, Wendy and Moira decided to take a turn round the grounds to admire Moira's new rose garden, created in a sheltered spot away from the wind.

They could see them now from the window, meandering down the path between the clipped yew hedge.

'She's an *awfully* nice girl,' Ginny said, looking from Wendy back to Robert.

'Yes, she is.' Robert didn't look at Wendy but sipped his coffee; however there was a note in his voice that made Ginny look sharply at him.

'Intelligent and . . .'

'Oh, Ginny, for God's sake.' Robert leaned over and put his empty cup on the table in front of them.

'Well, I'm sorry.' Ginny seemed nonplussed. 'But I do think she's charming.'

'The trouble is, she isn't you,' Robert murmured, so quietly that Ginny wondered whether she had heard him correctly.

'Robert, please . . .'

'I mean it, Ginny.' He placed a hand on her arm and looked earnestly into her eyes. 'I still feel exactly the same about you.'

'But, Robert.' Ginny looked anxiously around, aware that Simeon, apparently engrossed in conversation with Angus, nevertheless kept glancing at her. 'You've just got engaged.'

'It doesn't mean I don't still love you,' he whispered urgently. 'It was done on the rebound.'

'Well I hope Wendy doesn't know it.'

'She knows it. She didn't want to come over today; but she's a sport.'

Robert would need a 'sport' for a wife, the sort of person who would never make a gaffe or let a man down. She would have been like that too. Noblesse oblige.

'I suppose she'd be "sporting" enough to let you go,' Ginny said sarcastically.

'Yes, I suppose she would.' His eyes lit up with hope, but Ginny vigorously shook her head.

'No, Robert. *Never.*'

'I thought you seemed so pleased to see me today.' He kept his voice to a whisper, which made Varga look suspiciously at them again.

'I was pleased to see you as a friend. I was pleased that we could meet again, that you had brought your fiancée knowing I'd be here. But nothing else . . . never.'

'It's *him* I suppose?' Robert jerked his head in Varga's direction.

'It's *nothing* to do with him. You know you and I were finished ages ago.'

'Only after you met him,' Robert persisted. 'The rumour in the City, everywhere, is that you're having an affair.'

She shrugged noncommittally. 'What can one do about rumours?'

'Do you deny it?'

'In the time-honoured phrase: I neither deny nor confirm.' She smiled infuriatingly.

'He *is* a crook you know, Ginny.'

She raised her eyebrows in surprise.

137

'Really? Is that so? Yet your bank trusts him enough to lend him so much money.'

'The bank don't like it but they bent to pressure – mine. If he flops, out I go.'

'You *know* he won't.' She was beginning to sound angry. 'His business is rock-solid.'

'His methods are shady. He's so secretive. You should know that.'

'I know he plays his cards close to his chest,' Ginny's expression showed exasperation, 'but *I* respect him for that.'

'Not even *you* know what goes on.'

'I know a lot of what goes on because I have to do the PR. Tony Liddle knows everything that goes on because he susses it out in the first place. You can't question his integrity. I think you say what you say about Simeon because, frankly, Robert, you're jealous. You can't believe anyone can be successful so quickly. You . . .'

'Ginny.' She stopped suddenly as she heard Varga's voice near her, and looking up saw the expression on his face was strained. 'Angus and Betty would like us to go and see the farm.'

'What, now?'

'It will have to be now.' Angus, behind him, looked apologetically at his watch. 'We have to pick up the kids. We dropped them at friends as it's nanny's day off and we wanted to have lunch here on our own. Besides it will soon be time for milking. Simeon says he has some ideas about how we could increase our yield.'

Robert rose and, hands in his pockets, remarked dryly, 'Really, Simeon. A farming expert now, are we?'

'Business methods, Robert,' Simeon replied with a gentle smile, 'have universal application.'

When they returned from the visit to the farm it was nearly six. Pru and Douglas had left, taking Robert and Wendy. Gerald was in his study and Moira was in the sitting-room, knitting. As Ginny and Simeon entered she

138

looked up with a smile, glancing at her knitting gauge to note the number of rows.

'Well, successful?'

'Very.' Simeon sat opposite her with an air of suppressed excitement which in a seasoned man of business like him was quite unusual. 'I learned an enormous number of things I didn't know. I was most impressed indeed, but,' he shrugged and his expression changed, 'it is uneconomically run. I think Angus can make a number of improvements. Ginny agrees.'

'It's quite amazing.' Ginny, the enthusiast now, sat opposite her mother. 'Things *I* never thought of before, and Angus certainly didn't, Simeon sees at once.'

'It is obvious to the trained eye,' Simeon said modestly. 'As I said to Robert earlier, business methods are universally applicable.'

'In what way can Angus improve?' Moira looked at him curiously. 'Maybe we could do with some help here, too.'

'I'm sure you could.' Simeon leaned forward, hands loosely linked in front of him.

'I think I'll go and change,' Ginny said yawning, and looking at the clock.

'No need, dear, it's only supper.' Her mother recommenced her knitting. 'About eight, I thought.'

'I need a wash and that sort of thing.' Ginny gave her a smile. 'It will give Simeon a chance to explain his ideas to you, and Daddy if you like.'

Simeon rose and quickly preceded Ginny to the door to open it for her. As she went through he gave her a smile and then spontaneously leaned forward and pecked her on the cheek.

When he returned Moira had put her knitting yet again on one side and sat watching him with a speculative light in her eyes.

'You see, Lady Silklander,' Varga, instead of resuming his seat, took a stance in front of the fireplace which now had a large bowl of cut flowers in the grate, 'the economics of any business are the same. Take the manufacture of pharmaceuticals. It isn't only a question of maximizing profits . . .'

'Before you go on,' Moira said, lowering her voice, 'and while Ginny is out of the room, there's something I'd like to talk to you about.'

'Yes?' Varga bent his head forward attentively.

'Are you serious about my daughter, Mr Varga?'

Simeon seemed to consider the question and then replied: 'You have, if I may say so, a very old-fashioned way of thinking, Lady Silklander.'

'We are old-fashioned people,' Moira replied serenely, 'with old-fashioned standards of which we are not ashamed. You see we were *very* fond of Robert . . .'

'Yet *you* were not going to marry him, Lady Silklander.' Varga's tone, though polite, was steely. 'I understand it was *Ginny's* decision to break off and nobody else's.'

'And it had nothing to do with you?' She sounded sceptical.

'Not that I am aware.'

'Yet you gave her a diamond brooch, a Christmas present to someone you scarcely knew.'

Simeon appeared to hesitate as to whether to sit down or remain standing. Finally he sat down with a deep sigh and stretched his feet out in front of him as if he felt completely at home, a gesture not lost on his hostess.

'Lady Silklander, much as I appreciate your concern for Ginny, I must point out to you that she is a mature woman and not a child. Any decisions, I should have thought, were her own; but yes, you are her mother and I respect your anxiety. I do assure you that I esteem Ginny very highly and my intentions towards her are entirely honourable. If Ginny will have me, as soon as I am free to marry her I will.'

Moira suddenly stiffened.

'You are *not* free, Mr Varga?'

'Not at the moment, though I have been separated

140

from my wife for several years. I have asked her for a divorce.'

'I see.' From the frosty expression on her face divorce appeared as lamentable to Moira as the act of fornication. For a moment or two there was an uneasy silence; then, lowering her tone as if afraid of being overheard, she continued.

'May I ask, from what part of the world do you come, Mr Varga?'

'England,' Varga replied stiffly.

'You do not look English.'

'Neither does a man born in England of Jamaican parents look English. Yet he is.'

'You . . .'

'Lady Silklander,' his tone was patient, dignified, 'I am concerned with the present, not the past. I would *never* presume to question you about your family.'

'There is nothing to question,' she replied haughtily.

'Precisely. That is exactly the case with me. Now if you will excuse me I too will go and freshen up.'

And, without giving her the chance to reply, he left the room.

Stony-faced, he shut the door and strode through the vast hall to the great stone staircase, his air of urgency decreasing, as did his anger, as he climbed the stairs.

He was conscious that his overwhelming feeling now was one of sadness, of alienation, even of grief. For he realized that in this great warm family clan, however much he longed to join it, however much beloved he was by Ginny, he was forever destined to be an outcast: a man alone.

CHAPTER 8

Claudia sat in a chair in the centre of the room with her brothers Carlo and Matteo standing on either side of her like a pair of Praetorian guards, mouths set, faces grim. Claudia wore a cream suit, black stockings and shoes, and a black silk blouse with broad cuffs fastened by large pearl buttons. Her dark hair was swept smoothly back from her brow and her imperious Roman nose was raised in the air as though she had just detected a rather unpleasant smell. Her hooded, almost black eyes gazed malevolently at Simeon who wondered, not for the first time, how he could ever have imagined he loved her. This cruel, strange woman for a *wife*?

Yet the whole effect of the Bernini family thus pitted against him appeared both grotesque and frightening, even to him, and he swallowed twice in a determined effort to gain his composure.

They had assembled in Carlo's office at the back of the showroom, although Simeon had asked for the interview at his former home. The settlement of separation had barred him from visiting Mill Hill except to collect and return his children for the formal weekly visits when he was in London. They were occasions which both he and the children seemed equally to dread.

Simeon, composing his features as best he could, approached the triumvirate, pausing to shake hands with each one, first his wife then his brothers-in-law. Carlo pointed to the chair opposite and, as Simeon sat down unbuttoning his jacket, he said: 'Won't you sit down too, Carlo and Matteo?'

'We prefer to stand, thank you, Simeon,' Carlo said politely. 'Now, what is this matter which you wish to discuss?'

'I wanted to speak to Claudia,' Simeon replied. 'My request was made to her. I didn't expect this *formal* inquisition at your offices.'

'You know the separation prevents you from visiting Claudia's house.'

'Nevertheless, I don't see why we can't be amicable about this whole business, more grown-up.'

'It is not a question of "amicability" or being "grown-up",' Carlo, who seemed to have appointed himself the spokesman, replied in a tone weary with sarcasm. 'It is a matter of protecting Claudia.'

'I assure you, Claudia needs no protection from me.'

'Nevertheless you deserted her. *We* feel a need to protect our sister. Now what is it you want to ask her, Simeon?'

'Does Claudia have no tongue of her own?'

'Any more questions like that, Simeon, and we shall ask you to leave,' Matteo intervened threateningly. 'You will kindly observe the rules.'

'Rules!' Simeon exclaimed in disgust, then determinedly making a fresh effort he said: 'I have come to ask Claudia for a divorce. I see no point in continuing this charade. I want to be free. I am prepared to make a generous settlement; very generous if she will agree to do it quietly. A divorce by mutual consent is now possible and need not take long.'

'You know that the answer is *no*,' Claudia intervened without waiting for her brothers to reply. 'No, and no, and no.'

'Please, *cara*.' Carlo put a hand gently on her shoulder. 'You agreed we should conduct the conversation.' Then, turning to Simeon, he said: 'May one ask why, when you previously agreed to a separation, you have changed your mind?'

'I wish to be free.'

'Have you a *specific* reason, Simeon?' Carlo's eyes narrowed.

'No.'

'Do you wish to remarry?'

'Not at the moment.'

'There is gossip about you and a certain woman in your employ.'

'That is quite irrelevant.'

'You don't wish to marry her?'

'No.' Simeon's gaze fearlessly met Carlo's.

'Well then, we see no reason to alter the terms of the agreement.'

'Claudia?' Simeon looked directly at her but, avoiding his eyes, she said nothing. 'Very well,' Simeon stood up and fastened his jacket, 'if that is your attitude I can tell you I shall not forget it. I shall never forgive, or forget. I could make Claudia rich beyond her dreams; as it is she will get the minimum the law demands.'

Suddenly Carlo crossed the room and, seizing his brother-in-law by the lapel of his Savile Row suit, brought his face to within an inch of his own.

'Now see here, Simeon, no *threats*, do you understand?'

'I am not threatening, I am telling you,' Simeon replied. 'I don't care how you threaten me or what you do to me. The final settlement for Claudia and my children will be on the meanest terms I can get, and I will hire the best divorce lawyers in the country to ensure that that is so. There!' As Carlo released him he shook himself, carefully tightening the knot in his tie. 'You do yourself no good by your behaviour, Carlo,' theatrically he pointed a finger at the group in front of him, 'because I can tell you I will not stop with Claudia. I will do all in my power to make things very difficult for you too.'

Almost shaking with rage, Carlo moved rapidly back

to his desk and, pressing a button, spoke into the intercom to his secretary.

'Frances, would you please come in? Mr Varga is ready to leave.'

He looked as though he was about to make a fresh onslaught on his brother-in-law, but Matteo put a restraining hand on him.

'Calm yourself, Carlo. Two can play this game. If Simeon makes things difficult for us you can be quite sure that we can reciprocate. In Italy our ancestors were quite used to this kind of thing.'

Carlo then deliberately turned his back on Varga and remained there, looking out of the window. Varga seemed to hesitate, looked from Matteo to Claudia and then, with a shrug of his shoulders, went without another word to the door, not waiting for the secretary to open it.

After he had gone there was a profound silence, at last broken by Claudia.

'Why did you have to be so unpleasant? Why do you have to antagonize him? Why didn't you let *me* speak? I know him best, after all.' Carlo turned round and, going to her side, put a hand reassuringly on her shoulder.

'*Cara*, I was afraid you would weaken. I know you still burn for that man . . .'

'I do *not* burn,' she objected, 'but there was the possibility he may have wanted a reconciliation.'

Carlo vehemently shook his head.

'Don't deceive yourself, Claudia. If he wanted a reconciliation it would have been different, but his attitude was not conciliatory. He wants a quick divorce so that he can marry Silklander and disinherit you and your children.'

'He would never do that. He would have been generous, but now I'm not sure.' Anxiously she studied her long, carmine nails, but Carlo continued to shake his head.

'You persist in deceiving yourself, Claudia. He has

145

dishonoured you and lied to you. You have lost your place, your status in the community. Leave it to your brothers who love you to make sure that Simeon one day obtains his just deserts.'

The office was in one of those grey, anonymous back streets behind Paddington Station. At one time they had been full of Georgian town houses or neat Victorian villas, but now they consisted mainly of boarding houses or seedy hotels catering for a trade best described as dubious. There was a motley collection of shops, garages, and here and there a modern office building erected without style when planning regulations had been more lax.

The small office block backed on to the canal which ran between it and part of St Mary's Hospital as it had encroached on to the surrounding streets off the Edgware Road. The name on the glass door in gold letters was SESMAR AGENCY and it looked to Carlo like any other small office dealing with a variety of trades, with nondescript furniture, cheap carpet, walls hung with poor-quality reproductions and a general lack of intimacy shared by so many others like it.

The only thing that made it slightly different was the number of locks on the door and plate glass so thick it seemed meant to deter callers. Certainly unwelcome ones.

An elderly secretary sat at a desk using an electronic typewriter. There were no VDUs which, in these days, was unusual.

'Mr Thomas won't keep you long,' she said for the second time, glancing at the door behind her. Carlo began to tap his feet impatiently. He was not a man accustomed to being kept waiting.

At that moment the door behind the receptionist's desk opened and a tall, thin man emerged who went straight over to Carlo, hand outstretched.

'Mr Bernini? I am extremely sorry to keep you waiting. I am Edward Thomas.' His accent was classless, his tone clipped; he had close cropped hair, a ginger moustache and a military bearing.

'How do you do?' Carlo stood up and shook hands and Thomas gestured towards the door.

'Do please go in.' He then followed his client, pausing on the way for a few words with the receptionist before entering his private office and shutting the door. 'Sound-proof,' he said with a smile, tapping it. He then pointed to a door at the far end. 'So is that. Our clients often do not like to meet one another.'

Carlo had a feeling of unease and showed it.

'Please don't worry, Mr Bernini,' Thomas said jovially, placing a comfortable armchair covered in fake leather in front of him and taking a similar one opposite. 'I'm sure that you will feel happier knowing your visit here, and everything you tell me, is a matter of the utmost confidentiality. No records. Nothing to steal. All my information is kept in here.' He confidently tapped his brow.

'Quite.' Carlo joined the tips of his fingers and stared at him. Thomas was a surprise to him with his very Eng-lishness, so unlike the stereotype of the private eye. In his pin-striped suit and club tie he looked like a middle-ranking civil servant in some ministry or other, with regular working hours and a dull home life.

'I can see I'm not what you expected,' Mr Thomas said, with the smile of a person who could read minds.

'Not exactly.'

'Background Balliol, and then the Metropolitan Police, rank of chief inspector. Tired of the life. Now, how can I help you?'

He looked at a clock on the wall, noting down the time on a clipboard pad. Obviously, Carlo thought, charging by the hour.

'You were recommended to me,' he said, and paused as if trying to remember by whom. 'I am in the jewellery business and we have to be extremely careful about security, just as you do.'

147

'Quite so.' Mr Thomas doodled on the pad. 'Tell me,' he enquired looking up, 'is this a business matter?'

'Not exactly.' Carlo leaned back, clasping the arm rests with both hands. 'It is to do with my brother-in-law. You may have heard of him: Simeon Varga?'

'Ah!' Thomas nodded, but gave nothing away.

'I want him put under twenty-four-hour surveillance.'

Thomas nodded again and started writing on his pad.

'You're looking for grounds for divorce?' He twisted his lips. 'I'm afraid it's not exactly our line of business . . . I could recommend . . .'

'I want *you*.' Carlo pointed a finger at him. 'I don't want some second-rate seedy divorce private eye.'

Thomas looked instinctively towards both doors. 'Our business is almost purely commercial, covering if need be industrial espionage – for or against, you understand?'

'I want you to get Varga,' Carlo said. 'He has dishonoured my sister. He can't build up a business like that so quickly without making some dishonest deals.'

'His expansion has certainly been rapid.' Thomas looked knowledgeable. 'Is he – um, separated from your sister? I, um, don't *quite* understand what you mean by dishonour. Did he rape her? That is rapidly becoming a crime in the eyes of the law.'

'No he did not rape her. Merely wishing to divorce her is in our eyes, the eyes of a strict, honourable, well-brought-up Roman Catholic family, grounds enough to dishonour a woman. Henceforth she is diminished in status in the eyes of the community. In Mafia circles it would be sufficient grounds for . . .' he ran his finger beneath his chin.

'I see.' Thomas, his face expressionless, began doodling again. There was a feeling, however, that behind his insouciant manner there was a keen, alert brain ticking over.

'My sister, who is devout, will never remarry. She is doomed for the rest of her life to celibacy, to the miserable lot of a single, rejected woman.'

'I'm surprised in this day and age . . .' Thomas raised his eyebrows.

'Nevertheless that is how it is with her, with us as a family. We are true, loyal, communicant members of the Church.'

'Did she give Mr Varga any cause . . .'

'He denies there is any reason, but we suspect that he has a relationship with a woman who is a director of his company, the Honourable Virginia Silklander, the daughter of a lord. Have you heard of her?'

Thomas nodded again.

'Very capable, I'm told.'

'Then rake up all the dirt you can on *both* of them. I want to find out all about them; what they do, where they go and, particularly, about him and how he made his money.'

Thomas was still doodling and Carlo asked, a little impatiently: 'Have you taken all this in, Mr Thomas?'

'Yes.' Thomas put his pencil down and studied the face of his visitor with his innocuous blue eyes. 'I must tell you, Mr Bernini, it is not the sort of work I enjoy. We regard ourselves as an honourable, legitimate business employed, I may say, by some of the biggest and best firms here and throughout Europe.'

'You're still snooping, spying,' Carlo said contemptuously. 'What's the difference? Please don't try and pull the wool over my eyes. You pocket huge fees to try and give one company a march on another. Don't please expect me to respect you for it.'

'You tempt me to reject you, Mr Bernini,' Thomas said thoughtfully. 'However, as you say, one has to earn a crust. Our fees are quite high and we present an account weekly. You expect us to follow him?'

'Twenty-four hours.'

'And examine where we can his business transactions?'

'Yes.'

'Do we go out of the country?'

149

'No. That is too expensive.'

'It is *very* expensive.' Thomas drew a line under what he had written. 'Very well, I'll accept your brief and I'll put one of my best operatives in charge straight away. Incidentally it's a woman.'

'A woman?' Momentarily Carlo looked aghast.

'Oh, don't worry,' Thomas said reassuringly. 'She's one of the best in the business.' He leaned towards his intercom and spoke into it.

'Kelly, could you come in and meet our new client?'

He then sat with his hands folded on his desk looking expectantly towards the far door. A few seconds later this opened to admit a slight woman who carried a clipboard rather like the one Thomas had used. She was of medium height with brown tightly curled hair cut short, rather like a man's.

'This is Mr Bernini,' Thomas said. 'Mr Bernini, meet Kelly.'

'How do you do, Miss Kelly?' Carlo said, politely getting to his feet.

'No, not "Miss Kelly", just Kelly,' Thomas corrected him. 'Our operatives are known by one name.'

'Oh, I see.'

'Kelly will be in charge of your account, briefing surveillance operatives, examining Mr Varga's activities.'

'I see.'

'I hope this arrangement suits you, Mr Bernini.' Kelly had a lilting Irish accent. 'I assure you I'll keep a very personal eye on your account.'

'We pinched Kelly from the Met . . .'

'"Headhunted" I think would be a better and more accurate description, Mr Thomas.' Kelly's tone had a gentle reprimand.

Carlo was reminded of a nurse tucking in one's bedclothes and stroking one's brow. It was difficult to believe that someone as fragile as Kelly could operate in the tough world of industrial espionage. She was not beautiful, not even remotely attractive. She was plain, but her face was nice, her expression pleasant. Rather like Thomas, she would appear to have emanated from the corridors of power, a middle-grade civil servant, say, in the Department of the Environment: brisk, efficient, discreet.

'Kelly has business and law degrees as well as experience in the field,' Thomas said, as if to disabuse him. 'If you want to know what's going on, telephone this number and ask for Kelly.'

Thomas handed him a card and, as if signifying that the interview was coming to an end, rose to his feet. Carlo also rose, aware of Kelly's appraising glance as she took in details of his appearance.

'I'll see you out, Mr Bernini,' she said, also rising.

'We'll bill you weekly,' Thomas added following them to the door. 'Payment please within forty-eight hours. Scream when it starts to hurt.'

He gave Carlo a cheerful smile, shook hands and then opened the far door where he waited as Kelly escorted their client to the rear entrance where he could hear murmuring goodbyes.

Kelly came slowly up the staircase and walked back into her chief's room taking a packet of cigarettes out of her pocket and lighting one as she sat down. Thomas, at his desk, folded his arms and looked at her.

'Well?'

'A very odd tale,' she said, having heard the whole conversation through a two-way connection to her office next door. 'A tale of jealousy and revenge. Could it possibly be worth *all* the money he's going to spend to get at Varga?'

'There must be more to this than meets the eye,' Thomas said, scanning his pad. 'That's why I took the job. It can't *just* be a tale of jealousy and revenge for a slight to his sister.'

'Oh, you don't know the Italians,' Kelly puffed away at her cigarette. 'It's a wonder they haven't encased

Varga in a concrete overcoat by now and sunk him to the bottom of the Thames.'

'Come, come,' Thomas said reprovingly. 'The Berninis are not the Mafia, far from it. They're the aristocrats of jewellers, middle-class, sound family background. I'm astonished that they can stoop to something like this.

'Simeon Varga must have upset them very much indeed. Anyway I don't think this will tax your brain too hard, Kelly. Everything I've heard about Varga seems to suggest that he's tough, but in matters of business he's above suspicion.'

About twenty kilometres north of Tecpan in the mountains of the Sierra Madre del Sur, on the west coast of Mexico, there was a small airstrip which seemed almost to have been carved out of the mountains, the size of a football stadium but twice as long as it was broad. On one side of it was a series of ramshackle buildings and a control tower that had a more pronounced lean than the famous one in Pisa and looked about as old. The land around frequently trembled from subterranean tremors, but it was many years since it had suffered a major earthquake such as had devastated other parts of the country.

Aero Acapulco was the brainchild of one man, Diego Salinas, who had known a few years of glory when he had flown bombers for the Americans during World War II. Then he had been twenty, now he was over sixty and his airline barely survived. Give or take a year or two and he would be bankrupt.

But a saviour had appeared in the shape of a charming, courteous but, above all, *impressive* man from Europe, a Mr Varga of London, who had been introduced by a former buddy from the war, Sol Steen, now a banker in New York. It appeared that Salinas had saved Sol's life and Sol never forgot it, doing a less fortunate man than himself a favour whenever he could.

At one time after the war the veterans of the squadron

152

had met every year, but then it had become every five years, and now it was ten. Soon they would probably stop altogether as old comrades died off.

It had been a surprise, but a pleasant one, to receive a phone call from Sol announcing himself to be in Mexico City with a client who might be interested in purchasing his decrepit airline that had been going almost since the end of the war.

The first time Varga had come with Sol, but on this occasion he was accompanied by a man called Liddle, introduced as his financial director, who had immediately set to examining the books of Aero Acapulco, such as they were, with the help of a small desk-top computer which transfixed Diego: he stood, open-mouthed, watching Liddle punch the keys which caused a string of words and figures to appear on the screen.

'Gee!' he said, munching his cigar while the sweat poured down his face. 'Ain't that magical?'

Varga, arms folded, leaned against the wall of the hut which passed for an office, an amused expression on his face.

'You're cut off from the world here, Mr Salinas.'

'Sure am.' Salinas moved his cigar butt from one side of his mouth to the other.

Tony Liddle stopped and frowned.

'You're sure these crates can get across the Atlantic?' he asked.

'Crates?' Salinas looked puzzled.

'These ancient aircraft of yours. I believe one actually predates 1939.'

'Always well maintained,' Salinas said indignantly. 'Never had an accident, not even a mishap. Never failed a delivery.'

'Do you ever carry passengers?' Varga flicked a fly away from his face. Disliking intensely the hot, sticky atmosphere, he drew his handkerchief from the breast pocket of his white linen suit and mopped his face. Salinas shook his head.

153

'Freight, all freight. It's a hard world. Ain't licensed for passengers.'

'Mmm!' Liddle put his head on one side. 'You just about break even. Not much profit.'

'Huh, *profit*!' Salinas said in a derogatory tone of voice.

Liddle looked over to Varga and nodded his head so imperceptibly that Salinas, absorbed in his thoughts, failed to detect it.

'I want to purchase outright,' Varga said.

'You want to *buy* it?' Salinas could not hide his incredulity.

'Every last nut and bolt, the sheds, the personnel, the whole outfit. For cash.'

'For *cash*?' Salinas stumbled heavily and sat down in a chair.

'For cash *and* secrecy,' Varga added. 'Nominally you remain in charge, but it belongs to me.'

'Oh *yes*, Mr Varga,' Salinas said eagerly. 'For cash I'll do anything. Provided it's a good price,' he added as though anxious to retain a modicum of pride.

'I think you'll find it's a good price for what you've got,' Varga said. 'And it's unconditional. Only it remains in your name, but you have no control. Oh, and I don't want you about the place either. We have our own operatives.'

'You don't want the *crew*?' Mr Salinas looked more and more perplexed. 'They're about the only guys in the world who can fly these kites.'

'I want the crew, but we manage the place ourselves.'

'I *am* the management,' Salinas said with a chuckle.

'Which is what I thought.' Tony Liddle closed the ledger, put it back on the desk and sighed.

Aero Acapulco had the air of a place seen many times over in B movies of the pre-war era. There would always be an aircraft flying over the mountains and limping home to base, a blonde with tight curls waiting to greet the hero. The music would rise to a crescendo as they embraced and then fade. Yet, in so many ways, its appearance was deceptive. Despite the alarming angle of its control tower, its clutch of tin sheds, its ramshackle hangars, the fleet of ancient aircraft had been maintained in good condition. They specialized in long runs, mainly to South America, carrying mostly fruit one way and cheap consumer goods the other.

It was a poor, but apparently honest, venture – which, apart from the unbusinesslike character of its owner, was why it did not make much money.

Before they left, Varga and Tony, trailed by a bewildered but grateful Salinas, made a last inspection of the property they had bought and then they climbed into the limousine which had driven them all the way from Mexico City and waved goodbye.

Salinas, cold cigar butt still in his mouth, stood for a long time looking after them until the clouds of desert dust obscured the car from view.

Ginny sat in the small sitting-room in Varga's suite, a drink in her hand. She could hear him singing in the shower and knew that he was happy. The shares had climbed steeply again on the strength of universally good half-yearly results. Even the big institutions, run by the most cautious managers in the world, had descended from their lofty perches and were buying – a sure sign of approval.

The singing stopped and, after a second or two, Varga appeared from his bedroom, a towel round his waist. His hair was wet and tousled and his body shone with droplets of water. His skin was smooth, his chest practically hairless. She laid a hand on it as he leaned over and kissed her neck.

'Missed you,' he murmured.

'I missed you, too.' Their mouths met in a long, passionate kiss. His smell was sensuous and seductive and he began to undo the buttons of her blouse and, when she was naked, pressed her breasts to his chest. The towel dropped from his waist and, like that, they came together.

After the brief coitus she dropped to the floor and he sat down beside her, his arms round his legs, gazing at her.

'I do love you,' he said. 'I can't bear to be away from you.'

'Then why don't you take me with you?'

She reached out and stroked his thigh; silky to the touch, it was a sensation that made her tremble. She sat upright and he stroked her breasts, one after the other, his fingers lingering on each nipple. Ginny, though stimulated, began to feel cold and shivered, and he put his towel round her as he gently helped her up from the floor and led her through the door to his bedroom, her clothes left on the floor where they'd fallen.

He drew back the covers and she crept between the sheets and lay shivering until he had got into bed beside her and put his arms tightly round her.

'It's not cold,' he said, puzzled. 'The temperature is seventy-five. I checked.'

'It's not *cold* . . .' she trembled even more violently.

'Then what is it, darling?'

'I think it's fear.'

'*Fear*?' He drew away, concern showing on his face. 'Fear of what?'

'Fear of losing you.'

'But you won't lose me, precious.' He smiled and drew her even closer to him. 'Why on earth do you say that?'

'Because you go away more and more and tell me less and less. Sometimes I'm afraid about what you're up to, Simeon.'

'Oh!' He pursed his lips as though she had annoyed him and moved away from her. 'That is not a very nice thing to say, Ginny.'

'You're so secretive, Simeon.'

'I am and you have always known it; but I do nothing

156

of which I am ashamed, I assure you, and I always take Tony with me. Now, surely, you don't doubt his integrity?'

'Of course I don't. Nor yours.'

'Then what is the mystery?'

'I wish you'd take me with you when you go,' she said.

'But then the joy of homecoming wouldn't be like this.' He lay upon her and began the gentle motion back and forth, gripping her face, smoothing her mouth, her nose, her eyes with his thumbs, splitting her mouth open so that he could lick her teeth.

To be in heaven was to be in Simeon's arms.

Later they had supper at the kitchen table of his apartment, Ginny in a white robe, Varga in his striped towelling dressing-gown. They had smoked salmon, steak, a bottle of Fleurie, a salad lightly tossed with chives in a french dressing.

He had been away three weeks, in the States, South America. He had bought a bank in Venezuela and a huge cattle ranch in the Argentine. Details of all the deals had been faxed through to her and she'd got to work on the press releases straight away. After the good half-yearly results the share price rose sharply; each new venture was looked at, vetted and, finally, praised.

He didn't tell her about Mexico.

After the meal they filled the dishwasher and climbed back into bed, the TV flickering in front of them to catch the news. They continued to chat and Ginny brought him up to date with what had been happening at home; the successful press conference, the sales conference, the inspection of a new factory for Ace Pharmaceuticals on a trading estate outside Poole.

'Why Poole?'

'It's a very pretty part of the country. It's near the sea. I thought we could have a boat.'

'A boat in *Poole*?' He seemed to find it amusing. 'I

157

would much rather have a boat in Monte Carlo or Majorca.'

'A country house in Dorset, on the Isle of Purbeck. You'd love it, Simeon. It would soothe you, calm you.' She leaned over him and touched his cheek. He closed his eyes and she thought his sculptured face was of an ethereal beauty, like the statue of an Egyptian god.

'You must do what you like, my darling. I leave you in charge,' he murmured and, under the soft, soothing touch of her hands, he gradually drifted off to sleep.

CHAPTER 9

Varga's *pied à terre* at the top of the mews office was tiny but exquisite. It consisted only of bedroom, sitting-room, a kitchen with a dining area, toilet and bathroom. In a very small space the architect had performed wonders. Maggie Silklander had spared no expense in design and fine furnishings.

The bedroom was a pleasant place to sleep in, a pleasant place to wake up in, and for some time the next morning Ginny lay beside the slumbering form of her lover and thought that this, so far, was the peak of her happiness with him. Could it remain like this or might it, as had happened with Robert, go downhill?

It was only seven o'clock and Simeon was still fast asleep. She had picked him up at Heathrow the night before with the chauffeur and he had been travelling for twenty-four hours. Today was a Saturday and he had promised to rest.

Ginny got quietly out of bed, put on her white towelling bathrobe and went into the kitchen to make her morning tea, without which she could not function. The kitchen was small but everything was in place – dishwasher, microwave, even a washing machine. During the week one of the cleaners who came in daily dealt with Varga's personal laundry. His shirts were laundered at a Mayfair cleaners and delivered in crisp cellophane packets.

Ginny maintained her house in Kentish Town and did not consider Simeon's flat as in any way her home. It was a nest; a love nest, a place for intimacy and quiet talks; the occasional evening spent, as last night had been, over a meal in the kitchen: steaks or scrambled eggs, a bottle of wine, early bed and making love. Tonight they were eating at Lambert and Maggie's to celebrate the completion of the apartment, the half-year results and the fact that Lambert had had a good year too, thanks to the buoyancy of the art market.

Ginny made her tea, then took the tray into the sitting-room and dropped into one of the comfortable arm-chairs. On a table by the side of the chair was Simeon's briefcase and among the papers stuffed in at the top was a letterhead: Aero Acapulco. Thinking that it was rather an amusing name, Ginny leaned over and gently pulled the paper higher. It was a letter marked *Personal and Confidential* and addressed to Simeon: naturally she shouldn't have read it but, naturally, she did.

> Dear Mr Varga
>
> Further to your offer to purchase the above company outright for cash I am happy to confirm that I am in full agreement with your terms and await the despatch of a contract at your earliest convenience.
>
> I am sure that you will find . . .

Hearing movement from the bedroom she hastily stuffed the letter back and was sitting sipping her tea when Varga emerged and, walking quietly over to her, bent and kissed the nape of her neck.

'Good morning, darling.'

'Good morning, darling,' she replied, running a hand across his cheek.

'Sleep well?'

'Very.'

'Me too.' His lips lingered on her neck.

'Shall I get your coffee?'

'I'll get it,' he said and walked into the kitchen humming a tune under his breath. She listened to the sound of the coffee grinder, the running of the tap, the domestic trivia that made up a life together, as well as the sex and the excitement in bed. Soon Simeon came in with the coffee, black and very strong. Ginny shuddered.

'I don't know how you *could*.'

'Oh, but I can.' He smiled at her over the rim of his cup. 'Now, what plans do we have for today?'

'Well tonight we're eating with Maggie and Lambert.'

'I hadn't forgotten, and this afternoon I must see Tony.'

'But you've just *seen* Tony.' She looked surprised. 'You've spent days and days with Tony.'

'We have a lot to go over, my darling. We did a lot of business. By the way,' he gestured towards his briefcase, 'among the mail I collected from the office was a letter from your brother Angus.'

'Oh?' Ginny, surprised, put down her cup.

'We have been in correspondence.' He smiled mysteriously.

'Indeed?'

'I wrote to him from the Argentine. I have suggested some improvements to him.'

'You *what*?' Ginny sat forward on her chair.

'I think I can help him increase his profits five hundred per cent. I have been studying intensive farming methods and I pointed out that his methods are wasteful and old-fashioned. I . . .'

Ginny tried hard to stem the feeling of anger rising in her breast.

'*You* tried to tell Angus how to farm?'

'Now wait a minute, Ginny . . .' Varga looked nonplussed, but she swept on.

'You know *nothing* about farming!'

'But that's quite wrong, my dear. I know a lot. I have interests in cattle in South America. I have broiler

161

chicken farms in the States. I . . .'

'Intensive farming methods are *quite* out of character with the kind of farming Angus does.'

'Exactly. If he goes on as he is now in five years he'll be bankrupt.' Varga took another sip of his coffee and then leaned forward and stared earnestly at her. 'Probably less. Have you ever considered, Ginny, how near to bankruptcy your family is?'

'No I have not, and they are not. My father and Angus between them own thousands of acres . . .'

'Your father's tree-planting methods are also very old-fashioned. The timber I own in Brazil . . .'

'*Really*, Simeon!' Ginny got up and walked angrily to the window. The lights were usually on in the houses opposite, but as today was Saturday they were in darkness. She turned and gazed at Simeon who was watching her with an impenetrable, almost imperturbable, expression, a half-smile on his face.

'You *do* get excited, Ginny darling. For no reason . . .'

'Simeon,' she folded her arms and leaned towards him, 'you know *nothing* about farming as we know it, centuries-old traditions that have stood my family well. Bankruptcy! We are nowhere *near* it. I think your pursuit of riches is beginning to spoil you, Simeon. You are forgetting the important things.'

'I am *not* forgetting the important things,' he said coldly, suddenly abandoning his bantering mood. 'When you have been as poor as I have, Ginny, nothing is more important than having sufficient money not only to clothe and feed yourself but to lead a dignified life. Without money you have no dignity, no self-respect. And the Silklanders will find that to their cost if they don't take care.'

'But too much money can make you greedy, Simeon.' Ginny turned to face him again. 'And while we're on the subject, what is Aero Acapulco?'

'Aero Acapulco?' Simeon looked genuinely surprised. 'How did you know about that?'

Ginny pointed to his briefcase where the papers he

162

had stuffed into it before leaving his office two floors down could clearly be seen at the top.

'Oh. Well it's a company, a tiny company, I happen to be interested in,' he said flatly.

'In fact you've already purchased it?'

'Since you read my private correspondence, yes.' His expression was distant, unfriendly. She knew there were two sides to Simeon and she had to take care.

'I was intrigued by the name . . . I'm sorry, Simeon. I thought we had no secrets, no business secrets from each other.'

'Nor we have. No secrets at all.'

'Then why was I not told about Aero Acapulco?'

'Because it is not finalized. I was going to tell you on Monday when we have our debriefing session in the office.'

'Oh! Oh, I see.'

Ginny took her tray into the kitchen where she pottered about for a bit before realizing that she was not hungry. She went back into the sitting-room and said: 'I think I'll have my bath and then I'll go back to the house. See you tonight at Lambert's.'

'Ginny!' Simeon rose and came swiftly to her side. 'This is our first row. Our very first misunderstanding.'

'Yes, it is.'

'It is not pleasant for me.'

'Nor for me.'

He put his hand out and caressed her cheek.

'Don't let's row, darling. I'm sorry about Aero Acapulco. Truly it is nothing but a tiny fleet of six aeroplanes some of which go back to the war.'

'Then why buy it?' She looked puzzled.

'Because it is very cheap.'

'But why do you need an old airline, Simeon? I can't understand it.'

'It is useful for freight.' He looked vague. 'It specializes in freight, supplying goods to South America. It runs back and forwards between the Americas with well established routes. I picked it up for a song and I think it will be useful. Really, my dear. It is nothing. It is unimportant, trivial. It will not even appear in the balance sheets. It is certainly not enough to make us fall out.'

'Simeon.' Ginny hesitated, aware that she had to choose her words with care. 'Sometimes I wonder if you're going too far, taking on too much, getting – please don't misunderstand me – *too* greedy? I know how you love your business and how important it is to you. But lately your acquisitions seem to have become almost wild, lacking discrimination. You have forgotten your core business: pharmaceuticals, perfume. When you began Oriole seemed to have a great future, but you've lost interest. Since then you've acquired banks, oil wells, timber yards, cattle ranches. Simeon, *please* don't let your instincts, your common sense, desert you in what I can only call an unbridled lust for power. I hope you don't mind me speaking to you like this, but I happen to love you. Angus knows what he's doing. Advise him by all means; but don't impose too much. Do you understand?'

Simeon continued to look at her and she knew he resented her. Should she have used words like 'a lust for power'? Suddenly he caressed her cheek again. His expression was one of detachment rather than love.

'I hear you, Ginny,' he said softly. 'I hear you and I understand. I know you love me and what you say is out of love for me. But believe me, I know what I'm doing; every step is carefully taken. And as for your brother's farm, of course I won't butt in if that is what you want. I won't interfere at all as long as *you* promise not to come to me in two or three years' time and ask for help when he needs it.' He pinched her cheek so hard that it hurt her and then he drew her face so near to his that she felt like a rabbit mesmerized by a stoat.

'Promise me that?' he repeated.

*

To add to her other attributes Maggie Lambert was an accomplished cook. There was a daily woman who usually did the vegetables; but Maggie's standards were *cordon bleu* and she liked to do her own shopping, making her own selection of meat, fish and starters. She said it helped her to relax.

Of course she was helped by an emporium just around the corner called Harrods that supplied the finest ingredients and would deliver at short notice. Maggie would stride through the food section of the famous store checking off items on her shopping list, discussing the fish with the fishmonger, the meat with the butcher and, hey presto, it was all delivered later on in the day just before she got home.

By that time the table in the dining-room was laid with exquisite linen and cutlery, most of it wedding presents from the Silklanders or her own wealthy father.

That evening there had been huitres au gratin – fresh oysters with a velvety cream sauce – served with a fine dry Chablis; then côtelettes en cuirasse, boned lamb chops in pastry served with baby carrots, mange tout and pommes dauphines. With this Lambert had selected a Corton of the exceptional vintage of 1976. There was a very light tarte aux pommes which she had in fact bought from the patisserie at Harrods.

The quarrel of the morning was forgotten and Ginny, who always loved the company of her brother and his wife, the excellence of the cuisine, was relaxed and at ease. As for elegant, sophisticated Simeon, at home almost anywhere, who would not be proud of him? She knew that he and Lambert liked each other and she could see that Maggie liked him, found him attractive, and admired his taste in the fabulous antiques and objets d'art with which she had furnished his office and apartment. His good taste was instinctive, because it was obvious that his knowledge of art was negligible and not anywhere near the top of his priorities.

'That Lac burgauté table you bought for the sitting-room is fantastic.' Varga put his fingers together and kissed them. 'I never saw anything so exquisite. It fits perfectly, doesn't it, Ginny darling?'

'Perfectly,' Ginny replied with a smile, and in her mind's eye she saw the letter from Aero Acapulco lying among the papers on top of it. It was a funny name, almost like a joke, and in many ways it was a joke, buying a small, down-at-heel airline whose prime business was the transport of fruit.

'*And* at a price.' Maggie returned the smile and acknowledged the praise. 'Luckily you can afford it.'

'Tell me,' Varga leaned confidentially towards her across the table, 'how do you find these things? One never sees them in the shops.'

'Ah!' Lambert, looking like the cat who swallowed the cream, sat back in his chair fingering the stem of his wine glass. '*That* is the secret. It is a question of who you know.'

'And how much they want,' Maggie added. 'The world of antiques is indeed a devious one. You see, so many people want to avoid tax on their precious objects.'

'And some are not allowed to export them. Dealers in India, for example, which is awash with antiques, find it very hard to get a licence to sell them abroad.'

Varga sat back, a thoughtful look on his face.

'I suppose quite a lot of funny business goes on in the art world.'

'And how!' Lambert refilled his glass with the Château d'Yquem they had drunk with the sweet.

'Not, of course, among *reputable* dealers,' Maggie said hastily and then, glancing at Ginny, added: 'Shall we take a break to powder our noses?'

'Fine by me,' Ginny said, rising. 'I suppose it's the modern equivalent of passing round the port.'

Maggie smiled as Lambert drew back her chair, then she gave him a slight wave.

'See you in the drawing-room in about ten minutes.'

'Ten minutes, darling,' he lightly kissed her brow, 'and thank you for a wonderful meal.'

'Heavenly,' Ginny echoed.

'The food is some of the best I had in my life.' Varga patted his trim stomach in a gesture of appreciation.

In the hall Maggie said: 'Do you really want to go to the loo?'

'No, but I *would* like to powder my nose.' Both the women burst out laughing and ascended the stairs to the first floor where the master bedroom overlooked the garden at the back of the house.

This was an elegant, gracious room with pastel coloured walls and light modern furniture, most of it made by craftsmen to Lambert's specifications and design. Ginny sat down at the dressing table and gazed at her face in the mirror.

'I think I'm showing the ravages of age.' She pressed her fingers against her high cheekbones.

'That's nonsense.' Maggie stood behind her. 'You're only a year or so younger than Lambert.'

'I'm not far off thirty.' Ginny inspected her face again then, opening her purse, drew out her compact and dabbed at her nose. 'It's different for a woman.'

'You're thinking of kids?' Maggie perched on the side of the bed.

'I suppose when a girl gets near thirty she does think of kids.' Ginny concurred. 'That's what Robert always wanted. When I thought we were going to be married I decided that thirty would be about the right age. All that's changed now, of course.'

'Any regrets about Robert?'

'None at all. We saw him not so long ago. He's engaged to a nice girl called Wendy. I believe the wedding is quite soon.'

'Yes, we know Wendy. She's been here for dinner. Nice, but not like you of course, and I think Robert realizes it.'

Ginny got up, stretched, and began to walk round the room.

'I can't help what Robert does on the rebound . . .'

'And Simeon,' Maggie sounded as though she hardly dared mutter his name. 'Is it serious?'

'I guess it's serious.' Ginny flopped on the bed beside her. 'The thing is, he's not free. His wife won't divorce him and he has to wait the full five years.'

'Well that should be up quite soon.'

'There's also the fact,' Ginny leaned back and gazed at the ceiling, 'that he's never asked me.'

'Well maybe he's waiting until he knows he will be free.'

'Maybe and maybe not. Who knows with Simeon?'

Maggie detected an odd note in her sister-in-law's voice, and her expression changed from one of conspiracy to one of concern.

'Darling, I thought you were so happy. Tonight you seemed to have such rapport. I hope nothing's wrong?'

'Nothing at all.' Ginny continued her inspection of the ceiling. 'Only Simeon *is* a strange man. He refuses to discuss anything personal about himself. One never feels one quite knows him . . . and do you think it's wise, even if you got the chance, to spend the rest of your life with a stranger?'

Meanwhile, in the dining-room, Lambert poured another glass of the fine, sweet Sauternes and held it up to Varga.

'Here's to you, Simeon, and your continued success. I believe it's been a fabulous year for you?'

'Yes, it has.' Simeon, looking pleased, stared into the depths of the beautiful golden liquid. 'And getting better. Tell me . . .' he leaned back and jingled the loose change in his pocket, 'about the export of antiques. I am in the process of acquiring an airline. I don't know if that interests you at all?'

'Oh?' Lambert sounded if anything perplexed. 'How?'

'It's a freight line situated in Mexico.'

'Mexico!' Lambert whistled. 'Plenty going on in South America.'

'I thought there might be. There *everyone* is at great pains to conceal their wealth.'

'Oh, I don't mean anything illegal.' Lambert's eyes narrowed. 'I mean, no doubt, neither do you?'

'Look.' Varga held his glass in his hand and, screwing up his eyes, studied it as a merchant might a diamond. 'There is a blurred edge, is there not, between what is illegal and what is legal?'

'Not really. Legal means documentation.'

'But you told me that clients operate under assumed names . . . in order to avoid tax, presumably?'

'Well, I never know the reasons. They never tell me. That's their problem.'

'No, but if you make an invoice out in a false name how can the authorities get to know who it really is?'

'That's the customer's problem.'

'It sounds like a dodge to me, all the same.'

'I don't get involved.' Lambert sounded uneasy. 'I have to be very careful because I have a good reputation. I keep the books and pay my taxes.'

'And never ever get involved in any fiddle at all?' Varga's tone was vaguely suggestive.

'No more than any other businessman.' Lambert wriggled nervously in his chair. 'You, for example. I bet you have tax havens to avoid paying as much tax as you can.'

'Of course I do.'

'The Cayman Islands, and that sort of thing. Offshore companies?'

'Who doesn't?' Varga's expression remained bland.

'And Mexico, perhaps?'

'Mexico is quite a useful little place, actually. I'm just beginning to see its merits.'

'But how did you come to acquire an airline *there*?'

'I simply heard it was going. It's small,' Varga sounded dismissive, 'very small. No more than a few shacks, a control tower which looks as though a plane once collided with it.' He gave a short laugh. 'But the planes, six of them, are old but in excellent condition, capable of flying round the world, I would say at a guess, with plenty of stops to refuel. India for example . . .' his eyes flickered, 'places like that. Then back to Mexico. No questions asked.'

'You aren't *seriously* suggesting . . .' Lambert swallowed his wine and began agitatedly to play with his silver napkin ring.

'I'm suggesting nothing,' Varga said smoothly. 'I'm just saying that should you ever . . . if a client has a surplus of stock . . . the means are there and the risk is negligible. Now,' his manner became brisk and he glanced at his watch, 'the ladies will be wondering whatever has happened to us.'

Carlo Bernini was a man who loved his mother. It was not uncommon for Italians to venerate the matriarch – rather as they venerated the Madonna – but Carlo was more mother-dominated than most. Probably the reason that he had never married was that no woman had ever come up to the standard of his mother; thus he found it almost impossible to form a normal relationship and was forced to look to unusual sources for his pleasures, where emotions were not involved.

Carlo and his mother lived in some style in a vast, solid Victorian fantasy with gables and turrets at the top of Highgate Hill, which reflected the position of the Berninis and the scale of their wealth. Fortunata was a stickler for routine; her eldest son was expected at home for dinner every night and if he was ever late or absent he had to have a very good explanation.

Carlo and his mother had tried to get Claudia to move back into the family home after Simeon left her; there was plenty of room for her and the children and the matriarch loved to have lots of people round her to boss and organize, feed and dominate. As a widow she wore

170

black and her religious scruples drove her to Mass every weekday morning and twice on Sundays. She had no time for fashion and her clothes were weeds indeed; black dress and fine black stockings, sensible, not elegant, black shoes. She could have been any peasant woman from Naples, from where she had originally hailed, only she was enormously wealthy and instead of wasting her money made sure that it was well invested to pass on to the grandchildren and that generous contributions were made to church charities.

It was a strange household by any standards and was served by a Neopolitan couple, as cook and butler, and two Filipino maids. They all lived in the attics at the top of the house. In addition there was a chauffeur who lived above the stables which had been converted into the garages which could hold five cars. Now there was just Carlo's Mercedes in which he was driven to and from work every day, and his mother's comfortable Daimler, in which she was taken to visit the Italian shops in Clerkenwell and Soho where she could buy fresh pasta, Italian coffee and the various national delicacies so much beloved by herself and her son.

Carlo usually got home by seven and he and his mother drank an aperitif in the drawing-room and discussed the events of the day. Fortunata was an important shareholder and liked an up-to-date account of the progress of the business. At a quarter to eight dinner was announced and, sharp at eight o'clock, it was served: antipasto, soup, a meat or fish dish and a good but inexpensive Italian wine, Bardolino or Verdicchio.

They sat at either end of a long table in the dining-room in a style that could have come straight out of some costume drama, with the butler hovering at one end and a maid in attendance by the sideboard waiting for orders.

When the cheese course was served the butler replenished their glasses and then left the room. It was usually at that time that Carlo moved up the table to sit closer to his mother and they talked.

171

'Any news of Varga from the agency?' Fortunata demanded, spreading her cheese thickly on the *ciabatta*, Italian bread baked freshly by cook each day from flour and olive oil.

Carlo, similarly engaged, shrugged.

'They have searched the books, they find nothing irregular. He has a number of private offshore companies which, naturally, they can't touch. The figures are not disclosed. Officially the publicly quoted company, AP International, is very careful to obey the rules. His gearings, that is his borrowings, are low, he seems to have a plentiful supply of cash. He is most economical and lives, as he always did, apparently frugally.'

'What about the woman?'

'There he is discreet, too. Of course he has a flat above his office, so who knows what goes on there? But apparently she goes to her own home every night. Varga spends a great deal of time abroad, so there is not much to report.'

Fortunata, clad in black from head to toe, her grey hair piled on top of her head, her face chalk white, made a gesture of irritation and, putting her hand discreetly over her mouth, began to pick her teeth.

'There must be more to it.'

'In a few months he can divorce Claudia whether she likes it or not.' Carlo threw up his hands in a gesture of resignation. 'I really think, Mama, this vendetta of yours should stop. For one thing it is costing us an enormous amount of money.' He reached into his breast pocket and withdrew a small sheaf of papers. 'Five hundred pounds a day, Mama, for surveillance alone. It is a ridiculous sum of money.'

In a gesture of impatience Fortunata snatched the papers from her son and, placing a pince nez on her nose, began to peruse them.

'Five hundred pounds a day and they can find nothing! Ridiculous!'

'They're supposed to be the best. They are corporate

investigators with contacts all over the world. They've come up with nothing, Mama. Let us forget about Simeon Varga, take him to the cleaners by all means in settlement, and get on with our lives.'

'Over my dead body,' Fortunata said vehemently. They always spoke Italian at home, even though Carlo had been born in England. She looked at him scornfully. 'What kind of ninny are you, Carlo Bernini, son of Antonio, that you let a man as lowly as Varga, a peasant, dishonour your sister, condemn her to live the rest of her life a single woman . . .'

'She is protected by *us*, Mama, the family,' Carlo said in a voice so craven it would have surprised his many business acquaintances.

'It is not the same thing as having a man by your side. Someone to protect you and give you a status in the world single women are denied. Believe me, I know. I had strength of character and it was hard for me; for a woman like your sister, as weak as she is, it is harder still.'

'Claudia is not weak, Mama,' Carlo protested. 'She is making a great impression in the showroom; she has a good understanding of our business. She . . .'

'I don't mean weak in that sense, you fool,' his mother said scathingly. 'I mean in the sense that she is like so many modern women who have none of the toughness and strength of character of those of us who were born in Italy. She wants sex.' A gleam came into the brilliant black eyes. 'She wants to be admired as a woman. In the days of my mother if you lost a man you gave up all thoughts like this, but now . . . who knows how far Claudia will stray? Despite the strength of her religion she will be tempted . . . and it is for that reason I cannot forgive Varga, whom we helped when he was nothing. He was unworthy of my daughter and we should have done all we could to prevent him marrying her. Had she not been so headstrong *then*, she would not be so unhappy now.'

Then she swept up the bell from the table and rang it loudly in Carlo's ear, as if chastising him for his cowardice.

A low light burned in the corner of the room and it took a long time to become accustomed to the dark. After a while, however, it was possible to make out the outlines of the cruel instruments of torture on the walls, the chains, the leather thongs, the hooks and iron bars deeply embedded with sharp, ugly-looking nails.

In the centre of the room was a giant wheel whose circumference was the size of a man and in the centre was a hole from which the main spokes radiated out to the rim.

The man, naked, lay spreadeagled on the wheel facing downwards. His body gleamed with sweat and he was panting. There was blood on his head from a superficial wound and scratches on his back and buttocks, as though a tiger had run a giant paw over him. His hands were bound by thongs to the rim of the wheel, and so was his left ankle. A woman dressed in a black wetsuit was finishing tying his right ankle to the rim. Then, stepping back, she gazed for a moment with some satisfaction at her work and, selecting a long whip with a mean-looking thong from a set of instruments in the far corner near the light, she approached the wheel again, flexing and unflexing the whip in her hand with evident relish.

'Now,' she said, raising it above her head and, as it lashed down on the bare buttocks of the man he let out a scream of pain that anywhere else would have raised the roof.

But the chamber, like everything else in the house, was soundproof.

CHAPTER 10

From the forty-eight floor of the Empire State Building there was a magnificent view of the Hudson River sneaking through the city of New York, a distant glimpse of the sea. Yet even this mighty building seemed in danger of being eclipsed by others which were springing up around it. Far below the streets resembled nothing so much as tiny arteries wending their way through the amorphous body attended by parasites scurrying hither and thither with the determination of a swarm of ants.

Yes, people were like ants, Varga thought, gazing out of the window while behind him computers whirled, faxes and telexes clicked, telephone wires hummed. Yet, besides himself, there was only one occupant of the room and even then he wasn't sure he knew his real name.

The Empire State Building was a very easy place in which to take cover.

He'd given his name as Beaufort, Max Beaufort. Maybe he thought it had a fine medieval ring, striking a note of authenticity in a shiftless world, a world of distrustfulness and deceit.

Beaufort was Beaufort and Varga was Voitek, Samuel Voitek, with its Semitic overtones that might encourage the dealer to deal.

Tony Liddle had set the whole thing up during a recent visit to Mexico. He had met a man who knew a man who knew a man who wanted . . . It was intricate, furtive and undoubtedly illegal. It was a good thing to be Voitek, or Beaufort, or Smith or Cohen . . . to be anonymous, easily lost, unidentifiable.

There had been a lot of faxing, many telephone calls. Now there was the meeting and at first Varga had been unwilling to meet on the forty-eighth floor of the Empire State. It seemed a long way down to the ground. He suffered from vertigo and the higher he got the more uneasy he felt. He'd taken a Valium to steady his nerves, but even now he felt queasy looking down on those ants scurrying about and knowing they were people.

Varga turned to see that Beaufort was still poring over the map they had been studying on his desk, his stubby finger at some point in the middle of it. He was a short, thickset man of about fifty with a Brooklyn accent; his origins seemed about as vague, as cosmopolitan, as Varga's. In many ways they spoke the same language. There had been a mutual understanding, rather than mutual attraction, as soon as they met.

Beaufort was a chain smoker, however, which was one of the reasons why Varga had turned to the window – not for fresh air, because it didn't open, but for the illusion of air, of wide open spaces.

Beaufort wore his spectacles on his forehead, his shirt-collar was open and between the fingers of his puffy right hand was the inevitable cigarette.

'I can't see it,' he said, frowning. 'I can't see no corridor, Mr Voitek. From the Turkish border to the centre of Iraq I can't see no corridor at all.'

'The corridor isn't *marked*, Mr Beaufort,' Varga said patiently, leaning over the desk so that his shoulder almost touched Beaufort's. He stabbed the map some-where between Bitlis in Turkey and Masul in Iraq. 'It's about there. It's a corridor through the mountains that only experienced pilots know about. Of *course* it isn't marked on the map.'

His contemptuous expression seemed to upset

Beaufort, who huffily began to fold up the map.

Suddenly the phone rang and he answered it, speaking in a language with which Varga was familiar. He looked at him in surprise, and when Beaufort finished speaking he said, 'Armenian?'

'My parents.' Beaufort shrugged and lit a fresh cigarette from the stub in his mouth. 'You too?'

'Somewhere around there,' Varga said with deliberate vagueness. 'But I was born in London.'

'I could tell you weren't English,' Beaufort said with a smirk.

'But I am English.'

'I mean a hundred per cent.'

'And I could tell you were not American,' Varga said with a note of spite in his voice.

'But I was born in Brooklyn,' Beaufort looked offended, 'right beside the Hudson River.'

'I mean a hundred per cent,' Varga said in a whisper. 'I think we understand each other, Mr Beaufort.'

'Yeah, I guess.' Beaufort scratched his head, drew his spectacles down on his nose and began to work quickly with his calculator, his fingers running expertly over the keys. 'Right, Mr Voitek, you are going to fly my merchandise through this corridor you know about, but which isn't on the map, from Turkey to Iraq. How does it get to Turkey?' He leaned back and folded his arms and, momentarily, Varga was reminded of those gangster films, beloved since his youth, featuring Edward G. Robinson or Paul Muni.

'I thought you already had it in Turkey?' Varga looked surprised. Beaufort pointed his finger once more to the floor.

'The merchandise is right here in New York State.'

'Ah, then you have a problem. How *are* you going to get it to Turkey?'

'Can you help me, Mr Voitek?' Beaufort dropped his blustering manner and looked appealingly at him.

'Seventy per cent to you, thirty to me,' Varga said,

feeling an inner glow of satisfaction, the knowledge that he was on top of his opponent.

'Oh, no!' Beaufort vigorously shook his head. 'It wouldn't be worth my while.'

'I don't even know what your merchandise is.'

'Better you shouldn't.'

'In that case I'd better make it sixty–forty.'

Beaufort threw his arms into the air and, with an exclamation, stood up. The telephone rang again, but he ignored it. After a while it stopped, which made Varga think he had another office, or he subscribed to an answering service. 'I think the deal is off, Mr Voitek.' He held out a hand. 'Sorry I troubled you.'

'No trouble at all.' Varga picked up his briefcase. He extended his hand.

'I know where to find you if I change my mind.' Beaufort, seemingly discomfited by his attitude, clung on to his hand. Varga shook his head, a regretful smile on his lips.

'No, I'm sorry, that contact is closed.'

'Oh!' Beaufort, looking thoughtful, dropped his hand. 'No way I can contact you at all?'

'None I'm afraid.'

'That makes it difficult.' Beaufort sank back into his chair again and indicated that Varga should do the same. Varga, however, his irritation showing clearly, stood where he was, poised to make for the door. With an ostentatious gesture he looked at his watch.

'I'm afraid I can't give you much more time, Beaufort. You have to make up your mind. If you thought of shopping around to see if you could get a cheaper deal I have to tell you now that I don't think there's much chance of it.'

'There I have to agree with you,' Beaufort said, solemnly nodding his head.

'The contraband that you have is, as I hazard a guess, highly volatile. It could cost you, and me, thirty years in prison if it was discovered.' Varga eyed him gravely.

'If not life,' Beaufort intoned. 'Some states might give you the gas chamber.'

'Therefore I, a legitimate businessman, am taking a very big risk . . . and I want a big reward, Mr Beaufort. Sixty—forty, or there's no deal. I want the agreement now. I want half the money in US dollars, lodged at a destination of my choice, and the rest on deposit in a bank or banks I shall also nominate . . .'

'I need thirty days,' Beaufort whined. 'Give me at least thirty days for the balance.'

'You have the upfront money now?' Varga looked at him sharply.

Beaufort nodded.

'*All* of it?' Varga insisted.

Beaufort nodded again, this time more vigorously.

'On my daughter's life!'

The man even had a daughter. It was impossible to think of someone like Beaufort having any sort of family life, any uxorious feelings or fatherly devotion.

But maybe some people thought that about him.

It was the first time she had invited Varga to the house. Hitherto it had seemed a separate part of herself, literally a place apart. There she relaxed, unwound, read, watched TV, slept, day-dreamed.

And now he was here, strolling around poking his nose into everything: cupboards, corners, as if he were a prospective purchaser.

He was there because he was part of her life, too. When he was in London they spent each day together and, increasingly, each night, or part of each night; but he had never been invited to her house and never slept with her there.

She had met him at the airport on his return from the States and they drove to her house to pick up some clothes because the following day they were flying north for Christmas. Varga had just purchased an executive jet which he had been anxious to show her. For the first time he had flown to the States and back in it, and she had watched it landing in a corner of the vast Heathrow complex, a little frightened about what Varga was becoming.

Finally, now, he stood on the threshold of her bedroom, a frown on his brow, nose quivering slightly.

'I'm uncomfortable here,' he said abruptly. 'Let's go.'

He turned sharply, cannoning into her, unaware, perhaps, that she was so close. 'I'm sorry, my darling.' He clutched her round the waist. 'Forgive me. You know what it is. It's about Robert.' He kissed her cheek and she closed her eyes, aware of the aroma that was typically Simeon; spicy, pungent, sexy. His hand rested on her breast and their lips met.

'Let's get out of here quickly . . .' he said as they broke apart.

'But, Simeon, it's my home.' She felt affronted and annoyed.

'Your home is with me.' His clasp on her arm tightened. 'Don't you realize that, Ginny? I hate to think of you living here with Robert. This is in the past. I am your present and your future. Ginny, I've got details of a house in Gloucestershire. It's a large house, Purborough Park.'

'I didn't know you were looking for a country house?' She opened her eyes wide.

'Of course I am! This has been on the market for some time. There was some trouble with the estate of the last owner. It is in a state of advanced disrepair, but the outside is intact. It stands in seventy acres of grounds and looks lovely. I want you to come and see it with me. Darling, put this on the market. Get rid of it.'

'Simeon, I'm fond of it.' Ginny, uncertain about his meaning, followed him down into the sitting-room, where he stood moodily looking out of the window on to the patio where she had enjoyed so many happy hours with Robert.

Yes, the house was full of him, of them and the good

times they'd shared. She sank on to the sofa as Varga slowly turned round and gazed at her. He looked pale and tired from his journey, but to her he was so beautiful, almost ethereal, with his soft brown eyes and skin the colour of honey, his black hair waving softly back from his brow. He had one hand in his pocket and the jacket of his well-cut suit was fastened by a single button.

She thought he was the most attractive man she had ever known. He was in a different sphere. He seemed to sense her emotions and, coming to sit beside her, took her hand.

'Ginny, my weeks in America were interminable without you. I can't tell you how much I missed you . . .'

'I missed you too,' she murmured. 'What kept you so long?'

'There is so much to do in the States. I am negotiating to buy a bank, another TV station . . .'

'Simeon.' Ginny pressed his hand to her lips and then lowered it, still clasping it. 'Darling, I've spoken to you before about going too fast. You're in the fast lane and you can't seem to stop. Your borrowings must be enormous . . .'

'Robert has spoken to you,' Varga said accusingly, abruptly removing his hand. 'I can tell.'

'I haven't seen Robert for weeks, *or* spoken to him. But it's obvious to me you must be borrowing heavily. The faxes about your acquisitions continue to flood into the office. I can't keep up.'

'For your information,' he said coolly, 'I have kept my borrowings very low. I do not want to be at the mercy of the banks. They put up an umbrella when the sun shines and take it away when it rains.'

'Then how . . .' she looked puzzled.

'My cash flow is good. Besides, I have other resources . . .'

'Oh?' She gave him a curious look.

'Ginny darling.' He placed his hand once more on her lap. 'You know how it is. Tony is a very clever chap.

181

There are some off-shore trusts which enable me to pay for an acquisition, say, in the States without the authorities in this country or America, where they are just as nosy, getting to know my sources.'

'So you financed your Mexican airline like that?' Her expression was inquisitorial.

'Yes, and others. It is very easy to be an entrepreneur in Latin America. They have the right attitude to business. Here the Stock Exchange controls and in the States the SEC stick their fingers in every pie. Oh I assure you, my darling, there is nothing illegal. It is just easier to operate without for ever having to think of shareholders . . .'

'So some of these things aren't part of AP International?' She didn't know whether to feel worried or relieved.

'No, of course they're not. I have a profitable little airline in Mexico, several companies in the Argentine and Brazil, and they don't appear in our accounts. They are a nest egg, my darling,' his eyes looked deeply into hers, 'for you and me, in case anything ever goes wrong.'

'What could go wrong, Simeon?' Her sense of foreboding deepened.

'My dear, we could have a war, a recession, who knows? Do you think the boom will last forever? No, the boom won't and Mrs Thatcher won't, and when that time comes I want to know that I am not solely dependent on the whims of the banks and shareholders. Believe me, Ginny, I know what I'm doing.'

Now it was his turn to draw her hand to his lips and his kiss lingered. Then he stood up, hands in his pockets, and began to pace the room.

'My divorce is absolute in the spring.'

'Has Claudia agreed?'

'Claudia will have to agree. It is the law after five years' separation and we shall have been separated for five years. I am making a generous settlement. Even her brothers can't disagree about that. As for that mother of hers . . .' his brows angrily knotted together.

'Her mother?'

'Her mother is a fiend. Were it not for her we should have been divorced long ago. You know in Italy women rule the roost? Well, Italian mothers continue the tradition here. She has emasculated her elder son Carlo. He has never married because he has not found a girl of whom Mama approves. And yet he reigns supreme at Berninis, one of the most famous establishments of jewellers in the country. I tell you he is a tough opponent. However . . .' he paused, 'I am letting myself run on. By April all obstacles will be resolved and, Ginny . . .' he held out his hand and looked at her, 'I'm asking you to marry me.'

They sat together in the back seat of the car as it headed along Kentish Town Road towards the West End. Tomorrow they would choose the ring; later that day look at the house in the country; and at night they would fly to her parents' home. Ginny felt an exhilaration she had never believed possible. For a while they didn't speak, but she was aware of a restless movement as he kept glancing out of the rear window.

'What is it, darling?' She sat upright and looked out of the window too.

'I know it's absurd,' he said, glancing over his shoulder, 'but I have the odd feeling I'm being followed.'

'What?' Ginny looked out of the window again, but there were so many cars behind them with their lights on that it was impossible even to discern what makes of car they belonged to.

Varga leaned forward and tapped the chauffeur on the back. 'Peter, are you listening?'

'No, Mr Varga. I'm concentrating on the driving.'

'That's a good man, Peter,' Varga smiled reassuringly at Ginny, 'but I want you to keep an eye on the mirror. If you think you see a car that is tailing us, tell me.'

'It's difficult to make out any particular car at night, Mr Varga.'

'I don't mean now, but during the day as well. I want you to take particular care when the roads are wide enough for a car to pass us. By the way, can you use a gun?'

'Mr *Varga*!' The chauffeur's expression was impossible to see, but there was a note of fear in his voice.

'You have no licence I suppose?'

'No, sir.'

'Still, a gun in the glove compartment might be useful.'

'Simeon, you're *really* worrying me.' Ginny looked at him in alarm. 'Are you joking?'

'Not at all.' But his expression was amused.

'Then why should someone be following you?'

'My darling, I am a rich man. You've said it yourself. My shares are now the fastest rising shares in the whole of the UK. The news has got out about my personal aeroplane. As soon as we have a look at Purborough Park it will be in the papers. Agents do it deliberately with the hope of putting the price up.' He shrugged and, bending towards her, gave her a swift kiss. 'It is something which you will have to get used to from now on, beloved. But I can assure you, in time it will be worth the inconvenience.'

'Really?'

'Really.' He squeezed her hand. 'Together we shall conquer the world.'

Purborough Park was a magnificent mansion in Gloucestershire built in the style of classical Baroque probably by a pupil of Nicholas Hawksmoor, in about 1710. It was rectangular in shape, with Corinthian pilasters which accentuated the height of the building. The east and west façades had bays flanked by high columns, and above the frieze was a parapet which surrounded the building.

From the outside it was spectacular, but the inside of

Purborough Park told a very different story: one of years of neglect. The hall parallel to the façade smelt of damp and decay; there were holes in the floors and the ceiling plaster showed imminent signs of collapse. The staircase at the end of the hall rose to the full height of the house, but parts of the balustrade were completely missing and, on the instructions of the agent who accompanied them, Varga and Ginny trod with care along the bare boards of the first and second floors and into the huge bedrooms which similarly were in chronic need of repair and refurbishment. The attic was barred to them altogether as completely unsafe, and once they had descended the staircase they stood again rather disconsolately in the main hall looking out on to the lake which, similarly neglected and full of pond weed, lay between the house and the overgrown lawn.

However, much magnificence shone through: the shell beaded niches, the beauty of the ornate cornices and original plasterwork of the ceilings of the main salons, their quatrefoils, rectangles and octagons joined by loops and twists, rosettes, stars and *fleur de lys*.

The scope of the house was breathtaking and, by closing her eyes, Ginny could briefly envisage what it might look like after all the repairs had been undertaken — and how much it would cost. When she opened them she saw Varga looking at her with his gentle, loving expression. He held out his hand and she grasped it.

'Like it, darling?'

'Love it, but . . .'

'I've already had an architect to look at it.'

'The cost will be fantastic.'

Varga shrugged as if this were the least of his worries.

'I am more concerned about how long it will take.'

'Oh, I think it can be done very quickly with local labour. There is plenty of that about,' the agent, anxious to make a deal, said reassuringly. 'Basically the place is sound . . .'

Ginny looked meaningfully at the floor and then raised

her eyes to the ceilings where great gaps were apparent exposing bare floorboards and joists.

'No, I assure you . . .'

'I might say my family live in a castle,' Ginny said firmly, 'and its upkeep, even in good condition, costs a fortune. Central heating has to be installed. One would freeze to death in a place like this without it.'

'One would have to be very careful of the panelling.' Varga frowned and ran his hand caressingly along it.

'I would suggest *part* central heating, sir,' the agent said respectfully, 'but, of course, your architect and surveyor will advise you on that. It can warp the wood in these old houses.'

'But you like it, that's the main thing?' Varga seemed uninterested in the opinion of the agent and looked at Ginny for reassurance.

'I adore it.'

'Then you shall have it. It will be my wedding present.'

Varga smiled and the agent gave an almost audible sigh of relief.

'But it must be done quickly,' Varga said sternly. 'I shall want to bring my bride here before the end of next year.'

Edward Thomas looked at his client with a wry smile.

'I'm afraid we've drawn a complete blank on Varga, Mr Bernini. He appears as clean as a whistle.'

At his side Kelly, dressed in a navy suit and white blouse, nodded.

'We can't unearth a thing. Of course he has a relationship with Miss Silklander, but you already knew that.'

'He can't have acquired *all* these businesses without substantial borrowings.' Carlo thumped the desk between them in his annoyance.

'Surprisingly modest and restrained.' Kelly turned over the pages of a file in front of her. 'His gearing is very low compared to his assets. The banks, in fact, would like to lend him more. He is a very cautious, clever operator.'

She chose her words with care, anxious not to offend a client who was already paying well over the odds for their services.

'But then you knew that,' Thomas said. 'After all he was your brother-in-law.'

'*Is*,' Carlo snapped. '*Is* my brother-in-law.'

'But I believe you told me that very soon the five years would be up.'

'That's true.' Carlo bit his lip. 'The bastard can then be free to humiliate my sister.'

'Really today, Mr Bernini, divorce is not such a disgraceful affair,' Thomas said placatingly. 'It does not carry the stigma it used to have.'

'I am not asking you for your opinion, Mr Thomas. Doubtless in your profession you don't set much store by morality. But that is not the case with my family. We are Italian Catholics of the old school. For us marriage is for life. My mother goes to Mass every day. To get a scoundrel like Varga and give him his just deserts would only be considered fair by us, playing the game.'

'But I *don't* agree. I am sure that Mrs Varga will soon re-establish her place in society,' Thomas said dispassionately. 'Maybe marry again.'

'She will *never* marry again,' Carlo said grimly, 'not as long as my mother is alive.'

'So the five years since they've been living apart . . .'

'Three years,' Carlo corrected him.

'But I thought you said that the divorce was probable next year?'

'They moved into separate bedrooms; then he moved out. For five years they have not lived as man and wife, probably more.'

'Oh!' Kelly tapped her forehead and her normally pale, composed features showed traces of animation. 'Can it be *proved* that they had separate bedrooms?'

'Well they had. We all knew it.'

'But can you prove it? After all, if Mrs Varga were to deny it . . .'

'For another two years you have him on the hook.'
Thomas smiled delightedly at his assistant for giving him
this unexpected opportunity to earn his fee. 'I'm sure
that a little venial sin like a white lie would not disturb
Mrs Varga's sleep, or her religious faith, too badly.'

'You mean for another *two* years I can harass him?'

'Exactly. That should give you some satisfaction, sir,
and in the meantime give us more of a chance to discover
something about him.'

'You're following him?'

'Only in this country as per your instructions.'

'Maybe he suspects something?'

'I think not.'

Carlo tapped the desk impatiently and looked at Kelly.

'Maybe the lady should follow him. He would be less
suspicious.'

'Frankly,' Kelly rose to her feet and buttoned her
jacket, 'and to be honest, Mr Bernini, I think you're
wasting your money. I don't think you are going to find
anything to Mr Varga's discredit. He has offshore companies – who hasn't? – and these we can't investigate.
No one can. But I have examined the balance sheets
of his publicly quoted companies and the accounts are
scrupulously kept. He seems to go out of his way to keep
the law. Hound him by any means you think fit for
your own personal vengeance; but we have a number
of urgent cases to occupy us. Besides, I never do personal
surveillance work. Never.'

'You think I should put up with that kind of insol-
ence?' Carlo demanded of Thomas, who had begun to
look uncomfortable in the course of Kelly's speech.

'Maybe Kelly was a little too forthright, but I am sorry
to tell you that I do think she happens to be right. However, Mr Bernini, the last thing we wish to do is give
offence to a good client and I apologize if she overstepped
the mark. We will review the matter after Christmas, let
you know what we suggest. In the meantime you wish
the surveillance to continue?'

'Everything!' Carlo spoke bitterly. 'Everything. I want you to do everything you can. I was told you were the best, now show me you are.' And, without a handshake or even a nod of his head, he walked abruptly from the room.

'Pig,' Kelly said to his back as soon as he was out of earshot. She slumped down in the chair and cracked the knuckles of both hands. Thomas, still at his desk, lit a cigarette and blew a long stream of smoke in front of him.

'He's a very difficult customer. So ungrateful.'

'He's mad; the whole family's mad. Whoever heard of such an attitude in this day and age?' Kelly snapped. 'Did *you* ever hear anything like it before, Edward? Honestly?'

'It's very rare,' Edward acknowledged, 'but I have heard of it. I've heard of it particularly in Muslim communities where it is quite common, and families are often keen to exact revenge. I believe the mother here is the cause of the trouble, a very powerful and determined woman. The honour of the only daughter has been sullied. Varga must pay for it.'

'I even feel sorry for Varga,' Kelly said thoughtfully.

'I don't think there's any reason to feel sorry for him. You say his nose is clean. I think he can look after himself.'

'Yet we suggested that he should be shackled to that odious family for another two years. Shame on us.'

'I considered it cheap at the price he's paying me,' Thomas chuckled. 'After all we've already taken a small fortune off the Bernini family. But here . . .' suddenly he sat up and became practical. 'Let's take another look at the surveillance. Maybe Brown *is* getting tired. There's a new man coming in the New Year.' He consulted a document in front of him. 'Philips. He's worked with Pinkerton in the States. Why don't you take a break from your desk and have a go on the road?'

'Surveillance? You're kidding!' Kelly looked at him angrily.

'Not at all. It does us all good to go back to fundamentals from time to time. I shan't insist, but give it a thought, Kelly.'

As usual Kelly was the last to leave the office; last to leave and first to arrive. She lived alone in the lower part of a semi-detached house in Wandsworth with a cat and a dog, good companions for many years, and she travelled to her job by car every day, leaving it in a nearby multi-storey car park.

She had few friends and little life outside her job; no men friends, a couple of close women friends, no strong attachments. She visited her mother in Dublin every other year and each summer she took a holiday as part of a package tour to some part of Europe. She was careful with money and it was never anything luxurious.

Many people would have said she was a lonely, unfulfilled woman, but she loved her work. She was a graduate of Trinity College Dublin and the London School of Economics and, strongly against the tradition of that liberal institution, had entered the Metropolitan Police as a graduate trainee, rising quite quickly before she met Thomas and was intrigued enough to join the sort of civilian force which worked undercover.

She was Thomas's right hand; she could almost read his mind. She respected him but she didn't love him; she had never been in love and didn't think she ever would be. People, she supposed, would call her undersexed but she didn't mind. She was extremely indifferent to the opinions of other people.

When she got home the night was already half over and she was greeted with undiluted joy by the two beings she cared about most in the whole world apart, perhaps, from her mother. The cat and dog were getting old now, but she loved them. She fed them both, took her dog for a walk round the block, and by the time she got in it was almost time for bed. Sometimes she ate in the office; sometimes she bought a McDonald's and ate it in the car, very occasionally she boiled an egg or warmed up a take-away in the microwave. Tonight she had worked late in the office fuelled by coffee and a sandwich.

Another day gone. She always set the alarm last thing before putting off the light and sleeping the sleep that only the just, the contented and the pure of heart can know.

Her last thought before sleep claimed her was that it might, as Thomas suggested, be fun to go into the field again, to trail the elusive Varga herself and recapture the sense of those rather heady, exciting days when, as a young woman, she was on car patrol as part of the Metropolitan Force. Then she dismissed it as absurd, as her cat jumped up on the bed and cuddled snugly into a hollow beside her. Moments later they were both asleep.

CHAPTER 11

'Of course the engagement's unofficial,' Moira Silklander babbled excitedly. 'The divorce isn't through for three months.'

Pru Mactavish took another handful of nuts and began to pop them one by one into her mouth.

'You like him, Pru, don't you?'

'I only met him once,' Pru replied cautiously. 'The time Robert was here. I can't say I *really* took him in.'

'Well *we* like him,' Moira said firmly. 'He's unusual, but he's nice and he's absolutely head-over-heels in love with Ginny. You should see her ring.'

'Mother, you shouldn't judge a person's love by the size of the ring,' Pru said acidly, looking at the small solitaire which was all her husband Douglas had been able to afford to plight his troth to her. The Mactavishes farmed on the Border, half of their extensive farmland on one side, half on the other. The farm was heavily mortgaged, they sent their children to state schools, but they just about got by.

'No . . .' Moira paused awkwardly and looked at Pru who, she felt, although happy, had missed out on much of the excitement of life, as indeed had she. They had both married young, had grown up in rural communities, borne a number of children.

Pru had three – and had never had much money. There was more than enough for the necessities, but not as much as they would have liked for some of the luxuries . . . the sort of luxuries that Ginny was on the verge of acquiring, only not on her scale.

'He has his own plane,' Moira said with awe. 'They flew to Newcastle and hired a car from there.'

'Ostentatious,' Pru said offhandedly. 'Who *really* needs their own plane?'

'I can see you're determined *not* to like him, Pru. If you ask me it's unwise. Possibly within a year he'll be your brother-in-law and you and Ginny have always been so close.'

Not true, really, though her mother liked to think so. There was seven years between them and Pru had always been very much the older sister, Ginny one of the child bridesmaids when she married. She was nineteen, Ginny twelve. Now she was thirty-six and the gulf seemed to have narrowed, in age anyway; in interests not at all. Ginny had done what no woman in the Silklander family had ever done: gone to university, and led an exciting, super-charged life with her own house, a glamorous job, and now her engagement to a man who, by all accounts, was a millionaire several times over.

Yet Ginny had never been ostentatious or acquisitive; never desired or respected vast wealth. She must, therefore, be very much in love with Simeon Varga because she wouldn't want him just for his money.

It was Christmas time and once again the whole Silklander family had assembled at the castle for the festivities. Lambert, Maggie and Roderick had come up from London, Roderick with a new French girlfriend the family decided they rather liked. Lambert and Maggie arrived with a car loaded with goodies. Angus and Betty would come over for meals with their three children who would, as usual, play and quarrel with their Border cousins who were roughly their ages.

Varga was quite entertained by the whole thing, amused and a little envious. He compared his own lonely boyhood to this; a boyhood where Christmas came and went almost unnoticed and there were certainly no presents or toys to play with but, maybe, a little fatty pork for dinner on Christmas Day.

He and Ginny slept in her old bedroom, hugging each other tightly at night because it was so cold. Sometime before dawn a woman would creep in and light the fire, but even then it only warmed a tiny corner of the room. They would leap out of bed and, running to the bathroom, jump into the huge old-fashioned bath which had been big enough, at one time, for all the small Silklanders to bathe together.

They would dry each other after the bath and dress in front of the fire, anxious not to be late for breakfast. Moira Silklander was a stickler for mealtimes: breakfast at nine, lunch at one and dinner at half past seven, drinks beforehand in the drawing-room at seven. At Christmas they dressed every evening: Gerald shook out the mothballs from the dinner jacket which had belonged to his grandfather; Moira wore the good black lace dress that was at least thirty years old; and even the older children wore smart trousers or pretty frocks as, dressed in their finery, everyone gathered around the tree on Christmas Eve for carols in the hall.

Apart from the cold Varga loved it all. It was many years since he had been so cold, but the circumstances were so different that he could hardly compare them. Then he had been cold from want, poverty and neglect. Now he was cold because central heating would spoil the castle and, to people like the Silklanders, tradition was everything. Yet it all made Varga more conscious than ever of his difference from the Silklanders; he was not and never would be one of them, even when he and Ginny were married and had children. The children would be Silklanders, but he would not; he could never aspire to the centuries of breeding, the gifts they had from birth, at ease with themselves and the world.

Maybe that was why he needed Ginny so much:

because, more than anything in life, he wanted to be like her.

And here they were sitting round the table for Christmas lunch, the stately dining-room open for the occasion. All those who helped in the house were traditionally given the day off, having cooked and served the more formal Christmas Eve dinner the night before, and Christmas lunch was cooked with a great deal of giggling and surreptitious sips of sherry by the sisters and sisters-in-law, Pru, Betty, Maggie and Ginny, with Moira in overall command. Traditionally the men walked and then all came together for lunch which was served, with the minimum of ceremony, at one and broke up at about three, just in time for the Queen's speech.

Varga threw himself into everything with gusto. He walked round the estate with his future father-in-law and Angus; later they were joined by Lambert and Douglas (Roderick having slipped away somewhere with his French girl) for a stroll down to the pub and a few drams of malt whisky from a local distillery.

He loved sitting between excited Ginny and steady, jolly Pru, who impressed him with her good sense: the quintessential Englishwoman – calm, robust, motherly. Next to Pru was her eldest son Hamish, and next to Douglas their daughter Harriet, a year younger. Douglas was sandy-haired and the children took after him. Angus's three had inherited the dark good looks of the Silklanders.

Varga could envisage the time when his and Ginny's children would be sitting round the table with their parents, grandparents, aunts and cousins. With his money and their ancestry and breeding, what a satisfying combination that would be! As if reading his thoughts Pru leaned towards him and said, 'I must say, Purborough Park sounds *awfully* exciting.'

'It is,' he smiled at her. 'The countryside round is magnificent. It's hunting country, not as grand as this . . .'

'Oh, but I love Gloucestershire,' Pru cried. 'You don't

need to sell it to me. Tell me, when do you think all the alterations will be completed?'

'Just as soon as I can get someone to work on them,' Varga said. 'When I get back to London I complete on the purchase of the house, and my architect and surveyor are already at work on the plans. Then a huge army of workmen will go in and . . .' he paused and gave her a shy smile, 'it is to be my wedding present to Ginny. It is for her . . . and our children and you all. Perhaps if not next Christmas then the Christmas after we shall all be sitting round the table there enjoying a big Christmas lunch.'

'Oh, won't that be fun!' Pru clapped her hands and then stopped, a dubious look on her face.

'But we've always celebrated Christmas here, ever since we were born.'

'Time to change.' Douglas, sitting opposite her, had been listening to the conversation. 'Doubtless you'll have a full staff in a place like that, Simeon?'

'Oh, I expect so,' Simeon said casually, and at that moment the portable phone in his pocket emitted a loud strident signal and everyone stopped talking.

'What on *earth* was that?' Moira, from the far end of the table, looked round.

'Do excuse me.' Simeon took the phone from his pocket and rose as he drew up the aerial and spoke quietly into it.

'Could you hold on a minute please?'

He then walked swiftly towards the door and shut it carefully behind him, his actions followed by a dozen or so pairs of startled eyes.

'Good heavens!' Moira exclaimed indignantly. '*Who* would telephone someone at lunchtime on Christmas Day?'

'Fancy bringing a *thing* like that to Christmas lunch-eon,' Gerald grumbled with a sideways glance at Ginny.

'I'm very sorry, Daddy.' Ginny looked, and felt, embarrassed. 'He does have contacts all round the world.'

'So do we all,' Lambert said languidly.

'Yes, but not quite like Simeon. He's expanded terrifically in the last year. Time zones are different. Many of his business acquaintances are not Christians.'

'Well personally I think it's very bad form,' Roderick spoke decisively. 'Bringing a *telephone* to Christmas lunch! Imagine that happening on Yom Kippur or Ramadan. No decent Jew or Muslim would think of it.'

'It isn't exactly a *religious* festival any more,' Ginny said caustically, defensively. 'But I'll speak to Simeon. I'll ask him to leave it upstairs.'

'I do wish you would, darling,' Moira said gratefully. 'We like him very much, we really do, but . . . well,' she looked deprecatingly around as if seeking confirmation from her family, 'no one has ever behaved *quite* like that at Silklands before.'

Normal conversation resumed and, after a few minutes, Simeon sidled into the chair next to Ginny and squeezed her hand.

'I do apologize,' he murmured. 'It was an urgent call from Japan.'

'Don't they celebrate Christmas there?' Betty asked with a brittle smile.

'No, they don't. They have a different religion and Christmas Day means nothing to them. However,' Simeon's tone was abrupt and, as if sensing the disapproval of the company gathered around the table, he said, 'I will make sure it doesn't happen again.'

'Not at mealtimes.' Moira inclined her head graciously. 'Thank you *so* much, Simeon dear.'

'How much is it all costing, I ask myself?' Gerald said to Lambert in the sitting-room after lunch as he lit his son's cigar.

'What, Dad?' Lambert drew on it until it glowed and then, removing it, gazed at his father through the satisfying haze of smoke.

'That house. It's a ruin.'

'I should think a few million at least, especially as it's being done in a hurry.'

'You really think that they'll marry next year?' Gerald screwed up his face in the puzzled, obdurate expression his son knew so well.

'Well, that seems to be the plan.' Lambert lowered his voice as the room began to fill with people drifting in from the dining-room. From the kitchen girlish laughter could be heard as the women cleared away, aided by Angus and Roderick, who were more domesticated than the urbane Lambert.

'Can't say I feel at *ease* with the fellow,' Gerald said thoughtfully. 'Can't pinpoint *why*. I don't dislike him . . .'

'There's nothing to dislike about him.' Maggie, who had also managed to escape chores, drifted up to him stirring her coffee. 'He is very charming, has pots of money and is crazy about Ginny.'

'He also has a wife and two children,' Gerald said severely. 'What are *they* doing this Christmas?'

'I believe they're spending it with their Italian family, just as large as ours and, undoubtedly, having just as good a time. Don't be so old-fashioned, Dad. Varga lived apart from his wife for ages before he met Ginny. It happens in the best of families, even ours occasionally.'

Looking unconvinced, Gerald accepted a cup from his daughter-in-law. 'Thank you, Maggie. So you too find Simeon charming? And sincere as well?' He looked at her keenly.

'Why not?' Maggie seemed surprised. 'Clever, sincere . . .'

'Why doesn't he tell anyone where he came from?'

'He has a secretive nature,' Lambert confided. 'He wants to forget about the past, maybe expunge it from his memory.'

'Does *Ginny* know?'

'Oh you can be sure she knows. She will know absolutely everything about Varga. As well as loving him she

198

has worked for him for the best part of two years.'
Lambert put a hand consolingly on his father's arm. 'You
should be thankful she's going to be so well set up, Dad.
She'll be one of the wealthiest women in the country.'

Their naked bodies touched; a fire roared in the grate
and the heat reached out to envelop them. Their lips met
lightly at first and then more passionately; their bodies
entwined, flesh merged with flesh.

When they came apart the fire had died; only its
embers remained glowing in the grate and Varga tenderly drew the bedclothes over their bodies to retain the
heat that had ignited between them.

'I love you,' he murmured.

'And I love you.'

He stroked her hair. 'I want to devote my whole life
to you.'

'And I to you.'

'Never let us forget this moment and this vow, Ginny.'

'Never.'

Their beating hearts slowed and they lay together,
replete. He began to feel the cold creeping in beside them
and shivered. She put her arm round him and drew him
very close.

'It's a good thing we're not going to live in a fourteenth-century castle.'

'We're going to live in a palace.'

'I know. My family are very jealous.'

'I don't think so. I think the Silklanders are proud of
who and what they are. They aren't jealous of anyone.'

'Do you find them arrogant?' she wanted to know.

'In a way.' His face brushed hers. 'I envy it, though.
Ginny,' he rose on one arm and then snuggled down
again as the icy blast from the room met his naked body,
'I want to tell you a little about myself. I never have.'

'Don't if you don't want to,' she said quickly.

'But I do. I saw your father talking with Lambert and
Maggie today and I'm sure they were talking about me.'

'They like you.'

'Your father likes me less than the others. I can tell. He looks at me in an odd way . . .'

'Well he would, naturally, prefer someone from the Shires . . . it's in the blood. That doesn't excuse it but he's that sort of man. I hope in a way they're a dying breed. But he approves of the fact that you've got a lot of money. At least they won't have to support me.'

'Did I overdo it?'

'No!' She sounded surprised. 'You never talk about your money. They like that. It's terribly bad form to talk about money. But they know Purborough Park has cost a bomb and will cost lots more. They know that yours is one of the most successfully performing shares on the Stock Exchange. Such things speak for themselves . . . however, darling,' her hand touched his chest, 'they didn't much go for the portable phone . . .'

'That was a stupid thing to do.' He struck himself on the forehead. 'I forgot I had it in my pocket.'

'Is it *really* necessary to bring it on holiday at Christmas time?'

'Yes it is.' He drew apart from her, once again the coldness, the feeling of rejection. 'In a business which covers the international time zones you have to know what's going on.'

'I'm sorry . . . of course you have.'

'I suppose you think it was bad form in front of your family,' he said sarcastically. 'Can't you just *imagine* them all talking about it at the hunt balls?'

'No. They're not like that. They love me and they know that I love you.'

'They preferred Robert.'

'They'd known Robert since he was a baby. You can't compare your relationship with them with Robert's, but they don't condemn you for it.'

'I think they tolerate me rather than like me.'

'Darling, you're getting a complex,' she said soothingly. 'Tell me about your past.'

'Another time.' His voice was reserved, strange. Temporarily they had lost their intimacy, his need to confide in her. 'My eyes are beginning to close.' He then turned his back on her, an attitude of deliberate rejection, and in a few moments she heard his deep regular breathing.

But Ginny remained awake for some time, disturbed by the ease with which they could go from the deepest intimacy to a sense, almost, of alienation: the darker side of love.

Next morning Varga woke aware of the pale morning sun visible through the slits in the curtains, and that the place in the bed beside him was empty.

He lay for some time accustoming his eyes to the gloom and then, raising his head, saw that a fire blazed in the chimney, for which he was thankful. Looking at his watch he saw that it was eight-thirty and, springing out of bed, he knelt in front of the fire, reaching for his robe which he draped carefully around him like a rug. He then rose and went along to the bathroom, sitting on the side of the bath while it filled with boiling hot water. Thank heaven there was plenty of that.

When the bath was ready he returned to the bedroom and drew the curtains. The full glare of even the wintry morning sun made him blink. The trees, outlined against the sky, looked magnificent; the tall Scotch pines seemed to stretch before him in an endless carpet. His breath steamed up the window pane and, as he cleared it, he could see in the distance figures on horseback. One of them was undoubtedly the woman he had spent the night with. He looked at her lingeringly, lovingly, and sighed.

Why was he always so prickly, so much on the defensive about his family? If he became too vulnerable her love for him might fade. He knew that a woman like Ginny was as much fascinated by his power as his masculinity, his sex. He felt he was capturing a strong, vigorous woman rather as modern man's ancestors had captured their mates. Only, instead of hitting her on the head and dragging her into a cave, he was seducing her with power, physical strength and money; also, he hoped, by his arts, his skill as a lover. Yet he was still not sure whether he was in love with Ginny or her glamour, her family heritage and connections. He was not sure whether he wanted to marry her or the institution of the English nobility personified by her.

These speculations in the forefront of his mind, he took a leisurely bath, shaved and then dressed with his customary care, eyeing himself in the mirror each step of the way.

He was kitted out in cavalry twill trousers and a green tweed jacket from Daks, a check shirt and knitted tie from Harrods, plain silk socks, also from Harrods, and brogues handmade for him by Lobb's.

His dressing and toilet completed, he carefully patted aftershave on his smooth cheeks and then, tucking a handkerchief into his top pocket, he sat down on the bed and dialled a number on his portable phone which he had kept beside the bed. There was a great deal of static and then, as he was about to redial, a very faint voice answered.

'Beaufort?' he said.

'Oh, Mr Voitek. I can't hear you too well.'

'I believe the consignment has been made to our depot?'

'That's correct, Mr Voitek.'

'And another payment is due?'

'On its way.'

'I'm glad to hear it. The other was late.'

'It's a matter of credit transfer.'

'See it's not late this time.'

'It's on its way, Mr Voitek. Say, Happy Christmas.'

'Goodbye,' Varga replied coldly and switched off the phone completely. On his last day with his future wife's family he didn't want to risk putting a foot wrong.

When he got down to the breakfast-room he found

the only other person at the table was Ginny's sister Pru.

'Good morning,' he said, going to the sideboard and inspecting the dishes on offer, raising the lids one by one.

'Good morning, Simeon,' Pru said warmly. 'Did you sleep well?'

'Very well, and you?' He turned to smile at her.

'Oh, we always sleep well here. It's the family home.'

'Quite!' Varga helped himself to porridge, which he considered a most curious concoction, and took his bowl to the table where Pru passed him sugar and cream.

'You make your own toast in the toaster.'

'I know,' he said pouring cream. Then, gingerly, he tasted the porridge, watched with some interest by Pru.

'Have you had porridge before, Simeon?'

'Not until I came here. We had it on my first visit.' He lifted his spoon to his mouth and then, when he'd swallowed the contents, added, 'I like it.'

'We have it every morning except in the summer. It's very good for one. Roughage,' she explained unnecessarily.

'Quite.' Varga nodded understandingly. 'Maybe Ginny will introduce it to the diet when we live at Purborough Park.'

'Will you live there all the time?'

'I think so. It's only an hour along the M4 from London. That's why I chose it, apart from its beauty, because of the proximity. I shall keep on my flat in the office. These days you can have everything you need in the home. I intend to be a family man, Pru, a farmer too, perhaps.'

'An English country gentleman,' Pru murmured.

Varga, quick to detect hidden nuances, looked at her sharply, but further conversation was prevented by the entrance of Lambert and Maggie who, invariably, slept late. They called out 'good morning' as they too went to the sideboard.

'Sadie makes a jolly good breakfast,' Lambert said,

lifting one lid after the other. 'I wish we could persuade her to come to Cadogan Square.'

'We don't do so badly with Maggie Silklander,' Maggie said laconically, 'though there's not quite the choice.'

'Not quite, sweetheart.' Lambert leaned over to peck her cheek. 'Besides, who would want a breakfast like this every day? It's for treats.'

'Quite.' Maggie, who was dressed in a tweed suit over a turtle-neck sweater, brought her plate over and took her seat next to Varga.

'And where's Ginny this morning, Simeon? Still in bed?'

'Not at all! She's out riding,' Pru replied with a mouthful of toast. 'She, Dad, Douglas, and I believe Angus is with them. Do you ride, Simeon?'

'No,' Simeon hesitated, 'but I intend to have stables at Purborough.'

'Then you'll have a very good teacher,' Lambert said. 'Ginny's a first-class horsewoman.'

'I wanted to talk to you both about the house.' Simeon finished his porridge with relish. 'I might have a little work for you.'

'We hoped it would be a lot,' Maggie said with a cheeky smile.

'I think you can say it will be.' Varga leaned back thoughtfully. 'Shall we discuss it after breakfast?'

'Discuss it now,' Pru said, getting up. 'I've finished.'

'Oh please don't think you have to go.'

'Really I have. I must see that the children are all right.'

'Oh, they'll be all right,' Lambert said. 'How lovely it is not having them bawling into one's ears at breakfast time.'

'When are you off?' Pru ignored her brother's rudeness.

'Not until tomorrow. We're calling at Maggie's home on the way back to town.'

'See you later, then. And Simeon, when are you and Ginny . . .'

'Alas, tonight,' Simeon replied ruefully. 'We have so much to do.'

'Of course. See you at lunch then.'

After Pru had closed the door Simeon leaned across the table towards Lambert and Maggie, who were listening attentively.

'I would like you, Maggie, to oversee the decorations at Purborough as you did the office, and you, Lambert, to get me some of the finest pictures and objets d'art and statues in the market.'

'It will be a pleasure,' Lambert began, but Varga interrupted him.

'I want you to see the house first. It is early eighteenth century, about 1710, and I want it restored and refurbished to suit the period. I want the very best available. It will be my wedding present to Ginny.'

'It will cost.' Maggie raised her eyes to the ceiling. 'It looks a huge place.'

'It is. Money no object. You tell me how much you want to spend and I'll tell you how much you can have.'

'Sounds very exciting.' Maggie was still heavy-lidded with sleep; getting up, she put her plate beside Pru's. 'I really must go and see Moira. Will you sort it all out with Lambert, Simeon? We'll be ready whenever you want us.'

Simeon rose and, going to the door, held it open for her.

'Aren't we lucky to have you?' she said, pausing at the door to smile at him.

'And aren't we lucky to have you?' he said and, stooping, for the first time kissed her on the brow.

She took his hand, gave it a quick squeeze, and he watched her go down the hall before gently closing the door.

'She's very talented,' he said, taking the place next to Lambert who, unlike his wife, who had had toast and black coffee, was making a good breakfast of bacon and egg, with black pudding and sausages made at Angus's farm from home-produced beef and pork.

'She's the best.' Lambert broke his toast and dipped it into his egg. 'Seriously, I'm very excited about this job for you, Simeon.'

'Good.' Simeon turned to him and, crossing his legs, joined his hands together in his lap. 'And while we're alone, Lambert, I'd like to remind you of our previous conversation. That is, that there are ways and ways of buying works of art.'

'No need to remind me.' Lambert first of all chuckled, then frowned. 'At least, I *think* I remember.' He carefully put his knife and fork together and then, folding his arms, looked at Simeon. 'But what exactly are you trying to say?'

'Premiums, taxes, export licences . . . they can all add substantially to the price of a work of art.'

'You can say that again.'

'*And* not always necessarily. I know for the office you went to the best dealers and showrooms and I appreciated it; but Purborough is much larger and, although I want the best, I want to be left with some loose change in my pocket.'

'Naturally . . .' Lambert's frown deepened. 'But I hope, that is I'm sure, you're not suggesting . . . well,' he unfolded his arms and scratched his head, 'I don't want to do anything illegal, you know that, Simeon.'

Varga's expression remained hard to fathom.

'I'm not talking strictly of illegality; but there are ways of acquiring works of art that don't put too much money in the hands either of the taxman or the middleman. I'm sure you don't object to *that*?'

'Not at all.' Lambert broke into smiles.

'As I've told you, I've an airline.' Varga looked over his shoulder to be sure the door was shut. 'I'm sure it can be a lot of help to you. It's a small airline and the planes hop all over the place. Who knows – it might be of help to you in some other business activities? I mean we're not cheating anyone, except the Inland Revenue, are we? And surely they have enough already?'

'We'd have to be very careful,' Lambert said cautiously. 'But I do know what you mean.'

'You must know people, impoverished continental noblemen say, who would be glad to sell their works of art and retain most of the profits?'

'Oh, I know plenty.' Lambert smiled wryly.

'And you *too* keep all your profit?'

'Naturally.' Lambert placed a finger against the side of his nose.

'I guess you've done this kind of thing before?' Varga said swiftly. 'On a small scale perhaps? It is after all pretty prevalent in the art world.'

Lambert too looked nervously at the door.

'Unofficially . . . who hasn't?'

'Well, let's shake on it then.' Varga gave him a broad smile and extended his hand which Lambert seized across the table and shook vigorously.

'I say, Simeon. It will be jolly good fun to have you as a brother-in-law.'

Simeon Varga picked his way fastidiously between the cowpats in the wet and muddy farmyard. He looked rather incongruous in his well-pressed cavalry twill and tweeds, his immaculately shining brown brogues, among the rest of the party who wore anoraks and green wellies into which were tucked either jeans or corduroys.

Ginny and Betty wore headscarves against the keen wind, hands deep in their pockets, but Varga didn't even wear a coat, though the tip of his nose was rosy-tinged with cold.

To an outsider, which he all too clearly was, a northern farm on a cold winter's day was a bleak prospect. All the animals were cooped up in their sheds or pens, feeding on the fodder that had been grown for them in the clement summer months.

Lambert and Maggie, considering themselves townfolk, had eschewed the visit to Angus's farm in favour of a morning by the fire or, perhaps, the most undemanding of strolls through the grounds. Pru and Douglas had gone back with their children to their own farm to oversee the welfare of their own stock. Gerald said he had paperwork to do and a cold coming which was a good excuse to confine himself to his study, probably for a snooze.

But Ginny and her mother set off in a Land Rover with Varga at about eleven to visit Angus's farm. They were greeted by Angus and Betty and taken to the farm kitchen where there was a warm fire and coffee percolating on the stove.

Varga seemed glad to get indoors, though he smiled cheerfully at his fiancée, who had told him to wear a coat before they set out.

'I don't know what you're trying to *prove*,' she had said rather tetchily, but Varga had assured her, in his soft-spoken way, that he wasn't trying to prove anything, that his tweeds were if anything too warm. Now he looked frozen to death, but she knew that he'd never admit it.

Moira had watched the little contretemps from her vantage point of the front seat of the Land Rover but said nothing. Now, surrounded by yet another brood of grandchildren and the family pets – two labradors, three cats – she sat by the fire, a cup of steaming coffee between her hands.

'It's a very raw day,' she observed to Varga. 'Even for these parts. Don't think the weather is always like this here, Simeon. Or we shan't ever see you and Ginny when you're married.'

'I assure you I don't, Lady Silklander.' He sat carefully beside her. 'Don't forget I've been here before and the weather was beautiful.'

'I always forget you were here before.' Moira sighed as though she was thinking how fond they'd all been of Robert. As if to confirm this she saw him looking at her and gave him a guilty smile.

'Well, shall we go?' Angus eagerly rubbed his hands together. 'I've a lot to show you. Are you coming, Ginny? Mother?'

'I think we'll leave you together.' Ginny was standing with her back to the fire. 'We know it all and we'll only hold you up.'

'But, darling, if we're to farm . . .' Varga looked appealingly at her.

'We'll be coming up here often,' Ginny replied soothingly, 'and I think in the first place you should go round with Angus yourself. He's terribly knowledgeable; besides, Mummy wants to get back in about an hour and I'll take her in the Land Rover. Angus and Betty are coming over for lunch, anyway. You can come with them.'

'Oh, that's fine then.' Varga gave her a reassuring smile and, still without a coat, followed Angus to the door.

The farm was one of the largest in the area, a dairy farm with a herd of Redhorn beef cattle. There was, in addition, a vast acreage of coniferous forest which was always being replanted as the wood was felled. A profitable timber yard was attached to this which was run by a manager and served all the Silklander estates. In addition there was a creamery where cream and cheese were made, mostly for towns in the north-west.

Angus took Varga to the extremities of the estate in his Land Rover, bumping over the uneven ground, through the lanes of giant conifers, and across the moorland which was full of game birds.

'Do you shoot?' he asked conversationally.

'No. I never had the time.'

'When you come again we'll give you a pair of guns. We usually shoot on Boxing Day, but because you and Ginny were here for such a short time, Mother thought it better not to.'

'Oh I hope I didn't break a family tradition?' Varga looked at him anxiously. 'I want to fit in, you know.'

'I'm sure you do, but as you don't shoot it would have

been awkward. Mother was right. Incidentally,' he looked sideways at Varga, 'we're awfully fond of Ginny, Simeon.'

'So am I,' Varga replied. 'I happen to love her *very* much. Why,' he paused as if searching for words which wouldn't give offence, 'why did you feel it necessary to say that, Angus?'

'Well we are . . .'

'I thought I detected a note of doubt in your voice. Do you think, perhaps, that I am not capable of looking after your sister?'

'Not at *all*.'

'That I . . .' Varga went on in a steely voice, 'that I am, perhaps, not the right man, should I say not from the right branch?'

'I say, steady on, old man.' Angus swerved the Land Rover to avoid a pheasant confidently strutting out as though in the knowledge that the guns, this particular Boxing Day, were to be silent. 'Don't get a thing about it.'

'Not like Robert,' Varga said in a tone that seemed to echo Moira Silklander.

Angus stopped the car abruptly and then turned to face his passenger, his tough, good-looking face red with anger.

'You're not like Robert, Simeon; but you *are* Ginny's choice of a husband. That's good enough for us. We have tended in our family to marry people like us, mostly people we know, I'll admit that. Betty was a local girl. Douglas a local man. Lambert and Maggie met in the art world, and Roderick's girl won't last – they never do – but when he does marry I daresay it'll be someone we know. But that doesn't mean things have to go on like that. In many ways it's almost feudal and you've made us see another side. We live after all in a cosmopolitan society and Ginny, of all the family, has moved away from home most. It was natural that she should meet and fall in love with someone we wouldn't know. That doesn't mean we don't like you, and won't welcome you to the fold.'

'I'm sorry I brought it up.' Varga gave him his most charming, apologetic smile. 'I am oversensitive I'll confess. The Silklanders are rather formidable, you know, when you meet them all together. I have a feeling I don't fit in, but I want to. It's better when I'm alone with Ginny; but I want to like her family and have them like me. I shall never be an English aristocrat but I will be the best husband I can possibly be, the best father . . .'

'Right, let's get on with the tour.' Angus sounded embarrassed and put the big car into gear again.

The Redhorn bulls were a fine sight, contentedly munching the turnips that had been grown for them in the summer in a nearby field and harvested in autumn. The farm was almost self-sufficient, producing food for both humans and animals and some to sell in the market.

Varga tapped the flanks of several of the prize herd asking intelligent questions about their marketing, when they were ready and how much they fetched a pound.

He admired the creamery, now closed for the holidays, and the large vats which had recently been installed to comply with EC regulations.

'They're a curse,' Angus confessed when they were back in the car, 'but we have to obey them otherwise we lose our markets. Farming is tough, you know, Simeon. Sometimes I feel that if I were to start again I'd do something else. It's not the work; I love that. It's the regulations. Hundreds of farmers are throwing it all up or going bust, people who have farmed this land for generations. Our most profitable activity is the timber mill. We just about break even on the beef and creamery. Thousands of gallons of milk are thrown away because of the Community regulations. It's absurd.'

'It *is* absurd,' Varga nodded vehemently, 'especially when you think that two-thirds of the world are starving.' He paused for a moment looking straight in front of him. 'I can sense your frustration. However, I can't

211

help feeling that your methods are alarmingly wasteful.'

'What do you mean?' The burly Angus reddened again.

'They're not really effective. You're just ticking over, as you say, not making money. You own the farm and the land but you're not rich and you should be. *I* wouldn't work for nothing, which is in fact what you're doing.'

Angus put his foot on the brake and slowed down.

'Then what shall I do?'

'I think you should go in for intensive farming methods, as I already pointed out to you.'

'You mean factory farming?'

'Well, if that's what you call intensive, then yes.'

'No. I will not see animals tethered in stalls all their lives, living in artificial light, unable to roam freely.'

'Then you're a romantic, not a businessman. These animals know no different. They are born to the life; they are fed, they are warm, and they are well looked after. They are going to die anyway . . .'

'You can't have intensive farming of bulls . . .'

'You can of calves. They do on the Continent and the veal is delicious.'

'The idea revolts me.'

Varga looked round and spread his hand eloquently towards the open fields surrounding them.

'You could have battery hens, miles and miles of well-lit, well-heated, well-ventilated sheds. You could corner the market in eggs for the north-west.'

'Even if I wanted to I can't . . .'

But Varga, undeterred, swept on. 'You could mechanize your whole farm, and in a few years you would see the difference. You would make it pay.'

'I could never afford all the gear. We're just about to mortgage the farm for the first time in its history to get some money for the equipment the blinking EC demands that we buy.'

'Don't do that,' Varga said sharply. 'If you would like

212

to consult with me and my advisers I think we can help you.'

'Oh, no charity, thanks, Simeon,' Angus said politely, 'even if you are going to be my brother-in-law.'

'I wasn't talking about charity. I was talking about business. Believe me, I wouldn't invest in anything I didn't think would pay, not even for a member of Ginny's family. But, for the moment, not a word to her.'

After they left the farm, Ginny hunched over the wheel, Moira sitting beside her, for a while they said nothing as the Land Rover followed the familiar road to the castle. It was a wet and lugubrious day, the lowering clouds practically obscuring the surrounding hills, and odd sepulchral shapes seemed to emerge from the mist which rapidly gathered round them turning noon almost into dusk.

Ginny realized how much she loved this rugged un-bending countryside and, in a way, she wished Simeon would buy a place here, nearer her parents. Maybe one day he would.

'I do worry about Angus, Betty and the children,' Moira said after a while, interrupting her daughter's train of thought.

'But why, Mummy?' Ginny looked surprised. 'They're very happy. Tremendously happy.'

'I don't mean personally. Of course they're happy and it's a very good marriage; but they have so much worry. The farm doesn't pay, you know. Angus hates all the paperwork. Daddy does as much as he can, but he has all his own to see to. They're going to have to mortgage the farm because of some idiotic EC regulations and, of course, it has been in the family free of debt since there were Silklanders.'

'Oh, Mummy, that's awful!' Ginny sounded shocked.

'It's the only way of getting any money. We can't help him. We wish we could.'

'Well I hope Simeon doesn't think of helping him,'

Ginny said grimly. 'I mean, Mummy, I don't want you to feel Simeon is patronizing the family. Angus would hate it too.'

'Oh I don't mean *that*, darling. We certainly don't want any handouts. Besides, what makes you think Simeon would want to help him?' Moira looked curiously at her daughter.

'He'd do it for me,' Ginny replied. 'He wants you to love and accept him. But you can't buy that sort of thing.'

'Of course you can't and we should never accept it,' Moira said stiffly. 'But a little advice, now that you mention it, might be a very good thing. A farm, after all, is a business. You wouldn't object to that, would you, Ginny?'

The tone of her mother's voice made Ginny look at her askance.

'I hope I didn't sound offensive, Mummy. It's the last thing I meant to be; but money can create such barriers. You know what I mean?'

'I know perfectly well what you mean and I should hate Simeon to think we only liked him for his money. In fact the real reservation we have about Simeon *is* his money.'

'I thought it was the fact that he wasn't one of us,' Ginny said with a note of irony.

'Ginny, what a beastly thing to say.' Moira clutched her arm. 'Not true at all.'

'You don't really *like* him, Mummy, do you?'

'What makes you say that, darling?' Moira sounded distinctly offended. 'I really do take exception to that remark. We have done everything we can. We hardly know him. This is his second visit and you are already engaged to him. Then you can only stay two days.'

'Three nights,' Ginny said.

'Well what is that? Is it time to get to know someone? The next thing will be the wedding. That will be very quiet, I suppose, because he is divorced. Nevertheless you will probably have a large party.'

214

'Should you object to a large party?'

'Not in the least. Would you like to have it here? Or won't you be able to invite your London friends? You know, Ginny darling, all we want, the entire family, is your happiness and if Simeon makes you happy . . .'

'He does.'

'Then that's all that matters.'

'Mummy, it's your *tone*.' Ginny banged the wheel in frustration and the Land Rover slewed sideways. 'If you could only hear yourself you would know why Simeon feels uneasy with you.'

'Does he?'

'Of course he does! You have a slightly patronizing stare, and every time Daddy looks at him you'd think he was from Mars.'

'That's not *fair*, Ginny,' her mother sounded aggrieved. 'You must remember who we are. We're country people, rooted in tradition.'

'In prejudice you mean, Mummy.'

'No I do *not* mean prejudice. We are not prejudiced against Simeon, only he is *not* like us, is he, Ginny? Be reasonable.'

'Thank God he's not,' Ginny said heatedly.

'That's a hateful thing to say.'

'He's not *Robert* is what you mean, Mummy!'

'Well, he isn't is he?'

'No he isn't and he's glad he isn't. If you want to know . . .' Ginny appeared to hesitate and then went on rapidly, 'Robert raped me. That's why I split from him.'

'Oh darling, I can't believe that.' A hand flew to Moira's mouth and her pale skin turned pink. 'Not *Robert*.'

'Yes, Robert. Nice Robert. He made love to me against my will . . .'

'Well,' Moira looked doubtful, 'that's not really *rape*, is it, darling, if you were living together as man and wife? I mean a husband can't rape his wife, can he?' Obviously the experience had never happened to Moira.

'There's some difference of opinion on that. I say that if any man forces himself on a woman who doesn't want him, it's rape. I told Robert he'd raped me, and that was that.'

'You were awfully nice to him last time you saw him.'

'What happened happened two years ago. I could forgive him then because I knew I was in love with Simeon; but at the time . . .'

'Well, I'm shocked.' Moira removed her hand from her cheek. 'I'm sure there *must* be some explanation.'

'I wonder how many husbands of "our sort" rape their wives in marriage?'

'Oh, Ginny, please let's talk of something else. Now that telephone . . .' Moira, emboldened, decided on another tack. 'To bring a *telephone* to the table at Christmas lunch is the height of bad manners. You must agree about that, darling.'

'He forgot to turn it off.'

'Your father was terribly shocked. You see it's little things like that, Ginny, that no gentleman would do. I so wish I could make you understand what worries us. It's just strange to think of someone like you, who was so well brought up, marrying someone who quite clearly was not.'

'Mummy, you're the most frightful snob.'

'I don't mean to be, really I don't. And then there's his age,' she persisted.

'His age?' Ginny looked puzzled.

'He's *much* older than you, though I'll admit he doesn't look it.'

'Thirteen years between a man and a woman? It's not too much. As well as looks, he's young at heart.'

'It's all right now . . . but later on. You see, darling, it's this kind of thing that matters. The little things you don't think about that are so important.' She appeared to be searching around for something else to grumble about. 'We also consider the private plane a touch vulgar.'

'It's terribly useful.'

'But it does show off, doesn't it, darling? In this day and age? Daddy and I think it's just a bit too much, having a plane waiting round for your use. Really, and poor Angus having to mortgage his house for the first time in its history . . . well, you can see how we feel and why, can't you, Ginny?'

PART III

Gold on gold

CHAPTER 12

Anthony Liddle was the ideal assistant for a man with ambitions as big as Varga's. He was nothing, had come from nowhere, was without charm or personality, and had everything to gain by being the perfect henchman, unquestioning, loyal, as devious as his master wished him to be.

He was a north-countryman who had trained as an accountant and he retained strong traces of his Lanca-shire accent. Had other things been equal he would have spent his days as an accountant to a small-to-medium-sized business, as Ace Pharmaceuticals was when Varga bought it, living his life in anonymity with a medium-sized house, a wife and two children somewhere in the suburbs. Or he might have returned to his northern roots.

It had needed someone like Varga to bring him out. Varga could read a balance sheet, but Liddle saw the finer points, interpreted the signs, knew when a thing was doing well or badly and what its potential was.

It was he who had given the thumbs down to the Jacquets and who had counselled on the merits, or demerits, of every action or potential acquisition since.

It was he who had advised Varga to establish tax havens, offshore companies to husband his wealth; but it was Varga alone who had gone into criminal activities and then sucked Liddle in after him.

Were they criminal? Some people would have called dabbling in the art market a shrewd way of circumventing the tax man. Some might even have considered running guns to Middle Eastern tyrants an acceptable piece of business on the grounds that someone was going to do it, it was risky and if one was prepared to take that risk, well, good luck to them. Few, however, would have considered drug smuggling within the pale, or the ownership of a brothel whose speciality was bondage.

Only gradually had Liddle become aware what sort of man he was working for and even then he still admired him. He admired someone as dynamic as Varga, as urbane, as skilled in covering his tracks, as quick-witted, as cunning. He had concluded many years before that Varga was amoral; he was one of those people who had difficulty in recognizing the difference between right and wrong. He was a man from obscure, humble origins – even Liddle didn't know the whole truth – and he wanted to be among the great, one of the richest men in the world. No amount of lawful business could make him this, and even before Liddle had known him Varga had established that crime was the only way to get rich quickly but that the umbrella of a respectable business was essential.

Varga played with Liddle like an angler bringing in a fish, a little at a time. First he hooked him, then he gave him a little more line, then he pulled it tighter and as the barb gradually sank deeper Varga alternately tugged and slackened the line until there was absolutely no escape.

By that time Liddle didn't want to escape. He knew that if Varga were ever caught he would be involved too. But it would never come to that. Varga was too careful, too subtle, too adept at covering his tracks.

Or rather Liddle *had* thought it would never come to that; that the pair of them were immune. But Varga had embarked on an earnest courtship of a member of the English ruling classes and Liddle considered that a mistake.

He knew Varga's reason: he wanted respectability, and what was more respectable than the daughter of an English nobleman with a fourteenth-century baronial castle? But Ginny made Liddle nervous. She was so quick, so clever – it was amazing that she hadn't rumbled Varga already. He blamed her class for her obtuseness, or was it, as they said, that love was blind?

Liddle and Varga met frequently. They often travelled together and Ginny knew that the financial director was consulted about everything. Maybe she was a little jealous of him. Liddle often wondered.

He wondered today what were the views of the Silklander family about the engagement and the possible purchase of their farm and land by their future son-in-law?

'I would lease it back to them, rather like a mortgage,' Varga explained to Liddle, who sat opposite him thoughtfully stirring the first cup of coffee of the morning.

'You're going to buy the whole thing? Lock, stock and barrel?'

'The farm has potential. There are five thousand acres of trees, farmland, scrubland, a rich diversity. Frankly, it's a gold mine.'

'But you know nothing about farming, Simeon.'

Varga sat back, a pained look on his face.

'Not you too, Tony, please. How many times have people told me I know nothing about a certain thing? Electronics, perfume, oil, newspapers. Don't I have cattle ranches in the Argentine? The balance sheet of a good working farm is the same as that of an electronics company.'

'I'm sorry, Simeon.' Liddle inclined his head. 'I think I was wondering if it was really a good idea to let your personal life interfere with business? Does Ginny know?'

'Not yet,' Varga's tone was succinct, 'that's unless her brother has told her, but I asked him not to. We have to come up with an offer and that's why you're here.'

He thrust some papers in the direction of his finance

director, who leaned over and took them.

'The property isn't mortgaged or entailed or anything?'

'No.' Varga shook his head. 'Owned outright by the family. The father gave it to the son when he got married. Frankly it's peanuts compared to what it's worth, and it's helping them.'

'But do you think it's worth even such a relatively small outlay?' Liddle leafed casually through the papers. 'Two million pounds?'

'He will think it's a fortune. To him it is. He can invest it, do what he likes with it. The only thing I have to have is the father's consent for the sale of the land. He's an awkward old bugger and that may not be too easy.'

'I see.' Clearly Liddle wasn't keen.

'The son owns the farm and outbuildings outright, the stock and so on, but the land belongs to Lord Silklander. That's what I want because it's valuable. The north-east is short of housing and we may turn some of it into a housing estate; the rest into factory farms and so on.'

Liddle chuckled and finished his coffee.

'Will Ginny like that?'

'Well, Ginny won't know about it for some time and when she does she will be my wife. I doubt if she will consider it grounds for divorce.' Varga looked at his watch and tapped his desk in a businesslike manner. 'Let me know as soon as you can, Tony. I . . .'

'Simeon!' Liddle, who never liked to contradict or argue with his boss, shifted uncomfortably in his seat. 'Forgive me, but do you *really* think it's wise? Aren't you taking on too much? I know not a lot of money is involved but this kind of thing seems to me well . . . dangerous.'

'Dangerous?' Varga broke into a smile. 'You think this is *dangerous*? You must be joking, Tony. It can be absorbed in one of the trusts.'

'Oh, I know it can be absorbed in one of the trusts,

easily. No sweat. Cayman Islands or Guatemala. That's not the problem. But if I were you I would keep your future in-laws at arm's length. If Ginny ever *did* discover anything she might forgive you because she loves you; but I doubt that she would ever forgive you for involving her family.'

'Nonsense.' Varga airily waved a hand at him. 'Do it.'

'Right, Simeon.'

Liddle jumped obediently to his feet and was about to leave the room when Varga called him back.

'Tony.'

'Yes, boss?' Tony swung on his heels.

'I do have one small problem.'

'Oh?' Liddle perched on the arm of the chair where he had been sitting.

'I think I'm being followed.'

'Oh!' Liddle looked grave. 'Any idea by who?'

'No. But I *do* suspect that little twerp in New York.'

'Beaufort or whatever he calls himself?'

'Exactly.'

'But I thought he knew nothing about you. You even gave him a false name.'

'I know.' Varga gnawed at one of his perfectly pared fingernails. 'Then there are the Berninis. They don't want me to divorce Claudia.'

'But the divorce is automatic.'

'They still don't want it. They want to make it hard for me. They are liable to do anything. I have to be very, very careful.'

'You have.' Liddle felt a twinge of unease. 'And when did you notice this, Simeon?'

'Before Christmas. I couldn't be sure. Sometimes I feel a car is following me. Peter is looking out, but he too can't be sure.'

'When you're abroad?'

'Not as far as I know.'

'Well,' Liddle scratched his head, 'what do you want me to do?'

'I want you to find some discreet agency that will check it out.'

'Private investigation?'

'That's it. Someone not too smart, because I don't want them to find out too much. Someone to follow the follower.'

'I understand you, Simeon. I'll do what I can.'

'Get on to it quickly, Tony.' Varga ran a hand over his jaw. 'Frankly, it makes me nervous.'

The Villa Caracoli was beautifully situated in the hills above Florence in the town of Fiesole, offering a breathtaking view of the city lying beneath. This was almost always seen through a haze, making the view more mystical and beautiful, if that were possible, than it actually was. The cathedral, with its magnificent dome and the tall campanile beside it, was a well-known landmark. But that too was threatened by the pollution that affected the city. Now the centre of Florence had been closed to traffic and maybe one day the haze would eventually evaporate.

The villa was approached by one of the winding roads of Fiesole through a drive flanked by tall cypresses. By the standards of the Renaissance, when it had been built, it was not large, and it was tucked into the side of the hill like a priceless jewel. Inside it was light and airy, with marble floors and spacious rooms that housed the many priceless sculptures, tapestries, bronzes, paintings and other works of art that had been in the family for centuries.

Going from room to room was like visiting a small, perfect museum of exquisite proportions.

Alberto Caracoli sat in one of the tapestried chairs, his coffee cup balanced on his knee, his head tilted to one side. He was almost completely bald and had a large hooked nose and bright enquiring eyes which made him look a little like a hawk. A wise old bird. He was short, with the girth of a man who enjoyed his food, but his clothes were made in Rome and managed skilfully to disguise the ample proportions of his figure.

Opposite him sat Lambert and Maggie Silklander, who had spent the morning on a tour of the house, staggering even them by the magnificence of its contents, which various members of the Caracoli family had collected since they had built the villa in the time of Lorenzo de' Medici.

Yet outside a small circle of cognoscenti it was scarcely known. It was a house of treasures worth millions of pounds, millions of which the family was now sorely in need.

'As you see, beautiful though the villa is, it is falling into ruin,' Alberto said sadly, his mobile, expressive features creasing into a grimace. He spoke accurate English in a badly fractured accent due to lack of practice. 'A million alone needs to be spent on essentials, and I'm talking in pounds sterling, not lire. Then there are the gardens.' Alberto gave an expressive gesture of despair. 'How my poor father would weep if he were to see how overgrown parts of his beloved estate now are. There was once an arboretum that was only rivalled by . . .'

'You have, of course, thought of selling before?' Lambert broke in impatiently.

Caracoli shook his head.

'My father wished the collection to remain intact.'

'But your father is no longer alive,' Lambert said gently. 'I would have thought that the sale of a few pieces . . .'

'Alas!' Caracoli's expression became even more lugubrious. 'The Italian galleries are too poor to buy, and the state would never let me export. Besides I would not like people to know what pictures we have here or I would be forced to spend another fortune on security.'

That was true. The Silklanders had been surprised by the easy access to the villa which was apparently unprotected by any obvious form of security device.

Alberto's grandmother had been English, a very

227

distant relation of the Silklanders, as it happened, and it was Moira Silklander who had mentioned the connection during casual conversation that Christmas. Naturally, the conversation had been about Ginny and Simeon Varga, Purborough Park, and the commission to buy works of art for it. They had all been quite excited about the remote Caracoli connection and Lambert had lost little time in contacting a somewhat surprised cousin, several times removed. But the visit had not been easy to arrange and only with some difficulty and many delays had they penetrated the home of a man obviously reclusive by nature.

Lambert looked at Maggie and drew in his breath.

'Alberto, you know that I am a picture dealer. I explained that to you on the phone.'

'Yes, yes, I do recollect,' Caracoli said vaguely, 'but there is no possibility of my selling. There would be too much publicity; you would never receive a licence. Besides, my son,' he gestured again expressively, 'he would not like it at *all*.'

'But surely your son doesn't want the house to fall down?'

Caracoli sought for an explanation.

'He is a doctor, you know. They are not very interested in these things. As far as he is concerned it is a place to bring his children in the holidays. Not even then. They prefer the seaside.' He smiled at them mournfully. 'Since my wife died I am a man very much on my own.'

'Just one or two small items,' Maggie murmured, 'would fetch you a fortune. No one need *ever* know.'

There was a silence in the room, a silence accentuated by the ticking of an ormulu clock on the marble mantelpiece.

'No one need ever *know*?' Caracoli repeated her words in a whisper.

'That Mantegna for instance.' Lambert pointed to a picture on the wall. 'I doubt if people know of its existence.'

228

For a moment they all gazed at it, Maggie and Lambert slightly awestruck.

'It has probably hung on that wall since he was working for the Gonzagas in Mantua in the fifteenth century,' Alberto murmured. 'Luciano Caracoli, who built the villa, was a great patron of the arts and intimate with the family.'

'I could get you half a million alone for the Mantegna – pounds, of course.'

'Half a million!'

'That's almost half of what you need to restore the house. One small painting.' Lambert rose and, strolling with deliberate casualness over to the corner of the room where the painting was badly hung, peered at it.

'That's if it really *is* a Mantegna.'

'Oh, no doubt about it.' Alberto sounded offended. 'There is documentation.'

'It needs cleaning. That will cost a bit.'

'I thought I saw a beautiful little Pinturicchio in the dining-room,' Maggie ventured. 'There is a Dosso Dossi, and surely the bust in the hall is a Donatello?'

'You *have* been observant.' Alberto appeared childishly pleased, but then an expression of cunning came into his eyes. 'Are you trying to tell me you might be interested in acquiring some of my works of art despite the question of an export licence?'

'Very interested.' Lambert perched on a chair opposite him and tried to keep his excitement to himself. 'For a private client, an extremely wealthy Englishman who wishes to acquire works of art for a house he is restoring in the country. I could almost guarantee you two million now, with more if the deals go through and the scheme proves successful. You are sitting here, Alberto, on a fortune of about fifty million pounds. If we release a little at a time your financial problems are solved for ever. I agree you would be very unlikely to get an export licence for most of the treasures, even if you wished to part with them, and few people in Italy, particularly the galleries,

could afford to buy them. However, there are ways of
getting an export licence; there are ways and ways.' He
gave an elegant flick of his wrist and smiled mysteriously.

'How?' Caracoli looked bewildered.

'Oh, just ways, I can't be explicit. I can't betray my
trade secrets. Many Middle Eastern countries are glad of
the currency, Lebanon, for instance, Iraq maybe. However, that is a detail you need not concern yourself with.
Our greatest concern is getting you to agree.'

'I'd be breaking the law.' Caracoli continued to look
uncomfortable.

'I assure you the risks are minimal.' Lambert examined
his nails. 'My client has no wish to display his wealth or
treasures, for very much the same reasons as you. We
shall also choose items that are either not well known
or not known at all. Many in this fabulous collection
were painted for your family and have remained in the
house since their execution; paintings and sculptures
that have never come up for sale, that have never, for
all I know, been catalogued. But if you are worried I will
certainly see that valid export licences are obtained in
the event that one day my client may wish to sell them,
or his heirs in the event of his death.'

'May one ask who your client is?'

'Unfortunately, no.' Lambert stood up as if anxious to
get on with the inventory. 'I shall respect your privacy,
as well as his. You will not know to whom it goes and
he will not know from whence it came.'

'That will make everyone happy. It protects you both.'
Maggie smilingly produced a mini tape recorder. 'Do you
think we could now make an inventory, Alberto?'

'Is that wise?'

'It is necessary,' Lambert said. 'It would, of course, be
extremely confidential and known only to us; but you
see if we didn't have some record you could, in time,
accuse us of theft.'

'Oh, but I wouldn't dream . . .'

The Silklanders dismissed his protest with a reassuring

smile and, finally, Alberto was induced to smile too, if only because of the fortune he was sitting on.

Driving down the hill towards Florence the Silklanders remained silent for some minutes, apparently unable to take in their good fortune. In the boot of the car was the Mantegna hidden by the spare wheel. They would have it cleaned by a restorer in Rome who had worked for them before and then they would arrange for it to be picked up by Varga's private plane. The sum agreed had been half a million, of which twenty per cent would go to Lambert as the dealer.

He began to hum with satisfaction.

'I wouldn't be too chirpy if I were you, darling,' Maggie interrupted him after a while.

'But why not, darling?' He stopped humming abruptly and braked gently. 'We have just brought off the scoop of the century.'

'What we are doing or contemplating *is* illegal. We've never done anything quite like this before.'

'The Indian bronzes . . .'

'Were not in the category of an old master of the stature of Mantegna. I'm really quite worried, Lambert.' Maggie lit a cigarette and lowered the window of the car to release the smoke. 'In fact I'm scared stiff.'

'Darling, there's no need to worry.'

'Supposing somebody saw it? Varga will entertain.'

'We'll get the licence. There's a bureaucrat I know in Sofia who is desperate for cash. He'll sign anything. Up to now no one knows that Mantegna exists, except Alberto and us.'

'*And* his doctor son. He may be no fool. Also Forsci will recognize Mantegna.' Forsci was the restorer.

'He won't know we're exporting it. I trust him, anyway.'

'I don't like engaging in criminal activities for the sake of Varga,' Maggie said. 'I don't think he's worth it.'

'You don't like him, do you?'

'Not much.' She turned her head. 'Do you?'

'I think he's okay. Ginny's potty about him.'

'That I can understand. He's attractive.'

'I can't see it.'

'Animal magnetism, sexuality and also power. Power is very attractive to women. He can give Ginny everything she wants.'

'And he can give *us* quite a lot, too,' Lambert chuckled. 'Don't worry your pretty head about it, Mags. Tonight, with a clear profit of over a million bucks, we shall treat ourselves to a very good meal.'

Ginny stood in the outer office looking through the faxes that had come in over the weekend. She had got to the mews at about 7.30 because of the volume of work and the number of engagements she had, including a lunch with one of the more curious members of the press, someone who tended to be on the hostile side towards Simeon and who needed buttering up. Not every financial journalist considered him brilliant; but people who made a lot of money always had their detractors. Gloria Keane was a tough woman in a tough business who liked to think she was streets ahead of everyone else.

The faxes trailed on to the desk and on to the floor. They were from all over the world: Tokyo, New York, Moscow, Cape Town, Montreal, Rome, Buenos Aires, Mexico . . . the list was endless. Confirming this, asking about that, complex figures for the attention of Liddle that meant nothing to her. Usually Dorothy Richards dealt with them all so that when the appropriate member of staff got in they were on their desks; but Ginny was expecting a fax from Oriole about an impending visit she intended to make and she wanted to make an early reservation on the plane.

There was nothing from Oriole and she was about to let the continuous roll of paper fall back on the floor when a word, a name, caught her eye: Acapulco.

It had such a glamorous image: Mexico, the blue

waters of the Gulf, sand, sun and sex. Maybe she should suggest to Simeon that they went there for their honeymoon? Maybe Aero Acapulco could fly them. She started to giggle at the idea, but when she read through the message her brow furrowed.

'Consignment on its way; expect no delays at the border.' It was simply signed B.

She tore off this part of the fax and walked into Varga's office, knowing he wouldn't be there – he was in the States – but wondering if there was any clue in his diary.

She entered the office without knocking and, to her surprise, found Tony Liddle sitting at Varga's desk working. He jumped up when he saw her, a look of surprise, almost guilt, on his face.

'Ginny. I didn't expect you to get in this early.'

'I have a heavy day,' Ginny smiled. 'Isn't it early for you too, Tony?'

'I have to go over to Rome. Something's come up there,' Liddle murmured, sitting down again.

'What have we got in Rome?' Ginny didn't feel especially curious. One of the faxes had been from Rome; but they had business all over the world.

'Oh, this and that, nothing specially important.' Liddle, intent on his work, seemed reluctant to give her a straight answer.

'Rome has a very glamorous image.' Ginny sat down in the chair facing him. 'I'm always looking for a PR angle you know. Who do we deal with in Rome?'

'Our agent is Farnese.'

'And what has he got on at the moment?'

'You'd better ask Simeon.' Liddle appeared ill at ease. 'Look, Ginny. Do please excuse me, but I'm terribly busy.' He indicated the figures in front of him.

Ginny glanced down at the papers on his desk and suddenly she stiffened with alarm. For there before him undoubtedly were the plans of the Silklander estate. The castle to the left-hand side, the farm to the right and, in between and surrounding them, the acres of forest, the prime arable land, the fields full of grazing beef, cattle and sheep.

'Those figures . . .' she began, rising from her chair to take a clearer view.

'*Please* excuse me, Ginny.' Liddle made a half-hearted attempt to hide the large plans on the desk before him, useless because of their size.

'That *surely* is the Silklander estate?' she said, puzzled. 'Are the figures you refer to to do with that?' She placed a finger roughly over the side of the place where she was born.

'I thought you knew?'

'Knew? Knew what?'

'Well, you were there at Christmas. I thought Simeon discussed buying the place from your family in order to develop the land.'

'Buying the estate? All of it? The castle?' Ginny, normally so calm, sounded on the verge of hysteria.

'Not the castle.' Liddle checked his hand-written figures against a similar set of parallels on the screen. 'But the farm and the land, is my understanding.'

'Simeon has made a formal offer for it?' Her voice seemed to come from far away.

'No, that's what I'm working on.' He looked at his screen again and then down at the plan. In the light it was difficult to see what the columns on the computer stood for. 'I'm sure he wants to discuss it with you,' Liddle said hastily, 'that's why he wanted me to get the facts right first.'

'I see.' Ginny dropped into the chair next to the desk and looked at him.

'There are an awful lot of things going on that I seem to know little or nothing about, Tony.'

'I'm sure Simeon tells you all he thinks you should know,' Liddle replied diplomatically. 'He has so many irons in the fire, I don't know how he does it.'

'So it seems,' her tone was caustic. 'You're busy working on plans to sell my home . . .'

'Not *all* of it,' Liddle interjected.

'*And* you don't know why you're going to Rome?'

'Of course I do.' He looked irritated.

'As a director, shouldn't I know, too?' She tried to keep her tone pleasantly even.

'I'm going to Rome to see Farnese . . .' It seemed to Ginny that Tony hesitated, like someone desperately searching for an excuse, 'about some new offices we intend acquiring.'

'Doesn't sound very important to me.'

'Well it is,' Liddle snapped. 'And now do please excuse me. I don't wish to be rude.'

Ginny remained stubbornly where she was for a few minutes, aware of a feeling of unease.

There was little love between Simeon's chief lieutenant, his right hand, and the woman he wished to marry. Some said it was because they were jealous of each other; but it wasn't that so much as that, between them, there was an air of mutual mistrust and suspicion. Perhaps it was based on the fact that each occupied, in a different way, a place of special importance in the heart of the man who controlled their lives, to some extent their destinies.

Liddle of course had preceded Ginny and Varga had known him now for many years; but Ginny could never quite understand why Simeon trusted this rather nondescript man, lacking any interest or personality, whose vision seemed to go no further than his nose.

Simeon had told her it was not only because he trusted his discretion, but also because he was a wizard with figures.

As Liddle went on working, totting up columns with the aid of a calculator, Ginny rose and then suddenly remembered what she'd come in for.

'Is Simeon going to Mexico this trip?'

Liddle's eyes were instantly alert, wary.

'Why?'

'Because there's a fax from Aero Acapulco.'

'Let me see it.' Liddle peremptorily held out his hand, but Ginny clung on to the paper.

'I'm sure it would mean nothing to you, Tony.'

'I'd like to see it anyway.'

Their eyes met and Ginny knew instinctively how foolish it would be to add to that incipient hostility she already knew he felt towards her. She handed him the fax and his eyes rapidly scanned it.

'Oh, that's not important.' He put it on one side and got on with the process of addition.

'Tony,' Ginny perched on the side of the desk and stared fixedly at him, 'just what *is* Aero Acapulco?'

'It's an airline,' Tony said without raising his head. 'Very small and insignificant.'

'Then why is Simeon so secretive about it?'

'He isn't, as far as I know. Not to me.' Liddle raised his face with an air of assumed innocence.

'Maybe you know more than I do.'

Liddle ceased his calculations and with a deep sigh sat back, folding his arms across his chest. Even though it was early on a winter's morning his face was sweating slightly. Liddle was given to sweating just below the hairline, where beads of moisture always seemed to accumulate. Sometimes, too, there was a very faint body odour, as though he didn't use enough antiperspirant spray; yet he always looked clean, closely shaved and well turned out. He had a wife, but no one had ever met her; she was never brought to office parties or any social gathering even when Simeon suggested it. It made one think he was maybe a little ashamed of Mrs Liddle and kept her under wraps in case she dented his image of a tycoon. Yet he wasn't a tycoon; he was definitely a lackey, a subordinate, apparently without strong opinions of his own. He was Varga's shadow, a man without any real power or significance.

'Ginny, as far as I know Aero Acapulco is a small freight-carrying airline of no significance whatever. I

236

have heard you refer to it before and I have no idea why it makes you so upset.'

'It doesn't *upset* me a bit,' Ginny protested. She stroked the curve of her chin with a finger, presenting an image that was open, attractive, with a curious air of well-bred sexuality.

Suddenly the tension appeared to vanish from her brow and she gave him one of her dazzling smiles.

'I suppose it's because it has a racy name: Aero Acapulco.'

'Yes, I suppose so,' Tony smiled with relief. 'Well, it's nothing.'

'I think I'd have liked the chance to publicize it.'

'Oh, Simeon wouldn't like that.' Liddle's conspiratorial smile vanished immediately.

'Why not?'

'Ginny!' Once again Liddle dashed down his pencil on the desk and sat back. 'You must know that certain companies belong to Simeon's private, off-shore trusts. This is one of them.'

'Tax?' Ginny raised an interrogative eyebrow.

'Exactly; nothing illegal, nothing wrong, nothing to do with AP International. The airline is a fleet of old Dakotas and not the kind of thing you'd particularly wish to give prominence to. I imagine he'd think it would dent his image. They are well serviced, well looked after, but they're old and, maybe, one day one of them will fall apart, hopefully with no one in it. It's a very commercial, lucrative operation and Simeon wants to keep it that way. I'm sure he'll answer all your questions when he comes home.'

'I'll leave the fax on his desk.' Ginny felt rather ashamed of herself; of her attempts to bully and interrogate a close associate of her fiancé which indicated her own lack of trust in him.

'Dorothy will take care of it,' Liddle looked up again with a weary smile, 'and if she thinks he needs to do anything about it she'll let him know.'

'I'm sure she will. Thanks.'

Ginny walked swiftly from the room closing the door behind her, and for some minutes Liddle remained with his eyes on the VDU screen but not appearing actually to see anything, like a man in a trance.

Ginny spent the morning at her desk doing routine work, making various calls, many of them to do with Purborough Park, over which workmen were now swarming like flies. There was a call from Maggie about some wallpaper and curtain material she wanted Ginny to see, and some exciting news that Lambert had discovered a cache of art treasures in Italy.

Italy. Rome came to Ginny's mind for a few seconds, but there seemed absolutely no connection between Liddle's impending visit there and Lambert's find. She told Maggie it sounded exciting and arranged a meeting for the day after Simeon returned.

She telephoned her mother to see how she was, and returned several calls from journalists asking Simeon's reaction to the news that AP International's shares were among the best performing of the previous year.

It was a busy yet normal sort of morning and she left just after twelve for lunch with Gloria Keane, who was now the city editor of a tabloid with a high circulation.

Gloria was between forty and forty-five and enjoyed a rich life-style. She'd had a rapid career in Fleet Street and little went on in the money markets that she didn't know about. The lunch was on Ginny, who had chosen one of the new restaurants proliferating in the City to cater for the rash of wealthy aspiring bankers, stockbrokers and investment experts created by the deregulation of Stock Exchange controls.

Gloria was already in her seat sipping a drink when Ginny arrived, apologizing for being late because of a traffic jam round Ludgate Circus.

Gloria waved away her excuses:

'Don't worry. I was *early*. I only have a few yards to

walk. I ordered myself a bloody mary.'

'Good.' Ginny signalled to the waiter and ordered chilled mineral water.

'Not *ill* or anything are you?' Gloria enquired anxiously.

'I'll have a glass of wine with lunch,' Ginny said smiling as the *maître d'* appeared with menus which he gave to each lady, withdrawing while they made their choice.

'Or pregnant?' Gloria added with a superior smile.

'No, I'm not pregnant.' Ginny looked up from the menu at her guest. 'So you know?'

'I know about the engagement. Doesn't everybody?'

'It's not official. He doesn't get his divorce until spring or early summer.'

'I heard she was being difficult.'

'Very. Her family don't approve of divorce.'

'How quaint.' Gloria bent her head, absorbed by the menu. Although a decade or so older than Ginny she was a smart svelte woman to whom diet was important and she chose an avocado salad and warm breast of duck for her main course. Ginny decided to have the same.

'Wine?'

'A glass.'

Ginny ordered half a bottle of Sancerre. Then she joined her arms together and leaned over the table.

'Well, down to business.'

'Yes, to business.' Gloria took out her pad and put it on the table. 'One of the fastest growing shares ever. Simeon must be terribly pleased.'

'He expected it. It's all due to his hard work.'

'And very low gearing.' Gloria looked at some notes she'd made on her pad. 'A P/E ratio of twelve is excellent, and surprising.'

'But why does it surprise you?' Ginny sipped her drink.

'Because he's buying such a lot. How does he pay for everything?'

'He generates revenue by rationalizing the companies he buys.'

'Asset stripping?' Gloria commented, making a note.

'No, not asset stripping,' Ginny replied firmly. This charge was always being laid at Simeon's door. 'He is just terribly careful over what he buys and what he does with it. He usually buys companies which are overloaded anyway, where the management is poor and the shares under-performing. Sometimes he covers the cost of acquisition merely by getting rid of surplus staff or selling the expensive offices in which the company was housed.'

'Still very low.' Gloria drew a line under something. 'They say he uses a lot of private money.'

'Yes, he does.' Ginny felt a tiny warning bell ring somewhere inside her.

'Where does *that* come from?'

'From his private companies. He doesn't use shareholders' money in speculation but his own.' Ginny raised her glass to her lips. 'I would have thought you'd approve of that, Gloria.'

'Oh, I do. I wish I knew how to get rich so quickly and easily.'

Ginny had considered Gloria a friend. Now she wondered. A man's reputation could be destroyed by a mischievous article. She looked searchingly at Gloria.

'Is there something I'm missing out on? I always thought you were a fan of Simeon's?'

'Oh, I am,' Gloria answered. 'A very great fan. Just a little envious, maybe, of someone so talented. And now he has you. Now tell me,' Gloria shut her pad as though the business part of the conversation was over, 'are you going to stay on after the marriage?'

'That's the problem.' Ginny leaned back as their main course arrived. 'Naturally Simeon wants me to give up work.'

'Naturally.' Gloria smiled sympathetically but her thin, rather cruel mouth showed no real understanding. 'That place in the country looks vast.'

'It is; but I don't intend just to be the wife of a busy man.'

'Of course you'd like a family?' Gloria eyed her speculatively.

'In time. I haven't actually discussed it with Simeon – I mean about work – because I don't think he's thought about it.' Ginny took her fork to her salad. 'I rather thought I'd like to have a look at the perfume business. We have this company in France which is really not doing very much.'

'Oriole. There was trouble there to begin with, wasn't there?' Gloria flicked open her notebook to write an *aide mémoire*.

'It was the first acquisition after AP International went public and maybe he was a bit ruthless at that stage. But he has learned and I don't think he ever reacted quite that way after acquiring a new company again.'

'Sacked the proprietor and his son.'

'On extremely good terms.' Ginny's tone was defensive. In the dusk of the cellar in which the restaurant was situated she felt ill at ease. 'However, the point is that if Simeon agrees I would like to take on total control of Oriole and invent a new perfume.'

'Do you actually know anything about perfume?' Gloria, busy making a new note, didn't look up.

'I know something, but we employ a good "nose". I've had a few discussions with him already. The main thing is to iron it all out with Simeon when he gets back.'

'And the house, when will you move into that?'

'Hopefully in the autumn.'

'But it looked derelict!' Gloria exclaimed in surprise.

'No it's not derelict, but a lot does need doing. It could take years. We propose having a wing ready for our occupation by the summer. We'll live in Simeon's flat until that's ready and then use it at weekends. Ultimately we hope to live at Purborough and then use it as a base for making visits to other parts of the group.'

'A world-wide organization.' Gloria daintily dipped a piece of granary bread in the dressing of her salad. 'Aren't you the lucky girl . . . and isn't Simeon the lucky man. A very, very lucky man.'

Ginny watched the sleek, bent head of the woman opposite her intent on her meal, not sure whether or not she had unwittingly turned a friend into a jealous foe.

CHAPTER 13

'I missed you.'

'Me too.'

Their hands joined together in the subdued light of the rear seat of the car as the Jaguar took them swiftly along the motorway from Heathrow. To Varga, weary from a protracted foreign tour, the lights of London had never looked so good and, as they passed across the Hammersmith flyover, he leaned back and gave a deep, deep sigh, his hand tightening over Ginny's.

'When we're married I want you to come away with me every time. Every trip we'll make part business, part holiday. How about that?'

Ginny didn't reply and he moved closer to her, his expression of tenderness changing to one of concern.

'Wouldn't you like that, darling?' he insisted.

'Of course.' Her hand responded to the pressure of his. 'But I also like to be my own woman. I never want just to be your appendage, Simeon.'

'But you never will! That's an absurd idea.' He looked at her closely. 'What exactly *is* the matter, darling? Did something happen while I was away?'

'Nothing specific, except that I missed you. I was able to do a little thinking.'

'Tell me, Ginny.' He pressed his cheek against hers. 'You're really worrying me.'

'There's no need to worry, Simeon. I'll tell you over dinner.'

'Are we going out?'

'Dorothy has had Le Gavroche send something over for us. She thought we'd want to be alone.'

'Dorothy is an angel.' Varga leaned back again and sighed. 'Now she is a woman you really would have cause to be jealous of.'

By the time they reached the flat it was nearly nine and the table in the small dining area was laid for two. Dorothy had left written instructions that the starter was in the fridge and the main course could be reheated in seconds in the microwave. The champagne was in the fridge too, and she had decanted for them a Chassagne-Montrachet '78 to go with the entrée.

Simeon, palpably glad to be back, changed into grey flannels and a shirt and Ginny put on the kimono he'd brought her back from a recent trip to Japan. But there was a tension about her that disturbed him.

Like any normal couple after a day's work, they returned to the kitchen, where Simeon got the champagne out of the fridge, put some ice in a bucket and, after pouring two glasses, stuck the bottle in it. He leaned against the kitchen table and gazed at her, his glass raised.

'To you, Ginny.'

Ginny finished fiddling with the microwave and, turning to him, took her glass and raised it to his. Gently they clinked glasses and then, arms entwined, they drank. Their lips met; it was a sensual, thrilling sensation perfumed with champagne. He felt her unnaturally tense body relax as he put his arm around her and held her tight, conscious of the strong beat of her heart.

'What *is* it, Ginny?' he persisted, his eyes questioning. 'There is something the matter.'

'It's nothing.'

She took the plates of cold asparagus from the fridge and put them on the table.

'Bring the hollandaise sauce, would you, Simeon?'

Obediently he collected the sauce in a porcelain dish and put it on the table, then returned for the champagne and placed the bucket in the stand beside him.

Varga realized he was hungry and, dipping the succulent tips in the sauce, began to eat. Ginny ate with less relish. He pretended not to notice that she was toying with her food. He would wait. He had plenty of time.

The main course was boeuf en croute, underdone fillet in choux pastry, and fresh vegetables. He tasted the wine and, pronouncing the vintage superb, filled their glasses.

'This is a feast,' he said returning to his seat. 'The best food I had this trip was in Caracas of all places.'

'Caracas?' She looked up in surprise. 'You didn't say you were going to Caracas.'

'It was not on my schedule. The airline was running a consignment of oranges to Venezuela.'

'Aero Acapulco?' she smiled.

'Yes? Why do you smile, darling?'

'It's such a funny name.'

'Isn't it?' He leaned over the table and put his hand over hers again.

'I love you.'

'I love you too, Simeon.'

'Then tell me what upsets you.'

'I'm not upset . . . I'm just, well, surprised.'

'Surprised at what?'

'That you didn't tell me you were negotiating to buy the Silklander estate, after *all* I said on the subject!'

'My darling, there was nothing to tell. It's just an idea. I mentioned it to Angus, that's all. It's far from settled.'

'Don't you think you could have said something to me? After all it is my home.'

'Ginny!' Varga wiped his mouth and took a fresh sip of wine. 'What is the point of announcing something that may never happen? You know it's not my way. It's not the way I work.'

'But it's something so intimately concerned with me.'

'It's not concerned with you.' He looked surprised.

'*Of* concern to me, I should have said.'

'Why does it concern you, darling? I am only trying to help. I thought it might embarrass you if I mentioned it, that's all. You've made such an issue of it before.'

'It does embarrass me.'

'Then I was right. Angus might be forced to mortgage the farm. It has never been mortgaged before. Why borrow money at extravagant rates of interest when I can take the burden off him?'

'Not without advantage to yourself.'

'Ginny, please don't be so cynical.' Simeon frowned with displeasure. 'I assure you I should not lose on the deal, but the satisfaction for me would be in helping the family of my bride. Believe me, that's *all* I have in mind; but it will be done in as businesslike a manner as possible. I know that's what you would want. You would hate any hint of charity.'

'I should loathe it.'

'Quite. So should I. I think,' he began to draw an imaginary plan with his fork on the table top, 'that if Angus went in for intensive farming he could increase his profits tenfold.'

'You mean battery hens and factory farming?' Her lip curled with distaste.

'Exactly. Oh, I know what you think. "How cruel". But, my dear,' he reached out for the decanter and poured himself more wine, 'it is not cruel at all. These animals have never known anything else. They are warm, well fed and well looked after. I . . .'

Ginny put her knife and fork neatly together on her plate to indicate that she had finished, the boeuf en croute practically untouched. She reached for her glass, took a sip of wine and stood up. She walked across to the window and then back again, and stood facing him.

'Simeon, please don't lecture me. I am a country girl born and bred. The thought of rearing animals in these conditions nauseates me. And it would nauseate my brother, too.'

'How do you think the beef you've just eaten was raised?' He looked sceptically at her plate.

'I am not a fanatic. I don't want a certificate on every mouthful of meat I consume; but I know how I want animals to be reared and how my brother wants to rear them.'

'That's why your brother has to face the prospect of mortgaging his home.'

'You can be very cruel, Simeon.' She turned away from him back to the window and looked into the dark outside. Gradually, her eyes becoming accustomed to the dark, she could see the roofs outlined against the dusky red night sky of London where never a star was visible, unlike the clear crisp night air of the country. She thought of Silklands and then she thought of beautiful Purborough. The sky above that would be clear and frosty, too. And she knew that he had bought it for her. It was to be his wedding present. He loved her.

She turned round and he was looking at her; his steady gaze confirming what she knew.

Simeon loved her, but she must not try his love; she must not push him too far. He was a clever man, a businessman, a man driven by ambition and he always would be.

As if in perfect understanding he held out his hand and, as she reached for it, he drew her towards him on to his knee. His arms tightly round her, he embraced her and then murmured:

'You know I would never consciously do anything to make you unhappy.'

'I know.'

'The farm project will be dropped . . .'

'But what about Angus?'

'Well, you must decide that between you. If, when I have the figures, you want to be in on the discussions, you will be. If you want me to drop it I will drop it. It

247

isn't a bit important to me. But,' he put a finger against her lips, 'listen carefully. Only in something that concerns your family will I allow interference; never in anything else. I will never let you interfere in my business decisions or make me change my mind if I don't think it's right.'

'I know,' she said, 'and I won't.'

'Promise?'

'I promise.'

She knew then that, infatuated as she was by him, there was also an element of fear in her love for Simeon Varga.

Later in the night he cried out, a strange, eerie sound like the cry of a bird. It made her sit upright in bed and look at him; but in the light of the moon all she could see was a smile on his face as though he slept the sleep of the just.

It was incredible how much had been done in such a short time. Even on a Sunday workmen swarmed like flies over the house, along the scaffolding that covered the walls, up on the roof, repointing the stonework and the brickwork, replacing gutters and lost or broken tiles, repairing the chimneys.

Yet inside the restoration looked almost complete, although this was far from being the case.

'About a year,' Simeon murmured as they stood a quarter of a mile away from the house, gazing at it across the frost-covered lawn. 'They say in a year it will all be ready.'

'As long as that?' Maggie, one arm linked through Lambert's, a hand deep in the pocket of her sheepskin coat, looked surprised. 'I'm well ahead with my plans, then.'

'I mean the whole thing,' Varga said with an expansive gesture. 'Everything will be absolutely as it should be: the grounds landscaped, new trees and shrubs planted . . .'

'Goldfish in the pond . . .' Ginny gave him a sideways smile.

'Exactly.' Simeon glanced at her. 'Every last detail like that. *And* horses in the stables.'

'Oh, you're going in for horses?' Lambert looked impressed.

'Ginny loves riding. She's going to teach me.'

'That kind of stables. Not breeding or racing?'

'I wouldn't mind breeding fine Arab horses,' Varga said reflectively, his hand in Ginny's, 'but we'll see.'

In the cold frosty February day the house, its mellow stone in the process of being cleaned and restored, did look magnificent. The backdrop was the cerulean sky, the thick wooded copse surrounding it. In front of the house ran a terrace and a long gravel path leading to an obelisk, booty captured by some descendant of the Purboroughs and taken at great trouble and expense to his ancestral home. On either side were formal lawns, part of them covered with planks and scaffolding and, in the centre, a huge fountain, also scaffolded, standing in the middle of a pond overgrown and full of weeds, devoid of life.

To the left of the house, from where they stood, were the stables, long derelict and used as a storehouse and, further on again, was more woodland which clothed the slopes of a hill. On top of the hill was a cairn, visible for miles, which commemorated the Battle of Trafalgar in 1805, in which Ensign Eustace Purborough, the heir to the family title, had lost his life at the age of eighteen.

'How many years since the family lived here?' Lambert asked, shading his eyes.

'About ten. The last Viscount Purborough died in a nursing home in London without issue. By that time they hadn't got a bean and the place was left to rot.'

'No interest on the part of the National Trust or English Heritage?'

'There are so many places like this in England, if only one knew it,' Ginny said with a note of sadness in her

249

voice. 'They struggle and hang on but, in the end, they have to give up. They let the place go too far downhill and then no one's interested in taking it on. Besides, the Purborough treasures had long been sold, and the National Trust always requires some form of endowment.'

'I would love to fill it with treasures,' Simeon cried, with such enthusiasm that Lambert said: 'I believe you will. I think I'm on to something.'

'Oh?'

'A villa full of treasures in Italy, an owner rather like the Purboroughs who would like to get his hands on some money to restore his Renaissance house in the hills high above Florence.'

'How romantic.' Ginny squeezed Simeon's hand. 'Have you been there?'

'Yes I have, and talked with the owner. I believe that we could pull off something, if there's enough money.' His gaze wandered idly towards Varga.

'Oh, I don't think you'd find money a problem.' Varga released Ginny's hand and glanced at his watch. 'I have to go and see the architect. He's due here at twelve. Maggie, I believe you want to see him too.'

'I'd like to know when the walls will be ready. I'm having the wallpaper designed and made by hand. But first I'd love to see the stables.'

'I'll show you the stables,' Ginny began to walk in that direction, 'and then we can join the boys at the house.'

'Afterwards a pub lunch, I think.' Varga stamped his feet on the ground. 'I am hungry and thirsty. See you in,' again he looked at his watch, 'half an hour, darling. Is that okay?'

'Fine.'

'Will it give you time to do what you have to do?' Varga turned his head to Maggie.

'Should be ample. It's at a very early stage.'

'We'll split up then for half an hour.' Varga and Lambert began to stride towards the house and the two

250

women walked across the lawn towards the stables.

These were in a very derelict state, full of pieces of old furniture, farm implements, assorted paraphernalia to do with horses: bridles, saddles, ancient bales of hay and a horseshoe that someone had nailed to the wall before the luck of the Purboroughs ran out. There were huge cobwebs on the corners of the stone walls by the rafters and across the horse troughs, and ominous signs of rat droppings by the holes in the floor.

Maggie shuddered.

'Creepy,' she said. 'Fancy letting them get to this state! There's something sad about taking over an old house.'

Ginny moodily kicked a piece of leather, that could once have been part of a bridle, on the floor. 'It's a warning to me of what could happen to Silklands.' She looked gravely at her sister-in-law who, hands in her coat pockets, perched on a bale of hay.

'Silklands?' Maggie gazed at her in surprise. 'Surely you're not serious?'

'The estate is in a bad way. Angus wants to mortgage the farm. Daddy doesn't really know how to cope. Things are getting out of hand.'

'But I thought everything was going so well? Everyone seemed so happy at Christmas?'

'"Seemed" is the right word. I thought so too, but Simeon found out that Angus was making no money out of the farm and was going to mortgage the buildings which, of course, has never happened in the history of the family.'

'Good heavens. No wonder you look so pensive.'

'Did I look pensive?' Ginny gave a wan smile. 'I wasn't aware of it.'

'I knew you'd got something on your mind. It's nothing to do with Simeon, is it?'

Ginny kicked the bale of hay on which Maggie was sitting.

'Well, Simeon is involved. It was he who told me about Angus. I knew very little about it. Simeon has offered to buy the farm and lease it back to Angus.'

'But that's brilliant!' Maggie clasped her hands. 'Isn't it?' A look of doubt came over her expressive, mobile face.

'I'm not too sure. He wants the land as well; all the land belonging to the estate. He wants to develop it. Simeon is such an astute businessman, you know, he does nothing without a reason.'

'Well *I* would have thought this would have been for the family, and you too, of course. I wonder if Lambert knows?' Maggie frowned. 'I'll ask him. He can play his cards close to his chest too.' Maggie got to her feet and put a hand on her companion's arm. 'I'm sure Simeon's only doing what he is for love of you, Ginny. He's obviously crazy about you.'

'I think his motives are mixed. He loves me, wants to impress the family, can see a good deal. He told me the other night never to interfere in anything to do with business. I felt a bit afraid, that I didn't know him. I'm a director, after all. He can change from day to day . . . he's so volatile.'

'But you haven't *doubts*?' Maggie said nervously.

'None at all.' Ginny shook her head. 'This is an exciting adventure. Sometimes I'm a bit out of my depth; but underneath there's a solid core of love and trust.'

'Have you thought about what you're going to do *after* you're married?' Maggie asked, looking at her shrewdly.

'*Do*?' Ginny looked puzzled.

'You can't carry on working for the firm, can you?'

'No, not very well. I have got some ideas, but I haven't yet talked about them to Simeon. I think he imagines I'm going to be content with playing the lady of the house here; but I'm not. I think a woman should have her own life, don't you, Maggie?'

'Oh, definitely. But the trouble is men; some men like women to enhance their egos whether they admit it or not. It gives them a sense of power. Lambert's not so bad, but Simeon loves power. You can see he does.' She tucked her arm through Ginny's and drew her towards the door. 'We'd better get back or we'll be late.'

The two men came down the grand staircase very carefully. Around them was a chaotic scene, of builders' materials, ladders, breeze blocks, chunks and strips of plaster where the delicate cornices were being restored. A block of marble lay on its side ready to be hewn and polished.

Yet it was all taking shape; the walls were plastered and it would not be long before Maggie's wallpaper could be hung. The doors had been rehung or replaced altogether, and the painters were now beginning the decoration.

It had, in fact, all happened terribly quickly.

'It's surprising what you can do if you have the money.' Lambert gesticulated broadly around him. 'I didn't imagine you'd get so far in six weeks.'

'I gave them a time limit.'

'But you said a year.' Lambert looked puzzled.

'A year by when everything is *absolutely* complete. We shall move in this summer, hopefully. By next summer the garden has to be full of flowers.' He smiled broadly.

'And when will the divorce be final?'

Simeon didn't answer at once and Lambert looked uneasily at him. Finally he said: 'My wife is still making trouble. I have an interview with her brother some time during the week.'

'Trouble about money?'

'Just trouble,' Simeon said grimly as they reached the ground floor. Once again, an impatient man, he consulted his watch.

'Simeon, before we meet the women, could I have a word?' Lambert looked around to see if they were out of earshot, but a carpenter was working on a plinth at the far side of the hall. 'Perhaps we could find an empty room?' Lambert steered Simeon into the drawing-room. There, however, painters were at work on the ceiling, and eventually they found a room off the kitchen which would be part of the servants' quarters when everything was complete.

'This do?' Simeon looked anxiously at Lambert. 'I suppose you want to discuss your fee, hence the secrecy?'

'Not quite.' Lambert carefully shut the door. 'But I do want to talk money. It's about that hoard we found in Italy. But I have to be very careful.' Lambert put his hands to his head as if it ached. 'I can't *tell* you how exciting it is, Simeon. A simply priceless cache of treasures. It's worth an absolute fortune and the man who owns it doesn't realize it. Can you believe it, he actually has a *Mantegna*?'

'A what?' Simeon said politely.

'A picture by the Italian artist Andrea Mantegna, one of the geniuses of the Renaissance. It's a terrific find and I don't think he quite realizes what he has.'

'Will he sell it?' Varga looked fractionally interested.

'Yes I'm sure. If he can get the right price.'

'Then buy it.' Varga stopped. 'How much do you want?'

'At least two and a half million. He could get, maybe, four on the open market.'

'Then why does he want to sell it to us?'

'Because,' Lambert moved nearer Varga and instinctively lowered his voice, 'he would never get an export licence.'

'That should not be a problem.' Varga gave him a knowing look.

Lambert's voice dropped almost to a whisper. 'I can manage to get an export licence; but you must still be discreet. To have such a picture in your possession is an insurance risk.'

'The whole place will be insured.'

'It is more. The licence I can get will be a phoney licence. Now, what I want to know is, are you prepared to take the risk?'

Varga eyed him suspiciously. 'What does it involve?'

'It's very unlikely, but you may be found out.'

'Oh no!' Varga dug a finger into the chest of his companion. '*You* may be found out. You buy the picture for me, you get the licence.' Looking round, he too lowered his voice, despite the fact that they were alone. 'I've indicated the ways I can help you, generally speaking . . . as long as my name is not directly involved.'

'I see.' Lambert curled his lips. 'In that case we may as well forget it. Why should I risk my neck?' His voice grew cold. 'I *thought* you said you wanted the place full of treasures.'

'I do.'

'You would never get a Mantegna in the open market.'

'Then buy it, for Christ's sake, and get the licence. You mean we have to bribe the Italian authorities?'

'No, we could never get it in Italy; they are too proud of their treasures. But no one knows that the Mantegna is in Italy. It has never been recorded. It was probably painted for an ancestor of the present owner.'

'Who is?'

'It's better if you don't know.' Lambert put a finger across his lips, a gesture which made Simeon smile.

'Very well.' He too gestured with a finger across his throat. '*Omertà*.'

'I have,' Lambert looked deliberately vague, 'shall we say "contacts" who are prepared to issue a licence, and we do have to bribe *them*.'

'You have contacts in another country?'

'The Middle East is full of corrupt officials who are quite willing to sign a piece of paper saying that a certain work of art originated in their country. No one knows the difference.'

'I see.' Simeon looked interested. 'In fact we may have a very good little business going here. I once told you about the small airline I own . . .'

'We may well need that to get the picture and some other treasures out of the country and into this.'

'Easy. Then why do we need a licence?'

'Just in case. This is a large house. You will have visitors. I suggest the Mantegna is not very prominently displayed. The main thing is that you own this treasure. That is your source of satisfaction. Only a very few people would recognize it, anyway, as by the master; I assure you the risk is negligible.'

'Two and a half million!' Varga clenched his teeth. 'And this old master is really worth that much?'

'Every penny.'

'Can't you knock him down?'

Lambert, his heart torn asunder by greed, hesitated. 'I may be able to shave off half a million.'

'Do that.' Varga stuck his finger in Lambert's chest again, 'and include in it the export licence and you have a deal. Come on now, the ladies will be waiting.'

As he turned to leave the room Lambert grinned behind his back. Clever as Varga thought himself, he had his blind spots.

In what was to be the drawing-room Lambert and Varga found Ginny and Maggie poring over samples of wall-paper which had been flown from Italy the day before. Benjamin Spicer, the architect, wearing a duffel coat and what looked like an old college scarf wound round his neck, held a sample against the wall, his teeth chattering with cold. The wallpaper was of thin gold vertical lines against a cream background and he had managed to achieve just the right harmony with the decorations that Maggie had envisaged. On a box by the newly installed radiators, which were not yet in operation, were bolts of fabric which Lambert had carried from the car on their arrival.

'This design is perfect with that.' Benjamin pointed to one of the fabrics which was heavy silk shot with gold thread, a deep, voluptuous combination. Lambert took up the bolt and placed it against the wallpaper.

'Absolutely perfect,' he declared. 'What does everyone think?'

'Fine to me.' Varga, looking pleased, turned as always to Ginny for confirmation. She seemed less sure and, head on one side, arms folded, stood gazing at the wall.

'You don't think it's too, too . . .' she was making an effort to find the right word, 'too grand?'

'Not in this context.' Lambert shook his head and his eyes swept round the vast room. 'Imagine it full of people. Imagine paintings on the walls, a huge ornate mirror over the mantelpiece,' he gestured towards the beautifully restored Adam fireplace. 'I have found *just* the thing in Rome.'

'Italians seem to be doing rather well out of this,' Varga said with a smile. 'Now, as everyone's starving and freezing, why don't we all go and have a bite at the pub? Ben?' He looked enquiringly at the architect, who held up a hand and shook his head.

'Not for me, thanks, Simeon. I have to get back to London if I'm to get on with plans for the stables.' He glanced at his watch. 'Jesus Christ, I should be there already!'

'We'll let you go, then.' Varga held out an arm ushering him out and he walked on ahead talking to Ben until he got to his car. They stood chatting until the others joined them and then Ben got into his Aston Martin and, with a smile and wave, roared down the drive.

'He's done a first-class job,' Simeon said as they all climbed into a recent purchase, a Range Rover, in which he intended to play the role of country squire.

'No wonder he looks tired.' Maggie got in the back, followed by Lambert, and Ginny took the front seat next to Varga.

'You think he looks tired?' Varga put on his glasses, shoved the car into gear and followed in the wake of the architect. 'He always looks like that to me.'

'He works every hour God gives.'

'He earns his money,' Varga acknowledged and then, looking at Ginny, put a gloved hand on her lap.

'Happy, darling?'

'Very happy.'

'But you don't terribly like the wallpaper or material, or both? If not we shan't have it.'

'I love the materials, heavy silk, perfect for the curtains. I just wonder,' she turned to stare at Maggie in the back, 'if there's too much *gold*?'

'I don't think so,' Maggie sighed heavily, 'but if *you're* not happy . . .'

'We're going back to Italy next week,' Lambert said. 'We can have a look at alternative designs.'

'We can't waste much time, darling.' Maggie was clearly irritated. 'This has to be manufactured. All we have here is a sample.'

'It's being made specially for us?' Varga half-turned his head, looking impressed.

'Oh yes. And it's costing you, too.'

'What is money,' Varga again glanced at Ginny, 'when you want to please the most divine woman in the world?'

When they got to the pub, about two miles from the house, it was clear that lunches were nearly over, but the landlord nevertheless gave a fulsome welcome to his guests because he knew who and how important they were.

'Delightful to see you again, Mr Varga, so soon.' He steered them towards the deserted dining-room.

'I think we'd rather stay in the bar,' Varga said, 'if that's all right. By the fire. It's so warm, and we're so cold. I think soup and sandwiches round the fire. Does everyone agree?'

'Sounds marvellous,' Ginny began, peeling off her gloves. 'And a large scotch beforehand.'

'Immediately, Miss Silklander.' The manager looked ingratiatingly at the others.

'I think they seem to say scotch all round, hot soup, beef sandwiches and a bottle of red wine.'

'If we're having wine I won't have scotch,' Ginny said. 'I'll fall asleep.'

'So shall I,' Maggie agreed.

'I think, then, just a bottle of wine.' Varga laughed. 'Could we have it now?'

'Of *course*, Mr Varga.'

It was a cheerful foursome who consumed the excellent home-made vegetable soup, rare beef in wholewheat bread and Beaujolais Villages in front of the roaring fire while the pub slowly emptied of customers.

'So you think the summer?' Varga seemed reluctant to finish his meal and mopped up the crumbs on his plate with his finger.

'For what?'

'For completion?'

'The whole place?' Maggie looked worried. 'Oh no.'

'We do want to move in by summer.'

'Only into part of the house,' Ginny said quickly. 'We agreed on that, darling.'

'Well, the big rooms certainly won't be ready,' Maggie said firmly, 'especially if you're doubtful about the wallpaper.'

'Let's agree on the wallpaper, then.' Varga sounded like a man in a hurry. 'The sooner we can get it done the better. Do you agree, darling?'

'I agree.'

'Thank heaven.' Maggie took out her notebook and scribbled a few lines. 'One thing less to worry about. Tell me,' she looked towards the engaged pair, '*is* Ginny going to go on working?'

Momentarily Ginny looked annoyed and then, seeming to realize it was just as well if it came out into the open, the muscles of her face relaxed as she turned to look at Varga.

'It's a moot point,' he seemed reluctant to talk about it. 'I don't want her to work at all.'

'I agree, it would be most unprofessional to continue to work for my husband,' Ginny said, 'but neither do I want to become an idle woman, frittering away my time.'

'Darling, there is a lot for you to do here.'

'I know; but there's something else I'd very much like

to do.' She leaned forward, her eager face illuminated by the fire.

'Well, let's hear it.' Varga seemed reluctant to respond to her enthusiasm.

'I'm terribly keen to develop Oriole. We promised ourselves a new perfume and we've done nothing about it. As a company it's languishing.'

'You're right,' Simeon nodded. 'It hardly pays its way. I have it on the list of possible companies to dispose of. But I didn't know you were really interested in that aspect, darling?'

'Well I am. I think to have a lovely new fragrance, to make the plans for launching it . . .'

'And there are *all* sorts of spin-offs,' Maggie echoed her enthusiasm, 'maybe with an eye to the main chance, fashion accessories, stockings . . .'

'Right. What do you think, Simeon?'

'Well,' Varga tapped his glass, 'now that you mention it to me for the very first time, I must say I'm quite keen. If it's what you want to do, then I want to do it.'

'Morgan can take over the PR again,' Ginny went on. 'He's terribly good. The company is so diversified and there are so many things I don't understand.'

'Such as?' Lambert raised his eyebrows.

'I'm going into electronics a lot more,' Varga said, 'the components business. There's a steel firm in Italy I'm interested in; that is where the business is. Especially in the Middle East.'

'The Middle East?'

'Huge amounts of money.'

'You mean oil refineries and that sort of thing?'

'That sort of thing.' Varga looked vague. 'And there are others.' Then, as if on cue, he looked again at his watch. 'Well, we should be going . . .'

'What will you call your perfume?' Maggie asked. 'I like the idea enormously.'

'Have you any ideas, you're the creative one?' Ginny smiled encouragingly at her sister-in-law.

'How about ... how about *Silk*. It's so rich, so sensuous ...'

In her mind's eye Ginny suddenly visualized the lengths of heavy material lying on the floor near the window; those rich folds could have come from a painting by a Renaissance master.

'It's also an abbreviation of your name,' Simeon said with evident approval.

'Do you like it, darling?'

Already she could see the advertising campaign ... folds of rich, luxurious silk, everyone's idea of wealth and extravagance, the perfectly designed bottle in the middle. 'Silk ...'

'I like it,' she said suddenly. She nodded her head vigorously several times. 'I think I like it very much. It's slightly enigmatic.'

Varga raised the glass in which were the remains of his wine.

'Let's drink to Silk – the perfume,' he said.

'Silk, the perfume.' Glasses were raised and clinked together in the middle; then drained to the last drop.

CHAPTER 14

Paolo Bernini, youngest of the Bernini brothers, was the cosmopolitan *par excellence*, chameleon-like in character and personality. He could as easily be Paul in London and New York as Paolo in Rome, Madrid or Buenos Aires. He was all things to all men, a gentle, amenable creature with none of the warring instincts of his elder brothers Carlo and Matteo, the malicious revengeful nature of his mother.

He was a happy family man who lived with his wife and three children on the outskirts of Rome in a villa set amid olive groves.

Paolo ran the Italian end of the Bernini jewellery business; he was a trained craftsman, a connoisseur with a fine discerning eye. He had more talent than Carlo or Matteo, more flair, but less business acumen. While he indulged his craft and his hobbies of collecting vintage wines and fine paintings, he was content to leave the financial part of running the business to Carlo and his own highly paid accountant in the office above the elegant showroom in the Via Veneto in Rome.

Paolo's house was full of treasures, some inherited from his wife's wealthy and aristocratic family; but most of them collected by him since, in early youth, he fell in love with the painters of the Renaissance: Botticelli, Masaccio, Mantegna and the Bellini family, Jacopo, Gentile and Giovanni.

So well was the business run, and so profitable under the watchful eyes of his brothers, that Paolo spent much of his time in pursuit of his hobbies, tracing stores of his favourite wines, the great classical growths of Bordeaux, or visiting art galleries, private collections, and the premises of art restorers who were often able to put him on the track of some old or forgotten master.

Such a restorer was Leonardo Forsci, who operated from an atelier in one of the least salubrious parts of Rome not far from the station. There, in a small street, Leonardo used the delicate skills of his art to reveal the original work of a master behind the cracked paint of one less celebrated, or to restore it to its pristine colours without losing its subtlety. He worked for a number of the great galleries and museums including the Uffizi in Florence and the Museo Vaticano in Rome.

Leonardo was in his sixties and the years of closely detailed indoor work had worsened already poor sight; he worked with the aid of thick-lensed spectacles which had a magnifying attachment fitted to the frames.

In his studio was a kind of controlled chaos that, to him, was a form of order. He knew precisely where everything was, how long it had been there, when it was due to be returned, how long it would take to accomplish and how much it would cost. Always in the centre of his harshly lit studio was the easel holding the masterpiece on which he was working – and, because he was so skilled, they inevitably were masterpieces from some of the major galleries and museums in Italy.

Paolo Bernini and Leonardo Forsci had known each other since Paolo was a boy at school with Leonardo's son Marco, who had gone on to become a physicist, now attached to the University of Milan. It had been Leonardo's grief that his son had not followed him into the business of art restoration, but he was inordinately proud of him and what he had done. He knew, though, that when he died his little workshop would close and, inevitably, his skill as one of the great restorers of his time would be forgotten.

Leonardo was very fond of Paolo Bernini, and whenever he arrived at his studio, maybe two or three times a year, he would stop work for a few moments and offer him a glass of wine.

On this particular occasion they exchanged the usual pleasantries, reported on the health or otherwise of their respective families and then, putting on a pair of spectacles, Paolo began to saunter round the workshop, peering at canvases hanging on the walls or stacked on the floor, finally at the painting on which Leonardo was working at his easel. Half of it was clean and half of it was in the original state in which it had arrived at the Forsci workshop several weeks before. Paolo adjusted his glasses, stooped, and for some time gazed at it. After a few moments he raised his head, a look of amazement on his face.

'It looks like Mantegna,' he said, his face shining with excitement.

'That is my opinion.' Leonardo was cleaning one of his brushes carefully on a rag. 'It is undoubtedly one of his grisaille paintings in which he attempted to imitate sculptural reliefs. This is a singularly fine example of a true "guzzo", except that it has almost been ruined by varnishing which has destroyed the animal glue with which it was bound.' He replaced his brush on a table and came and stood by Paolo, bending to examine the painting so that their heads were level. 'You see the canvas is a fine linen weave with a thin layer of gesso toned with a red earth imprimatura. You can see in the part I have restored that the layers of varnish were never intended by the artist and have been added by a subsequent owner, perhaps in a misguided attempt to preserve it. Such paintings were never meant to be varnished but given a protective coating perhaps of egg glair. This is undoubtedly a very fine example of the artist's work, although the person for whom I am restoring it insists it is only *School* of Mantegna. But,' he pointed to the hand of a woman who carried a scroll, 'I cannot believe that this is not a fine example of the hand of the master.'

'And it is unattributed?'

'It is unattributed. I believe it may be a sister painting, or even the other half of the one entitled *A Sybil and Prophet*, which was acquired by Cardinal Pietro Aldobrandini in 1603 when Ferrara was absorbed into the Papal States. You may recall that Isabella d'Este was one of Mantegna's greatest patrons. He produced work for her studio. Alternatively it could have been bought by Margherita Gonzaga, the wife of Alfonso II d'Este for her private chapel. It is always thought that the existing picture, which is in the Cincinnati Art Museum, was one of a pair. The other has never been found.' He stood back and waved his hand towards it. 'Perhaps we have it here.'

'But this is amazing.' Paolo pushed his spectacles up his nose and peered at it even more closely. 'Where did you get it?'

'Alas, I am not at liberty to say. I think only someone with your specialized knowledge would have placed it so accurately. I was unwise to leave it on the easel.'

'Oh, you can be sure I shall say nothing.' But Paolo was aware of a sensation in his breast that he only ever experienced when he made, or was on the verge of, a discovery of spectacular importance; only previously felt on a very few occasions in his life. 'However, Leonardo, I would dearly like to know who owns it. I am quite sure this piece has never been seen or documented. This means it must have been hidden for all these years since the death of Mantegna in 1506.'

'Possibly it has remained in the same house with the same family, unaware of its significance or that it might be one of a pair.'

'You couldn't possibly ask . . . purely for the purposes of attribution?' Paolo's eyes glistened behind his gold-framed spectacles.

'To be truthful, I don't know the real owner myself.' Leonardo slowly moved away from the picture and recommenced the cleaning of his brush. 'I have not been told. All I know is the name of the intermediary who is a dealer. So perhaps it is for sale.'

'Then may *I*, a close friend of yours, not know?'

'I am sworn to secrecy.' Leonardo, beginning to look uncomfortable, shook his head. 'You can imagine if it is Mantegna . . . it is priceless.'

'There is always a price for a painting,' Paolo said grimly. 'I would never myself have the means to acquire it; but there are still very wealthy people in the world. If you think it is one of a pair, maybe it will be offered to the Cincinnati Art Museum?'

'Maybe.' Leonardo smiled ruefully. 'Only the Americans, after all, can afford this sort of thing. But I have the distinct impression it is in private hands and either the cleaning has been arranged through a dealer in order to hide the owner or,' he shrugged, 'maybe it will be sold privately, who knows?'

'There is no way you can tell me who?'

'All I can say is that he is a foreigner.' Leonardo smiled mysteriously. 'It would not surprise me if you have heard of him, maybe even had dealings with him. Now, my dear Paolo,' he clasped his friend and client by the shoulder, 'having tantalized you with that little mystery I shall have to pack you off because I have a lot more work to do on this painting. But remember, please, if you value our friendship, keep your counsel. I do not want to be overrun with curious art-collectors. And if I am I shall lay the fault at your door and should be reluctant to allow you to visit my studio unscheduled again.'

'My dear friend,' Paolo looked at him with a hurt expression, 'how *could* you doubt that I would keep something like this to myself? Besides *I* could never afford it. It will remain a mystery but if ever it *is* sold and you know the buyer, please let me know.'

'You will be among the first,' Leonardo shook his head,

'but I am sure I never shall. My client is extremely secretive. He would be very annoyed if he knew of your discovery.' He went to a pile of canvases stacked in a corner and began to inspect them one by one. 'Now, to change the subject completely, I have something else which I think *might* interest you. It is attributable and is possibly for sale. It is an early Giordano, from his Neapolitan period. The owner, who is short of money, might well be interested in an offer from someone who can keep it in the country.'

Paolo remained where he was, nodding from time to time, but he didn't take in a word, his eyes on the painting on the easel, his mind rapidly scanning the list of possible people of fortune to whom it could belong.

On the industrial outskirts of Frankfurt the Planz Steelworks Company occupied several acres, its rolling sheds stretching in an even line beside the complex of offices and the huge cooling tower.

Reconstructed after the war, the steelworks was not one of the largest but one of the most efficient, the most technically up to date in Germany. It had only fallen into difficulties because of a number of management mistakes over the past years. It always seemed to be replacing the managing director, and the highly qualified technical staff, growing restless, had started to leave in droves.

The advantages of adding a steel mill to his holdings presented to Simeon Varga a natural progression from the Yokkaichi electronic components company and other technical enterprises, to which he had added a Japanese company manufacturing TV sets, a machine tool company in Chicago making microchips, and various other technical companies scattered throughout the globe which, by now, far outnumbered the pharmaceuticals side. AP International was turning into an industrial conglomerate of vast proportions and everything he had read about, and was now seeing with his own eyes, concerning IC Planz he liked.

He sat in the boardroom with the chief executives drinking coffee after lunch. The strain on those Germans, forbidden to smoke their favourite after-lunch cigars or cigarettes, was clear for all to see; but they were under strict instructions and Herr Varga was much too important a man to offend.

Next to Varga sat Tony Liddle who had brought with him his inevitable desk top computer which was spewing forth facts and figures and into which he continued to feed fresh data.

Liddle looked grey with fatigue, having been without more than a few hours' sleep in two days. All night he'd spent working at the hotel, and the night before that. Varga, on the contrary, looked well rested; well rested and supremely confident of securing, after months of negotiations, his prey.

He liked the Germans. They were anxious to please, clued up and aware of the company's shortcomings. However they were not begging and were as determined as he to drive a hard bargain.

'I need sixty per cent of the company,' he said again. 'I need control.'

'Alas,' Herr Adler the managing director ran a hand over his smooth cheek, 'we would only part with fifty. Fifty—fifty. It's fair, Mr Varga. It's very fair. We have a lot to offer.'

'Sixty—forty,' Varga said again.

'How about fifty-five—forty-five?' Liddle said without looking up, tapping more figures into the keyboard and staring at the screen to see what emerged.

'Sixty—forty.' Varga looked at his watch. 'It seems all my efforts have been wasted. Could you ask your secretary to call my pilot and ask him to have the plane ready for,' he looked at Liddle, 'shall we say six o'clock?'

Liddle, quite used by now to the games his boss played, nodded. 'That's fine, Mr Varga.'

Herr Adler sat gazing at them rather as a poker player views his opponents. His expression remained inscrutable, his fingers tapping quietly on the table.

'If I could have a few minutes with you in private, Mr Varga,' he said, glancing at his companions, who appeared to understand him implicitly and nodded in agreement.

'Well . . .' Varga again pointedly looked at his watch.

'I think you will find it well worth your time, Mr Varga,' Herr Adler insisted. 'It may help you to see why we are so anxious to retain our fifty per cent.'

'Very well. Ten minutes.' Varga rose and looked at Tony, who started to rise too, until Adler hastily intervened.

'It will have to be just the two of us, Mr Varga. I think you will understand why.'

'In that case . . . I decline your invitation. Mr Liddle is fully in my confidence.'

'Oh, very well.' Adler smiled at Liddle, who carefully closed his computer and prepared to carry it with him.

'I'm sure that won't be necessary,' Adler said.

'I prefer it,' Liddle replied.

'Very well. This way please.'

Herr Adler preceded them out of the room and Varga and Liddle followed him into the white corridor which ran the length of the building. In the distance was the faint outline of the Taunus mountains where Varga and Liddle had been staying in one of the beautiful spa hotels of the area. As he shut the door behind him, Varga turned to see Herr Adler waiting for him with a curious light in his eyes.

'Now, Herr Adler?'

'I have something to show you and your colleague, Herr Varga. I think it will interest you. It will make all the difference to how you feel about sharing in a joint venture with us. Follow me, please.' Herr Adler beckoned, and began to walk quickly along the corridor, Varga hurrying to keep up with him.

'If it's so important, why didn't you show this to me before?'

'It was a risk I had to take. It is an extremely secret project. I had to know you were serious. I think you will be most impressed.'

Varga was intrigued and, eyebrows raised, glanced at Liddle. He respected the Germans, and the research facilities he had been shown were impressive. However he also thought them devious and cunning, but after dealing with the Japanese, to say nothing about the Arabs and the Americans, he thought he knew quite well how to handle them; never lose one's temper or show excessive emotion of any kind. Be inscrutable, be cool. His face was always mask-like, his expression detached, polite but unyielding of the secrets that lay behind that carefully controlled façade.

The two men accompanied Herr Adler through a series of doors, down a short flight of steps and into the laboratory they had visited only that morning. However there was obviously someone, or something, they had not seen. Herr Adler stopped outside a door that could only be opened by means of a security pass, and this led to another door which was opened in the same way. Simeon realized they were in a part of the laboratory block he knew nothing about and had not been shown. He began to feel uneasy.

'Why were we not shown this this morning, Herr Adler?' he hissed, but Adler put a finger to his lips as he opened yet a third door which led into a long laboratory which was entirely lit by artificial light. There were windows but they were all hidden by steel shutters which were firmly locked and barred.

'This is where we do our secret work, Herr Varga. *Most* secret.'

There were several technicians working at benches in the lab, but none of them seemed perturbed by the appearance of the MD and his guests. Some didn't even look up. One technician, masked and gowned, his hands covered with thick asbestos gloves, was turning something in a cabinet whose only access was through a tunnel which the highly protected operator had his arms in. Casually Varga glanced at it but could only see a circular dish with some transparent liquid in it bubbling away over a hidden jet.

At the far side of the lab was an office with glass windows, and inside this a man, also in a white coat, sat working at his desk. When he saw Adler he jumped up and came to the door just as they reached it. He was tall, thin, with steel-rimmed spectacles, a man of scholarly appearance, and he gravely shook hands with Varga and Liddle as they were introduced.

'This is Dr Helmut Schree. He is the head of research and development. Dr Schree, I may have mentioned Mr Varga to you in our brief discussions yesterday.'

'Yes you did, Herr Adler.' Unsmilingly Dr Schree shook Varga's hand.

'How do you do, Herr Varga?'

'How do you do, Dr Schree? My associate, Herr Liddle.'

'How do you do, Herr Liddle?'

Dr Schree politely indicated the interior of his office and the three visitors entered and sat down while Dr Schree returned to the chair at the other side of his desk. There he joined his hands before him and regarded them gravely.

'How can I be of assistance to you, Herr Adler?'

'I have decided to tell Herr Varga about our secret project.' Seeing the look of alarm on Dr Schree's face he added quickly, 'I know you may not consider it wise, but I think it will be the carrot that will induce Herr Varga to invest in this venture with us. Unless he has control he wishes to withdraw. Naturally *we* are reluctant to give him control because of our undertaking to our most important customer.' He turned to Varga. 'That stipulated total secrecy, Herr Varga. The project is known only to a few people in this company, and I must ask for your complete and total discretion on this matter.'

'I think you can rely on that,' Varga said with a trace

of impatience. '*If* it is tempting enough I shall soon be on the board of the company.'

'Well,' Adler made a gesture and Dr Schree rose and went across to a heavy steel cabinet in the corner which consisted of a single drawer operated by a dial. With his back to the visitors he turned the dial several times, first one way and then the other, and when the door opened he extracted from it a roll of plans which he proceeded to unroll on the desk in front of them.

Looking at the diagram, Varga's immediate reaction was that they were meaningless to him: a series of highly complex technical plans with equations on either side.

Dr Schree fastened the sheet by its corners to his desk and then held out a hand, inviting Varga and Liddle to study it.

'Take your time, Herr Varga,' Herr Adler said, with a smile for Dr Schree, and, with a slight feeling of unease at his obvious ignorance, Varga pored for some time over the plan in front of him.

'Make any sense to you?' Adler said after a while with a superior smile.

'I'm afraid not,' Varga said stiffly, sitting up. 'I am not a technical man, you know. Anything to you, Tony?'

Liddle shook his head without replying.

'What you are looking at, Herr Varga and Herr Liddle,' Adler said proudly, 'is a system of hydraulic cylinders for one of the biggest petrochemical projects in the Middle East. We are manufacturing these vast steel cylinders for an unnamed client.'

'Is that all?' Varga looked unimpressed.

'All?' Adler looked shocked. 'All, you say? This is a project of immense scope. It and its implications are vast. It is the most important project we have on hand at the moment and will net billions of marks. The scale of the project is incalculable.'

'Then why do you need my money?' Varga leaned back, his hands in his pockets. 'And who is your client in the Middle East?'

'That,' Adler turned to Schree for confirmation, 'we don't know. We act through an intermediary. The investment on our part is vast, hence the need for additional capital. But the profits are vast, too. When in place the hydraulic system will enable them to outstrip all their competitors in the supply of oil to the entire world.'

'I see.' Varga stroked his chin. 'Very impressive.'

'These giant cylinders you see are approximately a metre wide,' Schree went on. 'They are lined and capable of extension . . .'

Varga listened, understanding very little, while Liddle stared alternately at the plans and the two Germans.

'A completely new concept . . .' Schree droned on, 'operated hydraulically to speed the flow of oil.'

'It will double the output from the refineries,' Adler explained.

'Does this have government approval?' Varga interrupted the flow to look sharply at Adler.

'Naturally we have submitted the plans to the government, and in our experimental rolling mills,' he gestured towards one of the closely shuttered windows, 'we have already begun the process.'

'May one see them, do you think?' Liddle spoke for the first time, pointing to the plans. 'To the layman these mean nothing.'

The two steelmen looked at each other and then, at a nod from Adler, Schree opened the drawer in his desk and took from it a bunch of keys.

'Please come with me, gentlemen.'

Once again they trooped after him, out of another door, through a corridor, across a covered passage into one of the experimental rolling mills from which came the noises and hisses associated with the manufacture of steel. They were given protective glasses and asked to wear helmets and, as they were admitted, they stood for a while on the threshold of the building accustoming themselves to the noise and glare as the giant tubes were extruded from the presses.

It was a fascinating, almost awe-inspiring experience and for a time Liddle and Varga stood transfixed by the sheer size, complexity, and even beauty of the operation.

Shouting so that he could be heard above the noise, Schree explained that these were the liners for the pipes which were assembled in the shed next door.

'Would you like to see those?' Varga nodded and the party was led across another covered way and into a shed where a blissful silence prevailed. It was quite a sight to see the layers of gleaming steel pipes which awaited the insertion of liners before transportation to their destination. For a moment Varga and Liddle gazed at them, impressed by the scale of the operation.

'There's one thing I'd like to ask.' Liddle turned to Schree. 'In one of your plans the pipes appear to have a sharp elevation.' He lifted his arm at an angle of forty-five degrees or so. 'Does this mean they are intended to go uphill, or downhill perhaps?'

'Of course.' Schree looked perplexed as though only a fool would ask such a question. 'The terrain is uneven.'

'I thought it was just desert?'

'Oh no.' Both Adler and Schree looked amused. 'The country in question is a very *mountainous* one.'

'How mountainous?' Varga was interested because of the sorties his aeroplanes had to make from the Turkish border across to Iran and Iraq and he thought a knowledge of the topography would help him place the destination.

By this time, however, it was nearly five and his aeroplane had been ordered for early evening. He felt he'd learned all that he could from the steelmen for the time being.

'We'll give you a decision in a day or two,' he said, turning to go.

'I do think it will have to be now, Herr Varga,' Adler said uneasily as they left the shed without Dr Schree, who was talking to one of the technicians on the site. 'We have let you have access to *very* secret information.

You can see what a tremendous project it is. I think you have all the information you could possibly want.'

'Indeed.' Varga looked at Liddle, who nodded. 'I think in that case we say "yes".' He confirmed this with Liddle, who again imperceptibly nodded his head.

'Fifty–fifty, Herr Varga?'

'Fifty–fifty,' Varga replied. 'And then you can take the blame if anything goes wrong.'

'Wrong, Herr Varga?' Adler blinked in surprise. 'What can go wrong? You saw the scale of the enterprise, the excellence of the product.'

'Anything can go wrong.' Varga gave him a superior smile. 'So, in exchange for my money I want some indemnity. We'll send you the papers and the draft contract in a few days. Liddle will probably come over with them. Right, Liddle?'

'Right, Mr Varga,' Liddle replied.

'I'd better hurry or I'll miss my dinner date,' Varga said, smiling at Adler. 'Aren't I a lucky fellow? I buy into a profitable steel business and I am about to be married to a beautiful woman.'

'My felicitations, Mr Varga,' Adler said sycophantically, the relief on his face clearly visible as he shook hands.

A fast car took Varga and Liddle to the airport and they were only a little late for the plane, which had stood waiting on the tarmac. The car drove them straight to the aircraft after the briefest of customs formalities and the pilot stood waiting at the door together with a uniformed stewardess with her abnormally cheerful smile.

'Successful day, Mr Varga?' she asked, taking his coat.

'I think so, Karen,' Varga replied, entering the aircraft. 'Did you hear from my fiancée?'

'She will meet you at Luton, Mr Varga.'

'Good.' Varga looked relieved and turned to Liddle, motioning him to sit down and fasten his safety belt as, after the preliminary calls and checks, the Gulf Stream jet took off. They sat silently for a while, the inevitable

275

moment of tension, until told that the cruising speed had been reached and they could unfasten their belts.

The stewardess brought over to them a tray on which there were glasses and a bottle of whisky.

'Ah, just what I need,' Varga said, rubbing his hands. 'We have a little celebration, I think, Tony, eh?'

'Well,' Tony, assisted by Karen, removed his jacket and smiled as she took it away, 'if *you're* happy I'm happy; but,' his face clouded momentarily, 'what did you think of that operation?'

'What operation?'

'The hydraulic tubes allegedly for petrochemicals? I thought you climbed down from sixty–forty very quickly. You didn't even haggle. That's not like you, Simeon.' The accountant appeared mystified and gazed at his boss, who was looking at the night sky out of the aircraft window, an expression of satisfaction on his face.

'Those "tubes",' he said, turning to Liddle, 'didn't they remind you of something?' As Liddle looked puzzled Varga imitated the action he had made with his arm, tilting it at the elbow at an angle of forty-five degrees. 'I thought you were on to it.'

'On to what?'

'What about a gun?' Varga lowered his voice so that even Karen in the galley couldn't hear. 'Or a missile launcher?'

'A *gun*?' Liddle nearly choked on the word. 'That size?'

'Some sort of huge gun, or missile launcher, hidden in the mountains of Iraq or Iran. Dozens of them with projectiles that could hit all their neighbouring states. They are all at loggerheads with one another, and then there is Israel. I daren't even mention that.'

'You *are* joking, aren't you, Simeon?' Liddle moistened his lips.

'Not at all. Petrochemicals my foot.'

'You wouldn't *seriously* get implicated in anything like that?'

'I wouldn't know.' Varga smiled and took a gulp of his

whisky. 'I said I didn't know and I shan't ask any more questions. I shall simply refer to it as "the project" and if it ever gets out I shall be very angry and say I was deceived. I asked for indemnity, don't forget. In the meantime,' he raised his glass to Liddle, 'it is a very profitable project indeed and our investment is as safe as houses. Can *you* do better than that, Tony?'

'You're ingenious, Simeon. But I hope you're wrong. I think you're sailing close enough to the wind already.'

'You never get rich without taking risks.' Varga, looking completely at ease, smiled at him. 'Trust my intuition.'

'Intuition?'

'Beaufort is sending arms to Iran and Iraq. The Middle East is in ferment. Steel, guns, missile launchers – I don't care. It will be very nice and very profitable to be on the side of whoever wins.' He raised his glass again and winked. 'Cheers, Tony.'

'Cheers,' Tony said, but his eyes were thoughtful as he sipped his drink.

Thoughtful, apprehensive and, perhaps, just a little bit afraid.

CHAPTER 15

Ginny, having finished her tour of the premises, sat down dispiritedly and gratefully accepted the coffee which Roger Bennet's secretary had brought. Opposite her the managing director of Oriole looked just as depressed and smoked nervously, frequently tipping the ash from his Gauloise into an ashtray which was already full of stubs. How Simeon would have disapproved, Ginny thought, feeling a slight lifting of the spirits at this injection of a little humour into what had otherwise been a rather unhappy morning.

The premises of Oriole looked more derelict than when she had first visited them with Simeon over two years before. But worse, the atmosphere had degenerated, the laboratories were still old-fashioned and operated with old equipment, old methods. They even had ancient Bunsen burners which most modern manufacturers had discarded years ago.

In addition, Roger Bennet, who had at one time seemed a white hope, lured from another manufacturer to head the Oriole works, looked on the verge of a nervous breakdown with his tetchy manner and endless smoking, anathema to the true perfumer.

'I had no idea things were so bad.' Ginny sat forward on the edge of her chair.

'I'm sorry, Miss Silklander.' Roger ran his hands through his hair, rendering his appearance, if possible, even more wild. 'Mr Varga has not put a penny into this business since he bought it.'

'Oh come,' Ginny protested, 'I thought he had completely recapitalized it?'

'He saved it from becoming *totally* derelict,' Roger said savagely. 'That is, he gave enough to stop the buildings falling down. There was a certain amount of vital expenditure necessary to comply with French government and EC regulations, otherwise the buildings would have been unfit. But investment in new products?' Roger almost snarled. 'Not a penny.'

'But have you talked to him?'

'I have written to him, faxed him and spoken to him on the telephone, but,' Roger bowed his head and stared at his untidy desk, 'he is just not interested, Miss Silklander, I can tell you that. I think if he could get his money back he would sell the company.'

'In that case he would lose money,' Ginny said grimly. She stood up, went to the window where, for a few moments, she stood staring through the grimy pane at the outbuildings. Then she turned and came over to the desk where Roger sat morosely watching her. 'I must say, I'm quite shocked, Roger, by what I've seen.'

'I'm sorry.'

'I'm surprised that Mr Liddle even passes the accounts.'

'Maybe as a loss-making business it's good for tax purposes.' Roger seemed to be making an effort to sound helpful. 'I tell you, if I hadn't moved my family over here lock, stock and barrel I wouldn't remain a day more. As it is my children have settled at school, my wife likes Paris and French life. It would be a big upheaval.'

Ginny's first thought had been that this clearly bad appointment of Varga's would have to go, but something about his attitude, his dejection, brought out her natural human instincts, not exactly of pity, but concern. His qualifications had been good – a science degree and experience in cosmetics – and when she had first met him she had thought him just the man for the job.

'Look,' she sat opposite him once more and put out her hands, 'I propose to take over Oriole. I shall become chief executive and retain you as managing director at least for six months . . .' She saw the expression of incredulity break over his face, but did not give him a chance to speak. 'If you can prove yourself in that time, Roger, I shall give you a longer contract. I can see you've had a hard time, but you also have to prove you have the mettle to run this outfit. What I've seen today has not impressed me. You've no inspiration. You've let it go to seed. Now, if you will let me have details of *all* your correspondence with Mr Varga I will see what I can do to get a fresh and immediate injection of funds.'

'But . . .' Roger Bennet lit another cigarette while the smoke from the previous one still rose from the ashtray. 'Really, Miss Silklander, I don't know what to say. Mr Varga might have warned me . . .'

'Mr Varga knew nothing about it,' Ginny said briskly, 'except that he knows I wish to develop a new fragrance and intended to spend a few days here. However, as you have probably heard, we are to be married. I feel I can't continue as director of publicity on the main board of AP International, so I suggested that I took a closer interest in Oriole. Becoming chief executive just occurred to me this morning. Naturally, I don't wish to spend all my time in France. I must have a good MD here.'

'When are you getting married, Miss Silklander?' Roger stumbled over his words. Clearly the grapevine had not reached him on the outskirts of Paris.

'That is not yet decided. Probably later in the summer. However in the meantime I wish to establish a base at Oriole and see what I can do. With your help I think I can achieve a great deal.'

'Oh you'll have *that*, Miss Silklander.' Roger tipped the contents of his ashtray into his wastepaper basket as though he was symbolically making a clean sweep and his face actually broke into a smile. '*Every* co-operation I can give you and more.'

280

'Now, who is in charge of product development?'
Ginny produced a notebook from her briefcase.

'Well, I am,' Roger stammered.

'But who is the "nose"? Who succeeded Pierre Jacquet?'

'Well,' Roger nervously ran a hand over his chin, 'well, there we have a problem. There is currently no experienced "nose" employed in the factory, Miss Silklander. We didn't have sufficient funds to attract anyone of the calibre of Pierre, who was first class.'

'You mean we are simply trading on the old stock?'

'Yes. We are repackaging L'Esprit du Temps.'

'Well that's no good.' Ginny angrily stamped her foot, wondering if she had after all been too tolerant with Roger Bennet. Maybe a man who had failed as dismally as he obviously had to regenerate the company should have been fired immediately and someone else hired. Then she remembered the little Bennets happy at their French schools; Mrs Bennet, probably a young, good-looking woman, cheerful in her new apartment. Maybe she enjoyed shopping in the chic Parisian stores and maybe she attended French classes as well. She cleared her throat.

'First, Roger, we have to engage a really first-class "nose". Now I am returning to London tonight and I shall have urgent talks with Mr Varga. I will get him to put in a substantial sum of money to revitalize this business; enough to modernize the factory and employ the best possible "nose" in France.'

'You know who that is, Miss Silklander?' Roger said, with a slightly malicious gleam in his eye.

'Who is it?' Pen poised, Ginny sat ready to write down the name.

'Pierre Jacquet.'

'Oh, we can't have him.' Ginny had started to write down the name and then crossed out what she had written.

'He is the best. The very best.'

281

'But he will *never* agree to return.'

'I think he might.' Roger cleared his throat. 'His father is not well and he is looking after him. It is difficult for him to travel and find other work, though doubtless he has had plenty of offers. I also happen to know that the circumstances in which the family have been left are not good.'

'But the father was paid a large sum of money for this firm.'

'Not a very large amount, Miss Silklander. There were debts. A mortgage. As you know the firm had not been doing well for years. Madame Jacquet had been kept in a nursing home. She has since died, but now the father is there too.'

'Oh dear!' Ginny was suddenly overwhelmed with guilt, remembering how peremptorily Varga had dismissed the Jacquets from a business that had been in family hands for three generations. Yes, he was a hard man. Fair, but hard. She often thought that maybe her love blinded her to his defects. She put such thoughts out of her mind and hurried on. 'I really am very sorry to hear that. Has Pierre Jacquet a family?'

'He never married, Miss Silklander. I think he has devoted his life to his work and the care of his aged parents.'

A life devoted to parents and the family firm, and Simeon had destroyed both. Such were the tragedies of many a business venture which the onlooker couldn't see; couldn't possibly know.

'He didn't seem very old to me.' Ginny felt mortified.

'He was a gift to elderly parents,' Roger Bennet explained. 'I believe they were well into their forties when their son was born. He is not much more than thirty now.'

Ginny remembered Pierre Jacquet as tall, dignified, rather solemn, a figure standing in the background, someone with the air of an aesthete. Certainly not a businessman. Simeon's behaviour seemed even more calculatedly cold and cruel, dictated solely by business. And then, having destroyed the family, he had let the business go.

Well, this was the man she was going to marry. Maybe, in time, she would change him.

'I don't know that Mr Varga would like Pierre Jacquet to be reinstated,' she said. 'I have a feeling he has definite ideas on the matter.'

'Perhaps you needn't mention it to him at the moment, Miss Silklander,' Bennet said. 'I'm sure that, once you have established your new regime here, you will be able to do as you like.'

The man stood almost threateningly over Varga's desk; but Varga, unimpressed, continued his examination of the balance sheet before him, chin in hand, eyes registering disapproval.

'But this is the best blue chip stock in the country, Mr Varga.' The man brought his fist down on the desk in front of Varga.

'Then why is it so cheap?' Varga's eyes rose to meet those of the man who he had spent an hour grilling, doing his best to reduce his self-esteem to a very low level, partly succeeding.

'Because the company is in difficulties.'

'Well then?' Varga smiled at him. 'Blue chip, eh?'

'Our customers don't pay up.'

'That's your lookout.' Varga closed the file containing the balance sheets and threw it across the desk before turning to Liddle, who sat beside him.

'What do you think, Tony?'

'I should pay a little above par for the stock, Mr Varga. Not much more.'

'Right, two per cent above par,' Varga said, sitting back as though his interest had already waned and his mind was on something else.

'But that's ridiculous.' The man flopped down in the chair behind him as though he needed its support.

'Take it or leave it,' Varga looked at his watch, 'it makes very little difference to me. I'm afraid I have another engagement, Mr Wright. If the deal is agreeable my financial director will draw up the papers. If not . . .'

'Maybe I could have another word with Mr Liddle.' Mr Wright was clearly climbing down, his self-esteem very near rock bottom.

'Good. Fine.' Varga smiled at him and indicated that Tony should accompany him.

Wright leaned over to shake Varga's hand, his clasp very light.

'Nice to see you, Mr Wright,' Varga said amiably. 'I hope I have good news from Mr Liddle when you've had your talk.'

Varga, despite his brutal methods and the results he unfailingly got, was always polite.

Moreover, his apparent magnanimity earned him a good name in the City even if there were those who knew better. And those who did kept their silence, either because they didn't want to risk offending Varga or because they thought no one would believe them.

His image of a quiet, courteous, clever businessman, secretive but of unquestioned integrity, was carefully cultivated by Ginny and those who served him. His dislike of publicity was approved of. He was regarded as serious, cautious, above all sound.

The fifty per cent stake in a prestigious German specialist steel company had been pleasing to the City, and his shares had again risen sharply as a result.

In the next room he could hear Ginny busy on the phone and, rising, he went over to the door that divided them and gently began to open it.

'No, not one of the largest steel plants,' Ginny was saying, 'but one of the most respected. Special steels . . . oh, used for precision work, jobs such as petrochemicals. Yes, maybe a country in the Gulf. I'm afraid I can't say more. The shares rose another thirty pence on the news. Yes, of course I'll send you details.'

And now, Varga knew, another hastily assembled but perfectly produced glossy brochure would go out detailing the achievements of AP International and its most recent acquisition. The fact that he had only got half of Planz rankled, but then he remembered Oriole. He was a man who usually, in time, got his way.

Ginny looked up as he came through the door, noticing the glow on his face as he stooped to kiss her.

'You look pleased with yourself,' she said, clutching his hand.

'With good reason,' he perched on the edge of her desk and touched her hair, 'I have you.'

'I think there's another reason.' She planted a quick kiss on the back of his hand.

'One of the best cement companies in the country is mine.'

'Oh?' She made a note on the pad beside her.

'At least, I think it is. Confirm it with Liddle.'

'That is?'

'Polair Cement of Newcastle.'

'Sounds terribly unglamorous,' Ginny said, scribbling.

'But very profitable. At the moment I'm acquiring either outright, or an interest in, a company every ten days. I shall soon run out of money.'

'Oh Simeon, I hope not.' Momentarily Ginny looked dismayed before she looked up and saw the smile on his face. 'You're kidding.'

'Yes, I'm kidding. But I may have to have another rights issue. I don't want to overborrow at the banks. I never like being in their clutches. They are, you know, only fair weather friends.'

'But you have some very *good* friends in the banks.'

'Only as long as I do well.'

'Darling, you will go on doing well . . .'

'See anything of Robert?' He glanced casually at her.

'I wasn't even invited to his wedding.' She pretended to look dismayed.

'Oh good. He's married.'

'Well and truly. Simeon . . .' she reached out again for his hand, 'never *doubt* my love for you.'

'I don't, Ginny,' he said tenderly. 'Now, do you fancy a bite at Le Gavroche?'

'Well . . .' she glanced at the load on her desk. 'Why don't we send out for sandwiches? I've got a lot to do and there's something I want to talk seriously to you about.'

'Suits me,' Varga said, lifting up the phone. 'We can dine somewhere nice tonight. Oh, Dorothy, get us some sandwiches would you? And coffee. Coffee, darling?' Ginny nodded. 'A pot of coffee, please, Dorothy. Thank you.'

He replaced the receiver and, getting off the desk, sank into a chair by the window, his eyes on Ginny.

'What is this important thing, my darling?'

'Simeon.' Ginny left her desk and, drawing up a chair sat down next to him, turning her face towards him so that she had his whole attention. 'It's about Oriole.'

'I guessed it might be.' He smiled encouragingly at her.

'We've hardly had time to talk about it since I got back. But I am very concerned about it.'

'Ginny,' he leaned forward and took her hand, 'I am really completely uninterested in Oriole. I think you know that now. I have so many new really big, important ventures, they transcend any interest I have in a has-been perfume concern. I have progressed a lot in the past two years.'

'You destroyed a family for a whim,' she said accusingly.

'What on earth do you mean, Ginny?' His brows knitted fiercely together.

'It was a well run family business.'

'It was not well run.'

'But you didn't really want it.'

'At the time I thought I did. What's got into you, Ginny? At the time it was your idea.'

'The Jacquets were not left well off. They had debts . . .'

'That's their fault, not mine. Darling, you can't be *sentimental* in business. If you are you won't succeed. That's lesson number one.'

'And lesson number two?'

'Follow me and you can't go wrong.' He leaned towards her. 'I know it's chauvinistic and you won't approve, but you look so lovely when you're angry.'

'I'm not angry. I was upset about the Jacquets; but I suppose you're right. Anyway, my suggestion is that I take over Oriole completely.'

'You do such a good job here,' he said, looking at her desk, 'I can't bear to lose you. On the phone just now . . .'

'Simeon, it will simply *not* do for me to remain here as your wife, you know that. It looks bad and it is bad.'

'Then the house. There is plenty for you to do *there*.'

'You know I don't *just* want to be a housewife.'

'Ginny,' he drew her hand up to his lips, 'you know I would like family . . .'

'And I would too,' she faltered. They had only ever discussed the matter once and that seemed now a long time ago.

'You're thirty, my darling,' he put his face close to hers. 'It's not *old* . . .'

'It's not old . . . but certainly it's not something I should leave for too long,' she replied. 'However, being a wife and mother would not be incompatible with my running a perfume business. I have even suggested to Bennet that I become chief executive and he stays on as managing director.'

'Oh, really?' Varga looked up as Dorothy came in with a tray on which there were sandwiches and a pot of freshly made coffee.

'Excellent, Dorothy, and book at the Caprice would you for tonight, please?'

'Certainly, Mr Varga,' she glanced across at Ginny, 'for two, of course?'

'Of course,' he said with a smile, 'and no telephone calls while we have lunch, Dorothy. We have something important to discuss.'

'Of course, sir. Oh, Mr Liddle asked me to tell you that the deal was on. Mr Wright left a few minutes ago.'

'Excellent. I thought it would be.' Varga gave a smile of triumph to Ginny. 'See?'

As his secretary slid out of the room, Varga jumped up and passed a plate to Ginny with a sandwich on it. 'That is *excellent* news. I played him like a fish on a very long line.'

'How much is it costing?'

'A few million.' He took a sandwich and began to eat it hungrily.

'Oriole needs a few million.'

'That's no problem.'

'Then it's on?' She looked relieved.

'Of course it's on, if you wish it!'

She knew that the change in his humour, his attitude, was because of the cement deal. He thrived on deals. The adrenalin flowed and the blood sugar rose. Deals were meat and drink, regardless of what they were about. Cement, steel, airlines, pharmaceuticals, and now perfume.

She owed his rapid change in attitude to the new deal and she welcomed it.

'For a *while* I can do both jobs.' She would compromise to show her appreciation.

'Good. Incidentally, I am going to see Carlo about the divorce.'

She felt the pace of her heart quickening.

'Oh, *Simeon*! It's really happening?'

'It's really happening, darling, and I can't tell you how excited about it I am. This is emphatically going to be our year.'

*

288

The marble portals of the Bernini frontage in Albemarle Street had never daunted Simeon Varga, even when, regarded as an impoverished exile by Claudia's family, he had first been summoned there for his interview with Antonio, Claudia's formidable old father who had a face like wrinkled parchment.

Signor Bernini had made it quite plain that he thought Varga was no suitable match for his daughter but, as she was of age and, according to Claudia, deeply in love, he had no option but to agree. However there were stipulations: he had to move into a house of Claudia's choice, for which her father would pay, the children had to be brought up as Roman Catholics and there would be no question of divorce, ever.

At that time Varga had considered the conditions easy to fulfil and was only too willing to comply. However, to a man deeply burdened by a sense of insecurity, Varga's marriage had the effect of weakening rather than strengthening him. He felt continually dominated and oppressed by the wealth, the disdain of the Berninis, and maybe it was because of them he had striven so hard to succeed. Maybe for this he owed them a debt, he thought, as his car deposited him at the kerb outside the building and, as it purred away, he stood for a few moments, hands in his pockets, gazing at the plate glass windows with their fabulous but discreet display of priceless jewels.

The Berninis were still a force to be reckoned with. But so, now, was he.

The uniformed commissionaire had sprung to open the door and, as Varga strolled through it, he saluted smartly.

'Mr Carlo is expecting you, Mr Varga.' Still the old-fashioned reference to Mr Carlo, Mr Matteo, as if the older man, always Signor Bernini, were still alive.

Varga crossed the spacious salon with its deep pile carpet, its antique bureaux and easy chairs to the lift and was taken to the second floor, to the office overlooking the backs of the buildings facing Old Bond Street.

Carlo stood waiting for him in the corridor outside the lift and, as Varga emerged, amiably stretched out his hand.

'Hello, Simeon. Good to see you again.'

Seeing no need for such hypocrisy, Varga made no reply, but tepidly shook his brother-in-law's hand, rather puzzled at his affability. He stiffened himself for an astronomical figure to be placed on the divorce settlement.

Carlo was alone and, once inside his office, he carefully closed and locked the door, a normal precaution in the jewellery business. He then pointed to the pair of bergère chairs and Varga chose one with its back to the windows, so that he would have the light off his face. As Carlo sat opposite him he reminded Varga of a painting of a medieval pope, his face set in grave lines – adamant, devious and cunning.

'I have asked for coffee to be sent in, Simeon. Would you care for a cigar? Oh of course not . . .' Carlo put a finger to his mouth and smiled. 'How could I possibly forget? I shan't smoke, then.'

'Thank you.' Varga minimally inclined his head.

'You know, Simeon, we don't see you. One forgets these things.'

'I suppose any moment you're going to tell me that you miss me.' Varga glanced impatiently at his watch, his mind already on his next appointment.

'I think in a way we do miss you. And I think Claudia misses you, the children as well . . .'

'I hope we're not here to discuss a reconciliation.' Varga stared aggressively at his brother-in-law. 'If so, we are wasting our time.'

'Ah . . .' Carlo paused as there was a discreet knock on the door and got up to admit his secretary with a coffee jug and cups on a silver tray, undoubtedly sterling.

'Thank you, Frances,' he said. 'Mr Varga and I will look after ourselves.'

Frances said nothing but went to the door, followed

by Carlo, who opened it for her and locked it again afterwards.

'Black as usual, Simeon? I think I remember that.'

'Please. No sugar.' Simeon began to feel restless.

'You find the children well?' Carlo brought the delicate porcelain cup over to him and placed it on the table by his elbow.

'I think so, and doing well at school.'

'Yes, despite the fact that you and their mother are separated.'

Varga took a sip of his coffee, and his arm shot out again to examine the face of his watch. 'Now, can we come to the point, Carlo? I have a very busy schedule. I expect you have too. I am here to inform you, officially, that it is five years since Claudia and I have lived as man and wife and that on those grounds I am petitioning for divorce. As I've indicated, there will be a generous settlement. She only works here because she wishes to. Now if you, she and the family are in agreement, my solicitor has worked out the details.' Varga reached inside his breast pocket and, producing a long legal envelope, handed it to Carlo, who however shook his head, his hands remaining in his lap.

'Here, take it,' Varga said, edging it forward.

'No thank you, Simeon. You see I think you have your facts wrong.' Carlo appeared to settle more comfortably in his chair and stretched out his legs before him, hands joined at the fingertips.

'What do you mean, I have my *facts* wrong?' Varga's scowl deepened.

'According to Claudia it is only three years.'

'It is *five*.' Suspecting a trap – maybe he had always known the byzantine Berninis would think of some last-minute hitch – Varga stood up, slapped the document down on the table next to him and, arms folded, confronted his brother-in-law. 'What are you trying to say?'

'According to Claudia you did not live apart for those two years that you say you did.'

'Of course we did! We had separate bedrooms. You know that. I remember how upset your mother was when she found out.'

'Ah yes,' Carlo held up a finger, 'separate bedrooms, but was there not the *occasional* conjugal visit to the next bedroom?'

'No, there was not,' Varga replied. 'Claudia and I had no marital relations from that day on. In fact we'd abandoned them some time before.'

'She says you had not.'

'Well, we had!'

'She remembers a wedding anniversary. For old time's sake.'

'She remembers wrong. She is making it up and you know it. Probably you put her up to it.'

'She will swear.' Carlo examined his well-kept nails. 'It is your word against hers. That of a deeply religious woman against a known unbeliever.'

'You're not suggesting . . .' Varga leaned threateningly over his brother-in-law.

'All I'm *saying*,' Carlo leaned back in the chair, his expression bland, 'is that there will be no divorce under the present laws of this country for at least another two years; by which time, of course, we all hope there will be a reconciliation. Claudia loves you; the children love you . . .'

'Balls . . .' Varga roared. 'Claudia does *not* love me.'

'She insists she does. She is anxious for the children to have their father at home again. She swears this time she will do everything she can to make you happy. She will give up work. I believe you are buying a home in the country . . . she would like that.'

By this time Varga was so angry that he felt the room had started to revolve. Concerned for the effect on his health he sat down again.

'This is blackmail,' he said, shaking a finger at Carlo. 'This is just to get some more money out of me. Well then you can have it,' he threw up his hands, 'name your figure. As long as it doesn't take every penny I have, you can have it.'

Now Carlo rose and, as if forgetful of Varga's dislike of smoking, he carefully peeled the band off a cigar and put it in his mouth. But before lighting it he stood there gazing with unconcealed pleasure at his visitor.

'It is not money we are after, Varga,' he enunciated his words very carefully, 'it is justice. Justice for my wronged sister, my nephew and niece. Justice for the honour of our family. My mother has aged ten years in these few years. You promised our father there would be no divorce, and for women as religious as my mother the situation is almost unendurable.'

'Your mother is a vicious, tough old bird,' Varga pointed the accusing finger at him again, 'so don't try and take me in. I know you and your family, Bernini: hypocrites, the lot of you. Not one of you is really the least bit religious, especially Claudia. It is just form, habit, tradition . . .'

'Well, we happen to like form, habit and tradition,' Carlo said, lowering his voice. 'It is what we were brought up on.'

'You know perfectly well I won't come back, so why do you try and stop me? If it's not money what is it?'

'Money is of no real concern to us,' Carlo said loftily, 'you know that. We have plenty, if not as much as you *appear* to have.' He emphasized the word 'appear' in a suggestively insulting tone. He looked behind him and carefully sat down again. 'It is simply our intention to make life as difficult as possible for you, Varga; to deprive *you* of the beautiful, aristocratic wife you have set your heart on for as long as we can. I'll be frank with you. It is, if you like, a kind of vengeance for all the harm you have done, the suffering you have caused.'

'It is totally futile,' Varga replied coldly. 'Ginny and I will never split. We are together for ever.'

'Didn't you say that to Claudia?' Carlo asked with a sneer.

'The circumstances were different. We were both young. I was scarcely tolerated by your family, never mind liked. I am surprised that you're not anxious to be rid of me; to get me out of your life so that, while she is still young, Claudia may perhaps marry again, a man of whom your family will approve, though I don't expect there are many paragons around, even in the Italian community.'

'My mother would never permit her to marry again. In our religion it is for life,' Carlo said loftily.

'In your religion, yes,' Varga stabbed his finger at him again, 'your antiquated version of Catholicism, yes. But in the modern church, in the modern day, I thought these things were better understood. Mistakes made when one was young can be rectified.'

'Not by the Catholic Church. It does not recognize divorce and would not remarry a divorced Catholic. Such a person would be denied the sacraments, the comfort of her faith, and Claudia would find the situation intolerable.'

Varga was silent. He knew that in fact what Carlo was saying was right: brainwashed since childhood, Claudia went to Mass and received the sacrament. She obeyed the rules. The days on which they made love had been regulated by a calendar so that they could practise, successfully as it happened, birth control. Maybe this as much as anything had made his marriage that much more difficult, more intolerable, than it would otherwise have been. Maybe her religion had helped to cool his ardour and drive a wedge between them as much as anything else.

Suddenly he felt in the grip of a sense of despair, as though a great pit had suddenly opened and he stood on the side of it peering down. The plans for the house, for Ginny, for a family of their own . . . well, they would only be postponed. Two years. He put his hands over his face. Two years. At the moment it seemed like a lifetime. It *was* like a lifetime. Who knew what else could happen, what other dastardly plots the Bernini family would not dream up in two long years?

He rose and for a moment or two he and Carlo stared each other out. Carlo was the first to lower his eyes. He too stood up and shrugged his shoulders, his mobile features moulded in an artificial expression of regret.

'I'm terribly sorry,' he said, 'but there it is.'

'I will not forget this, Carlo,' Varga intoned. 'I will not forgive, or forget. One day you will be very, very sorry for thwarting me.'

'My dear Varga, if there was anything I could do, I would . . .' Carlo shrugged expressively again. 'It was just my unhappy task to convey to you the decision of the family. If you would like to see Claudia maybe you too would have a change of heart?'

'Tell Claudia,' Varga leaned forward and touched him on the chest, 'I never wish to see her again or, for that matter, my children either. As far as I am concerned they might as well all be dead. But that won't be the end. You will suffer. You, personally; believe me, I'll make sure of it.'

As Varga's Jaguar drove up to the pavement again and the chauffeur alighted to open the door for him, Carlo Bernini peered down from the window, his eyes fixed on the figure below. He had lit his cigar and he puffed furiously at it, aware of an emotion in his breast that was part anger, part fear.

Sometimes it didn't do to battle with the beast. He felt in a way that he had been placed under some kind of curse and that, one day, Varga would indeed carry out his promise to destroy him.

Some new, intangible quality that he had never known before now made him for the first time in his life afraid of Simeon Varga. But it was too late. A Bernini would never, could never, go back on his word.

His mother would never allow it.

CHAPTER 16

Ginny had been feeling tense and tired all day. Maybe it was the time of the month, or maybe it was the important meeting that she knew was taking place between Simeon and his wife's family. The divorce should be automatic now. Why then did she have this uncomfortable feeling that something would go wrong? Maybe it was because she feared that Carlo might want to attempt some last-minute reconciliation.

It was silly to worry. Whatever happened they would be together. There was a commitment on both their parts; a commitment for life. Whether in this day and age one was married or not was not supposed to matter. But it mattered to her, it mattered to Simeon, and it mattered a whole lot to her family.

Family.

Maybe it was the letter on her desk from Angus that was at the root of the trouble. She had known it was a mistake for Simeon to get involved; yet he did it from the best of motives. Though now these were being questioned.

> Dearest Gin (Angus had written, the affectionate diminutive that most of her family used from time to time)
>
> Did you know that Simeon wants all the land as well as the farm and outbuildings? He says he

is only doing it to help us and we appreciate it; but my initial understanding with him was that he would buy the house and lease it back to me to save me taking out a mortgage. The leasing back terms just received from his accountant are really generous and we appreciate it, so please don't get me wrong. The rent is a peppercorn rent. However as you see the payoff is that Simeon wants to buy the entire estate, except the castle, and develop it according to methods which he thinks will produce more money. Perhaps he's right, but they are methods with which Father and I don't agree. We have always been in favour of organic methods and against intensive or factory farming.

We feel therefore, Ginny, and I hope this won't upset you, that we are not going to take up Simeon's offer, however well meant. We would rather get a mortgage from the building society than sell our precious land, our heritage, and be in a position where we are told what to do.

I hope it won't upset the relationship between you two, and that you agree.

There was then some family news and, after reading this and the whole letter through again, Ginny sat back and studied the proposals which Tony Liddle had set out as only he knew how.

Reading them made Ginny's blood boil. In her own mind she felt quite certain that this was Liddle's idea rather than Simeon's.

Impulsively she lifted the phone and tapped out her brother's number. The telephone rang for so long that she was on the verge of replacing the receiver when she heard Betty's voice at the other end.

'Hello. This is Betty Silklander speaking.'

'Betty, it's Ginny.'

'Hey, Ginny.' Betty's rather anxious, preoccupied tone sounded pleased. 'How are you?'

'I'm fine; but Betty, I'm not very happy about Angus's letter.'

'Oh!' Betty seemed immediately to know what she meant.

'Do you know what Angus wrote?'

'Yes.' Betty's voice sounded flat and as though she were reluctant to discuss the matter. 'You'd better speak to Angus, but he's not here at the moment.'

'I just wanted to tell him that I'm *not* involved. I never was.'

'We know that.'

'I think Simeon meant well, Betty, I really do.'

Silence.

'He loves me, likes you *very* much, and he wants to help. Honestly. Betty?'

'I'm here.' Ginny could imagine her sister-in-law making a characteristic gesture of sweeping her hair back from her forehead. 'I don't know what to say. Oh, here's Angus.' She sounded relieved to be able to pass the telephone to her husband. 'I'll say goodbye now, Ginny.'

'Goodbye, Betty. How are the kids?'

'They're fine.'

'My love to them.'

'I will.'

'Hello, Ginny.' Angus's voice sounded strained. 'You got my letter?'

'I've just read it. I was telling Betty, Siméon only meant well.'

'I'm sure he did, according to his lights.'

'You mustn't be so . . .' Ginny paused angrily in mid-flight. She was going to say 'patronizing', but her brother had a short fuse and she didn't want a row. 'Well, I'm sure Simeon would give up the idea of buying the land.'

'We're just turning down his offer, Ginny. We don't want to argue.'

'I'll speak to him.'

'Gin,' Angus's voice sounded increasingly irritable, 'please don't become involved. I've written to Simeon or, rather, my solicitor has. We don't want to go any further. We'd rather have a straightforward mortgage. In fact we've applied for one. We want to keep our dignity, *and* our land.'

'I'm sure you do. I'm sorry.' Ginny felt humbled and angry.

'Ginny, speaking as your brother I must tell you I'm sorry you're involved with someone like Simeon. I'm really sorry . . .'

'Angus, you mustn't equate a business offer with something personal.'

'I can't help it. It's the sort of person I think he is. Not like us. Not with our standards of fairness. We wish very much you'd . . .'

'Stuck with Robert,' Ginny finished for him.

'Well, someone like Robert. You knew where you were with Robert. He was one of us.'

'I'll say goodbye now, Angus,' Ginny said in a voice taut with tension. 'I'm really sorry. I didn't want him to interfere and I'll keep right out of it. But I do love Simeon, you must accept that.'

'I'm glad for you, Ginny.' She could sense that Betty was tugging at his elbow, urging him to terminate the conversation. 'Hope to see you soon.'

'Lots of love,' she said and rang off, slowly putting the receiver back in its cradle.

She sat there for a while, visualizing the scene in the old farmhouse, a place familiar to her since childhood with the rugs on the old stone flags, fires roaring up the chimneys, cats sleeping contentedly in various places where they shouldn't be and the dogs scampering up and down impatiently waiting to be let out, or lying with their noses on their paws staring into the fire. In the yard the free range hens pecked busily and the geese ran up and down like people in a hurry who had nowhere in particular to go.

The cows would be grazing in the field by the river and the beef cattle ekeing out a long life beyond on the opposite bank. Just now the trees would be burgeoning, the daffodils pushing their way up through the earth and the landscape would take on a totally new aspect as it began to abandon winter and welcome the spring.

This was in her blood, in her bones, and she knew that Simeon had no part of it. To him it was an inefficient way of life, one he simply didn't understand.

But despite or because of this she loved him. She loved him the more just because of this attitude of her family based on class, privilege, centuries-old tradition. Much as she loved her family she sometimes hated what they stood for, resented their conservatism, which only made Simeon more vulnerable and, therefore, more lovable in her eyes.

Forgotten were her doubts about his business practices, his ruthlessness towards the Jacquets. Rising impulsively from her desk, taking Angus's letter with her, she went up to the top floor where Anthony Liddle was beavering away over his computer screens. He was drinking from a mug of coffee as she walked in and, putting it hastily down, began to rise from his chair.

'Don't get up, Tony, please.' Ginny flapped a hand towards him, holding out the letter. 'I've just had this from my brother.'

'Oh yes!' Tony reached out for a letter which lay on top of a pile of others. 'We heard from his solicitor. He doesn't want to go ahead.' He joined his hands together and grimaced. 'I guess that's it, then. I don't think Simeon will be too pleased, he did a lot of work.'

'*I'm* not too pleased.' Ginny perched on the side of his desk. 'I never wanted my family to be involved in this in the first place.'

'I'm sorry, Ginny, you'll have to sort that out with Simeon.' Liddle was obviously anxious to return to his computer screen and Ginny, knowing that it was unfair to badger him, was just about to drop the subject when she saw the distinctive letter-heading of her other brother Lambert and attached to it a document in a foreign language with which she was unfamiliar.

She leaned across the desk and said, 'May I ask what this is?'

Liddle, his eyes on his screen, shook his head.

'It's some export document. I think it's some art stuff your brother Lambert has bought in Italy for the new house.'

Ginny gazed at the accompanying letter.

'Do you mind if I read it?'

'Go ahead.' Tony began tapping at the keys.

> Dear Mr Liddle
>   Attached is the export certificate issued by the Bulgarian authorities for the picture by Mantegna which Mr Varga has purchased, among other items, for Purborough Park. With it I enclose my own invoice and, on settlement of this, I will discuss delivery to you of the picture which is at present in the vaults of my bank.
>   Kindest regards and good wishes.

Attached was an invoice for just under two million pounds, which represented the purchase price, the cost of the export certificate, and Lambert's commission.

Ginny let out a whistle.

'Oh dear!' Anxiously Liddle turned round. 'Maybe that wasn't meant for your eyes. Here,' he held out his hand, 'you'd better let me have it.'

'But if it's for the house?' Ginny looked curiously at him. 'It may be a wedding present or something . . . And this certificate, why Bulgaria? I thought it was found in Florence?'

'Really, Ginny, it's none of my business,' Liddle rose and almost snatched the letter from her, 'and, honestly, I don't think it's any of yours. It's a matter between Lambert and Simeon. Please don't mention to him that

301

you saw it. He'll be furious with me. And really, if you don't mind, I must get on. Simeon's due back this evening and I've an awful lot of work to get through.'

In the sunshine of early spring the house looked superb. Already the scaffolding had been removed from the front, which had been repainted. The stone had been newly cleaned and the woodwork of the doors and windows freshly painted white.

Varga left the car in the drive in front of the imposing portico and stood, his arm linked through Ginny's, gazing up at it. Inside the lights were on and workmen could be seen scurrying about, running up and down ladders and along the internal scaffolding. Already the rooms were changing colour as the painters began to finish their jobs: deep pinks and yellows to reflect the taste of the Georgian era.

'Let's go inside,' Ginny said excitedly, but Simeon, pressing her arm tightly, didn't move.

All the way down in the car, which he'd driven himself, he had had a preoccupied air and there had been periods of silence while they listened to music on the stereo. Not that this was unusual. Varga wasn't a chatterer, and for Ginny just to be alone in his company was enough.

'What's the matter, darling?' she asked.

'I have to talk to you,' he said and, abruptly turning his back on the house and still closely holding on to her arm, he began to walk along the path towards the obelisk. Around them the trees, surrounded by clumps of bluebells and daffodils, were beginning to burst into bud, but he took no notice of the beauty of nature.

'What *is* it, Simeon?' Ginny forced him to stop and looked at him closely. 'What is it you can't tell me?'

'We can't get married this summer,' Varga said abruptly.

'Oh!' She gazed at him gravely. 'I wondered why you said nothing about your visit to Carlo.'

'Claudia won't agree to the divorce.'

'But I thought it was automatic after five years?'

'I have only been living separately from her for three. For two years before that I remained in the house because of the children. I had my own room, and there was absolutely no intimacy of any kind between us.'

'But of course she can deny that if she wants to be awkward.' Ginny began to understand.

'It's not just her, it's her family.' Varga viciously kicked the gravel at his feet. 'They have always disliked me. Now they feel I've humiliated their daughter and will stop at nothing. There is literally nothing I can do,' he looked appealingly at Ginny, 'for the moment.'

'Two more years, then,' she said, gulping. 'Mummy won't be pleased.'

'But what about you, Ginny darling?' He gripped her arm so hard that it was almost painful.

'I'm in it already, for better or for worse.' She leaned forward to offer him her lips. 'In a way it gives us more time.' She looked towards the house.

'How do you mean "it gives us more time"?'

'Time to get the house ready. Time for me to get Silk off the ground. We can launch it to coincide with our wedding.'

'Can you *really* wait two years?' he asked.

'Yes.'

'I love you.' He bent forward to kiss her.

'And I love you,' she replied as they broke apart. 'That's all that really matters.'

After that he seemed more cheerful and they walked slowly up the path back to the house, arriving on the main steps just as another car drew up. Parking beside Varga's Jaguar, Lambert waved as Maggie lowered the window.

'What *fun*!' She opened the door and tumbled out. 'We didn't think you'd be here too.'

'It wasn't scheduled.' Ginny went up to her and kissed her cheek.

'Oh?' Maggie gazed at her. 'You both look rather solemn. Has something happened?' She looked anxiously towards the house, but Ginny shook her head.

'The house is absolutely okay.' She turned enquiringly to Varga and he nodded. 'It's the wedding. We can't go ahead as planned.'

'Oh dear!' Maggie clutched her arm as Lambert came towards her more slowly and pecked her cheek. 'That is terrible. Is it something to do with the divorce?'

Ginny nodded and Varga added:

'My wife is being difficult about the time factor. She won't agree to a divorce on the grounds that she is a practising Roman Catholic, so I have to wait five years, after which it becomes automatic.'

'He didn't move out of the house soon enough,' Ginny explained, suddenly embarrassed about the whole thing. 'Anyway, it changes nothing between us. Come on,' she pointed anxiously towards the house, 'let's go in.'

Inside it looked, if anything, even more chaotic than when they had been there before. There seemed more internal scaffolding, more men, more cans of paint and builders' materials littered about, and part of the ceiling of the drawing-room was covered with a white sheet.

'Just as *well* we're not getting married this summer,' Ginny said with a smile.

'They're all scheduled to be out in twelve weeks.' Lambert consulted a clipboard in his hands. 'July, it says here. There's a penalty if they default.'

'We can still move in, darling?' Ginny looked at Varga, who was glowering disapprovingly at the mess.

'A very *strict* penalty,' he added, not heeding Ginny. 'I'm paying way over the odds for this.'

'But, Simeon, we knew the *whole* thing wouldn't be ready.' Ginny clasped his arm. 'Lambert and Maggie have so much to do.'

'The workmen are meant to be out in July,' Varga tapped his foot, 'and at this rate it looks as though they'll be here for the rest of the year.'

Ginny and Maggie exchanged glances, but Varga, it appeared, didn't want to be pacified and went over to speak to the foreman. Very soon their voices could be heard raised in anger.

'He gets very uptight,' Maggie whispered. 'Can't we slink away somewhere?'

'I think we'd better stay here to prevent open hostilities breaking out,' Ginny said grimly. 'In the mood he's in it will take very little for Simeon to bash the foreman on the nose.'

'Perhaps I'll intervene.' And without waiting for a reply Lambert went over to Varga and, taking his arm, said with some urgency: 'Simeon, do you think we could have a word? There's something important I have to ask you.'

'Well?' Varga looked at him angrily.

'Besides,' Lambert smiled at the foreman, 'you will be all out by the scheduled date, won't you, Sam?'

'I was telling Mr Varga it would be *before* that.' The foreman pointed angrily at the disorder. 'This looks worse than it actually is.'

'There!' Lambert released Varga's arm. 'What did I say? Now if I could have a few moments of your precious time . . .'

'Well . . .' Varga glared at the foreman again and then, reluctantly stuffing his hands in his pockets, walked away, trailed by Lambert who gave the two women a wink.

'I wonder what he wants?' Ginny asked as, followed slowly by Lambert, Maggie and Ginny, Varga walked through the drawing-room, still obviously angry, not looking to right or left, and then out of a door at the far end which led to a small hallway. Off this hall, which had once been the administrative offices of the large house, and probably would be again, were a number of small rooms, none of which had been touched except for the installation of central heating. Ginny shivered. But Varga appeared unmoved and looked sharply at Lambert.

'Now, what is it you want?'

'I can understand that you're upset about the wedding,' Lambert said in an apologetic tone of voice. 'And perhaps this isn't the right moment to bring it up.'

'Bring what up?'

'About the Mantegna.'

'The what?' Varga looked puzzled.

'The picture by Andrea Mantegna that I have bought on your behalf.'

'Oh!' Varga still looked vague, as if he hadn't an idea what Lambert was talking about.

'I need the money to complete the purchase, Simeon. I have paid for the export licence . . .'

'You have to *pay* for an export licence?' Ginny looked at him in some astonishment. 'So that's what I saw on Tony Liddle's desk.'

'You saw it where?' Varga, still in a bad humour, turned to her.

'On Tony Liddle's desk. I thought it strange because it came from Bulgaria. You found a Mantegna *there*?' She looked at Lambert with a mixture of incredulity and excitement. 'How absolutely thrilling.'

'Oh, you've heard of him.' Varga, momentarily, seemed to have regained his good humour.

'Of *course* I've heard of him. He's one of the most famous painters of the early Renaissance.' She turned enthusiastically to her brother. 'Lambert, how very clever of you to have found a Mantegna. You're sure it's genuine?'

'No doubt at all. In fact I think it's one of a pair.'

'What a coup,' Ginny said. 'Lambert, why didn't you tell me anything about this before?' She turned to her sister-in-law. 'Maggie, did you know?'

Maggie gave her a mysterious look. 'I *think* it was meant to be a surprise,' she said.

'You think he's worth the money?' Varga looked critically at her. 'Two million?'

'It certainly is an awful lot.'

306

'Well if you think this guy is worth it, I don't mind paying it.'

'I thought you went to Italy.' Ginny turned to Lambert, an odd expression on her face. 'Now you say you found this in *Bulgaria*?'

'Some old villa high up in the mountains.' Lambert looked slightly uneasy. 'Lots of treasures that had been forgotten for years.'

'And it's all above board and everything . . .' Ginny's voice trailed off, remembering how unforthcoming Liddle had been. She never quite trusted Liddle.

'Of course it's above board – why shouldn't it be?'

'Usually governments won't grant an export licence for that kind of thing.'

'Oh, Bulgaria . . .' Lambert said with a grin, but Simeon suddenly got very uptight again and, taking Ginny by the hand, said:

'For God's sake let's get out of this place . . . Look,' he stopped and turned to Lambert, 'do what you like. See Liddle about the money, but don't bother me about it. I've got quite enough on my mind as it is.'

Ginny shrugged, grimaced and went over to her brother and sister-in-law, kissing them goodbye.

'I'll give you a call,' she whispered to Maggie. 'He's in a hell of a mood because of the divorce.'

'Of course.' Maggie smiled understandingly.

'The Mantegna is terrific.' Ginny squeezed Lambert's arm as she hugged him.

'You've got to keep very quiet about it,' Lambert hissed.

'Why?' Ginny, looking startled, hissed back.

'The insurance will quadruple on this place.'

'Oh, of course.' Ginny nodded understandingly.

'Come on,' Varga said impatiently and, without looking at Lambert and Maggie, he seized Ginny's hand and made for the door.

''Bye,' Ginny cried and, with a wave, disappeared.

'Well . . .' Lambert sat on an upturned box and

thankfully drew his cigarettes from his pocket. 'That man is a weirdo.'

'He's not weird, he's rather extraordinary.' Maggie nudged him to move up and then sat next to him, accepting the cigarette which he'd lit for her.

'He's got more on his mind than the divorce,' Lambert said darkly, inhaling deeply.

'What do you mean?' Maggie looked at him sharply.

'If you ask me, he's engaged in some sort of underhand activities.'

'Oh darling, how *could* you say that?'

'He looks and, to me, behaves like a worried man. And the trouble is that we'll be getting it in the neck too. He'll drag us down.'

'I did warn you, Lambert,' Maggie said sharply. 'I warned you not to get involved with Alberto.'

'Well I won't get involved any more. I won't take any more from that source besides what we've got already. I think when we've finished in here we'll steer clear of Mr Varga.'

'But what about Ginny?'

'What can we do about Ginny? Either she knows, or she'll find out one day in her own way.' Lambert paused and smoked silently for a while. 'She's absolutely obsessed by him. Won't see reason.'

'Really?'

'He's into all kinds of things, and I *bet* half of them aren't legal.'

'That doesn't make him a criminal.' Maggie put her arm tentatively through his as though she suddenly felt in need of comfort.

'He offered me his tacky little Mexican airline to export art purchases all over the world. No questions asked.'

'Oh my God!' Maggie put a hand over her eyes.

'There is definitely more to Mr Varga than meets the eye.' Carefully Lambert ground out his cigarette on the bare boards beneath his feet. Then he stood up and held a hand out towards his wife.

'Come on, old girl. Let's have another talk with Sam. Smooth his ruffled feelings.'

'I'm dying of cold.' Maggie also heeled her cigarette out on the floor.

'Better be careful. We don't want to burn the place down.' Lambert chuckled and, putting his arm through hers, they walked slowly together towards the side door. Opening it he stopped and looked through the trees to the distant outline of hills, sighing deeply. 'Varga is worried. He doesn't seem to have the fine, incisive mind he had before. Still,' he turned and carefully closed the door behind them, 'what can you expect from a man who's never heard of Mantegna?'

Laughing, they set off down the path towards the front of the house.

The drive back to London was as solemn and silent as the one down. Only this time Ginny knew the reason for it and occasionally, by touching his arm, would show that she understood.

They arrived in Mayfair at about seven o'clock and as he was garaging the car Varga turned to her:

'Do you want to eat out or in?'

'I'll have a quick snack with you and then I want to go home.'

Even the word 'home' produced a wounded expression.

'Home? Your home is with me, Ginny.'

'You know what I mean, Simeon.' She put a hand out to caress his brow. 'I have all my clothes in Kentish Town and tomorrow I'm leaving for France.'

'Oh!' He frowned and, instead of parking the car, reversed back into the street.

'What are you doing?' she asked.

'In that case I might as well take you home.'

'It's not necessary. I can get a cab.'

'I've a lot of work to do anyway,' he said.

'Right.' Ginny sat back with an air of resignation as he

309

headed the car north towards Kentish Town.

It was still light when they stopped outside the house and, after switching off the engine, he sat there drumming his fingers on the wheel.

'Do you want to come in?' she asked.

'Well,' he shrugged, 'if you have a sandwich.'

She got out and, after locking the car, he followed her.

She threw her things on to the sofa in the sitting-room and, still followed by Varga, went into the kitchen where she took a bottle of white wine from the fridge.

'A drink is what we need,' she said showing him the bottle and, with a nod, he got the corkscrew out of a drawer and, sitting on a stool, put the bottle between his knees.

Ginny remained in front of the fridge critically inspecting its contents.

'Salami and ham. That do?'

'That will do fine,' Varga said, finally extracting the cork and filling two glasses Ginny had placed on the table with wine. She could sense he was beginning to unwind and, as she took the rye bread from the bread bin she dropped a kiss on his forehead.

'You're sure it's all right about the Mantegna?' She began to cut the bread into thickish slices for open sandwiches.

'I'm sick of hearing about this Mantegna.' Varga tensed up again, rubbed his brow.

'Sorry I spoke.'

She turned back to look for lettuce and tomatoes.

'Is he really that important?' Varga looked up, sipping his wine.

'He's one of the old masters. Still, I would have thought two million pounds was a lot to pay.'

'I suppose your brother does know what he's doing?'

'I suppose he does. Oh, he's sure to.' She tossed her head and began to arrange the thinly sliced salami on the buttered bread. 'I was just surprised there would be a Mantegna that no one knew of in a country like Bulgaria.'

'What do you mean, "like Bulgaria"?' he demanded aggressively.

'Well, it's a poor country, under Communist domination since the war. I would have thought that all the exportable treasures would have found their way to the west long ago.'

'Well, they obviously didn't.'

He took another sip of his wine and then looked critically at the open sandwich Ginny placed in front of him.

'That okay?' she asked.

'That's fine.' He took several large mouthfuls and then smiled.

'I was hungry. We should have stopped for dinner on the way home.'

'You've been ratty all day.' She sat opposite him sipping her wine. 'It's the divorce. Really, it doesn't bother me in the slightest.'

'It bothers me.' He took another bite of his sandwich. 'I wanted us to get married this summer, to have all the ends tied up.'

'We will get married the summer after next and the ends will be tied up eventually. In the meantime it makes no difference to us at all.'

'I was looking forward to entertaining at Purborough. To having kids . . .'

'Darling . . .' she stretched out her hand, 'you have already got two kids and in two years' time I shan't be too old.'

'I told Carlo I no longer wished to see my children,' Varga said harshly. 'Neither them *nor* their mother, ever again.'

'Oh, *Simeon*.' Ginny sat back, her expression one of dismay. 'Surely that's cruel?'

'My dear, if I thought the children had any interest in or affection for me you can be sure I would have continued to see them, whatever the cost. But it has been obvious for a long time that the children only see my visits as a bore. It is a duty they don't enjoy. They have obviously been brainwashed by their mother's family.'

'But you don't really know that, Simeon.'

'I do,' he said angrily. 'I know my own children, please give me credit for that, Ginny.'

Ginny sat back, suddenly off her food, although she too had been hungry. This was a man with black, dark moods that she didn't really understand. An impulsive, irrational man, capable of rejecting his own children. Somehow an imperceptible barrier appeared to have arisen between them.

'I'm sorry,' she said and then, rapidly, his mood changed once again.

'Darling, forgive me . . .' He rose from his chair and went round the table to stand beside her, leaning over her and putting his arm round her shoulder. 'I'm in a bad mood. I'm upset. It was a shock; it was unexpected and it seems there is nothing I can do about it.'

'That's what irritates you,' she said. 'You can usually control events, but this you can't control. Believe me, darling, I quite understand your frustration. Now let's be positive . . . Simeon,' she said as he sat down again.

'Yes, darling?' He looked up expectantly.

'About Silk . . . the perfume.'

'Oh, do you still want to go ahead with it?'

'Of course I do.' She could hardly conceal her surprise at his statement. 'Whyever not?'

'Well, you can stay on if we are not to marry yet.'

'Oh no.' She shook her head vigorously. 'I think we've gone too far along the line. Besides, once we set up home at Purborough we're as good as married, and we will do that, won't we, darling? Some time this year?'

'I suppose so,' he said.

'You only "suppose" so?'

'Well those builders, who knows if they'll keep their

promise? Also Maggie and your brother,' his brows knitted together again, 'I'm not sure they were the right choice.'

Ginny felt a sense of despair. All at once she wanted to get out, get right away.

'You'll have to sort that out while I'm away,' she said briskly. 'For I am going on with Silk and the reorganization of the company. We've gone too far. Morgan is actively looking for someone to take my place.'

'Take your place?' Varga looked at her in astonishment. 'I'm not going to have new people sniffing around.'

'Simeon, I don't understand you!' She looked at him in amazement. 'We have to have someone to replace me.'

'Oh no we don't.' Having finished his sandwich he rose and began to walk round the room. 'I like a small, tightly-run ship. Liddle is my key man. The smaller the head office staff the better. I don't want new people finding out my secrets.'

'Secrets? You'd think you had something to hide.'

'Yes, I have things to hide,' he replied. 'I have a large organization to run and many people would dearly love to know how I run it, what is the secret of my success. Haven't you heard of industrial espionage? Well . . .'

'But, darling, even *I* don't know any of your secrets, as you call them. My job is to promote the image of the company, and whoever replaces me will do just that.'

'No one will replace you.'

'Very well.' Ginny rose and began to stack the dishwasher with the few plates they'd used. Then she stood by the table finishing her wine. Outside now it was quite dark and the distant hum of the traffic seemed to emphasize the silence. She knew that now was quite emphatically not the time to reintroduce the subject of Pierre Jacquet.

But, more disturbing, was the new dilemma he'd created in her mind. Did she, in fact, really know the character of the man whom she was going to marry and whose children she would eventually bear?'

CHAPTER 17

Pierre Jacquet smiled at Ginny with polite formality.

'I was expecting you, Mademoiselle Silklander. Do please come in.' He swept her inside with a courtly gesture and led the way along a rather dark corridor in the suburban house into a surprisingly light and airy room. On two sides there were floor to ceiling bookcases and opposite the door were french windows leading into an attractive garden. One could have been in the heart of the country, Ginny thought, instead of in a rather dreary house on the outskirts of Paris about ten minutes from the factory.

'Do sit down, mademoiselle.' Pierre pointed to a comfortable chair near the open window, but Ginny walked instead to the steps leading into the garden and looked out.

'It's very charming.'

'Not what you expected?' He smiled politely.

'Not really,' she smiled back and, turning round, sat in the chair he had indicated, putting her gloves on the bag on her lap. 'It's so unexpected.'

'Built years before this once beautiful spot in the country became just another Paris suburb, indistinguishable from the rest.' Pierre paused to offer her a cigarette from his pack, but as she shook her head he said: 'I suppose you have the same kind of thing in England.' He glanced at her. 'You don't mind if I smoke?'

'Not at all. It's . . . most kind of you, in the circumstances, to see me.'

Noticing the pause he put his head on one side.

'You didn't expect it?'

'Hardly. You weren't very well treated by Simeon Varga.'

'And you, as well as being a director of his company, are engaged to marry him?'

'Yes, eventually.' She lowered her head. 'He's not yet divorced.'

'Oh, I see.'

Pierre took a long drag from his cigarette and she realized that he was as nervous as she was, perhaps even more.

'How is your father?'

Pierre fluttered his hand.

'So-so. He was an old man, of course, when he sold out. You can't blame everything on that.'

'Nevertheless,' Ginny paused again, not wanting to add to his discomfiture by being tactless. 'I hear that you have not been left very well off financially.'

'That's true. However we have the house, there is a small pension – enough to take care of my father's medical and nursing needs – and enough for me. We own the house, at least.'

'You know why I'm here?' Ginny thought that frankness was the best policy.

'Is it something to do with the new perfume?'

'It is to be called Silk.'

Pierre nodded approvingly.

'Very nice. *Soie.* Sounds good in French too.'

'My family originally came from France many centuries ago. *Soie terre.*'

'So.' Pierre smiled out of mere politeness, rather than interest, Ginny thought.

Suddenly, placing her bag and gloves on the table next to her chair, Ginny stood up and walked once again over to the french windows, arms akimbo. Every move was carefully followed by Pierre Jacquet, who lit another cigarette but remained in his chair watching her.

'Monsieur Jacquet,' Ginny said, spinning round, 'I won't beat about the bush. I need you.'

He acknowledged her remark with a nod of his head, as though he'd been expecting it, but said nothing.

'You are the best "nose" for our business, one of the best in France.'

Again he seemed to acknowledge the correctness of her remark but, again, remained silent.

'I would like you to come back and work for Oriole on an exclusive basis. I understand you have some consultancy work.'

'A little.' Once more he tilted his head sideways.

'I would like you to give it all up, and work for us again. You will report directly to me. My plan is to revitalize the company and introduce the new perfume, maybe to coincide with my marriage in two years' time. But we do need *you*.'

'Why then, mademoiselle, were my services dispensed with?'

'Because Mr Varga knew, and still knows, nothing about the perfume business. Since he took the company over he has expanded rapidly into other fields he didn't envisage at the time.'

'And so he took away our livelihood, our pride, and did nothing with it?' For the first time a note of bitterness entered Pierre's voice. 'I am surprised that you could be associated with such behaviour, Mademoiselle Silklander. I would not have thought it of you.'

Ginny suddenly recalled the hard, obdurate man sitting opposite her in her kitchen a few days previously and thought to herself that, had she not been so blinded by love, she might admit that, in retrospect, it surprised her too. Was her natural humanity being eroded by Varga's hard-nosed business ethics?

'Do you have full authority to make this offer, mademoiselle, may I ask?' Pierre began delicately to stub out his cigarette, and she wondered that someone who prided himself on his sense of smell smoked so much. As if reading her mind he said:

'If I do join you, all this goes.'

'I was wondering.'

'Unfortunately the tragedy to my family affected my nerves.'

'Not surprisingly. But, in answer to your question, yes I do have full authority. I am to become chief executive of the firm and I have power to restructure it.'

'But does Mr Varga know that you are thinking of recruiting me?'

'Not yet.'

'Don't you think you'd better ask him?'

Suddenly she made up her mind to take a decision that would have been impossible even a week ago.

'No. I have full authority to do as I please. I shall only tell him if and when I think I need to, and by that time Oriole will have become the company it once used to be, and a new fragrance will be in the making.'

Gus Damian slouched in the seat of his motorbike, arms folded, head jogging in time to the music from his Walkman. He was dressed in a yellow helmet and black and yellow leathers and on the pillion there was the despatch box, also yellow and black, of a courier.

Gus was one of the new breed of private eyes, far removed from the stereotype of the down-at-heel, slouched-hat, heavy-drinking type beloved of B movies and pulp fiction. He never drank; he was also quite young and, before he took up his profession, totally inexperienced.

After all, you got what you paid for, and Anthony Liddle had decided that the engagement of a private investigator to spy on whoever was spying on Varga was not one of the top priorities of AP International. Where he could he cut corners and saved costs; he was scrupulous with the firm's money – scrupulous up to a point, that is.

Liddle had got Gus Damian's name out of Yellow Pages, astonished to find that it was so easy, that so many agencies were listed who promised adoption enquiries, investigations into internal theft, lie detector tests, insurance investigation and verification, and, of course, surveillance. The proliferation had been bewildering and Tony Liddle, short of time, eschewed the more expensively boxed ads in favour of a one-liner: *G. Damian, Confidential Investigations*. The telephone number had been that of a London borough well south of the Thames, his enquiry taken by an answer-phone system was soon returned. At £75 a day plus expenses Damian's fee was ludicrously cheap. But it suited him and it suited his employer, neither of whom gave top priority to the job.

He was paid weekly from the petty cash and made a brief report to Liddle. The conclusion, reached very rapidly, was that Varga was being followed, but Damian couldn't say who by or why.

The team changed weekly and once or twice he had lost the bait. The cars changed, and the personnel changed, the methods also changed, but now he knew the latest operative keeping Varga under surveillance was a woman. She was about forty, slight and with brown curly hair – well past sell-by date as far as trendy young Damian was concerned. He was not particularly interested in her nor what she did, merely in his weekly collection of his fee. One day soon Liddle would have had enough, but by then Damian would be able to afford a short holiday in the South of France. It was always a mystery to him the number who wanted to employ people like him just for doing nothing.

Suddenly the person in the car on the other side of the road sat up. Damian sat up. Varga and Miss Silklander were coming out of the AP headquarters. Both carried briefcases, and as Varga's Jaguar purred to a stop by the kerb outside the office they stood for a few moments in animated conversation, as though they were having a row. The chauffeur stood by the car waiting patiently and then finally Varga, with an exclamation, a shrug of his shoulders, turned his back abruptly on Miss Silklander and, handing his case to Peter, jumped into the back of his car.

Miss Silklander stood for a few moments as if undecided what to do. Then, as the car remained stationary with the engine ticking over, as though Varga were waiting for her to make up her mind, she abruptly turned and made her way in the direction of Park Street.

Varga's car started, the car on the opposite side of the street started, and finally Damian kicked his bike into life.

He could weave in and out of the traffic, bringing up the rear, riding alongside or, if he wished, taking the lead for a few moments, keeping careful surveillance on them in his mirror.

It gave him an advantage over them all.

Later that day Kelly drove the small Fiat she used for surveillance into the garage beside her ground floor conversion and, with a sigh of relief, took the shopping from the car and then locked it. Inside her dog started up a commotion, intended to be a sign of welcome; after she had fed her, and poured herself a drink, she would usually take her for a short walk.

Sometimes the cat accompanied them, sometimes it didn't; but she knew that she would get a welcome from both that would, in its way, be her main reward for her solitary life. The dog would jump up and down, and the cat would slide around between her legs purring. Then she would jump on the kitchen table and sit waiting to be fed.

The cat and the dog were females; it was an all-female establishment and men were only tolerated occasionally as guests.

Not much was known about Kelly's love life, or even if she had ever had one. Edward Thomas undoubtedly knew, but the details were locked in his safe together with other personnel records. Kelly was a loner to the few people who knew her with any degree of intimacy, a mere handful, and as she got older they got fewer and the numbers dropped off.

She was a career woman, married to her work; in love, perhaps, with its secretive, clandestine nature. A mysterious, unfathomable woman, for whom the symbolism of the dumb cat and dog was perfect. They were the ideal companions.

Kelly put her key in the door, and even before she had time to put down her things the welcome assault began. She put on the lights, laughing with pleasure at such a welcome, and then she took the shopping into the kitchen, chatting all the time to the animals. And as she talked away to them, unpacking her bags, the routine went on as usual, the jumping up, the rubbing of the legs, the perch on the kitchen table while she stacked away her shopping and opened the various cans of food, putting before them a choice.

While they ate Kelly lit a cigarette and poured herself a gin and tonic with a slice of lemon and two cubes of ice. Then she slumped on a kitchen chair and watched them. Her family. Perfection. She thought the trouble with dumb animals was that they couldn't tell you anything; their affection, or lack of it, was expressed by their behaviour; their wants and desires had to be guessed by their moods.

That night after the walk, during which the cat decided to accompany them round the block and a nearby square, she returned to her flat, heated up a Marks and Spencer ready-made dinner and then, with another gin and tonic by her side, the cat curled up beside her, the dog at her feet, she looked at the Polaroid pictures she'd taken that day, the close-ups of Ginny and Varga together.

They seemed to have been quarrelling.

She looked at the photographs with care: the dark, good-looking woman, her expression slightly pained.

And Varga. She studied his face for some time; attractive, enigmatic, the sort of man that, when she had had time for boyfriends, might have appealed to her. Then she took from her briefcase a stack of photographs that had been taken a few months before and which showed them happy, laughing, and together.

What had the strain of the past few months done to them? And what was the point of the surveillance, the very expensive surveillance, the agency had been keeping on them?

If nothing happened in a week or two she would advise Thomas that the time-wasting exercise ought to stop. There was nothing more they could find out about the activities of Simeon Varga except that many of his business deals were done through private offshore companies and that very occasionally, and perhaps surprisingly in the circumstances, he visited a brothel.

These days Varga's anger seemed to spill over everything, Liddle thought, as he ranted on about some insignificant point of detail to do with one of his many overseas operations. The structure was getting too vast; it was difficult to control. He himself was working a sixteen-hour day. His long-suffering wife was talking of an extended visit to her mother in the north, taking the children with her.

Liddle had developed a tremor and he smoked too much, feverishly extinguishing the weed whenever Varga appeared and, with an oath, went and flung open the windows.

Maybe that was why he was so bad-tempered now.

'And as for the builders and that *house* . . .' Varga banged his fist down on a sheaf of bills that Liddle had presented him with for payment from his private accounts, 'they are way, way over estimate.'

'That is because of all the special work the architect and the Silklanders have asked them to do. It's all itemized.' Liddle resurrected another set of accounts which he'd tactfully tucked underneath the pile on top.

'I can believe it. You know . . .' Varga sat back, his eyes narrowing. 'That Lambert Silklander is a crook. We have all this upper-class image to the eyebrows,' Varga indicated his own with two fingers, 'but it's all shit. Did *you* ever hear of a painter called Mantegna?'

Liddle's brows furrowed.

'No, I thought not,' Varga went on, 'neither did I. Not like Van Gogh or what's the name of the other bloke?' He clicked his fingers together in the air. Liddle knew nothing about art, didn't even pretend to like it, and his mind remained a blank. 'Picasso,' Varga said at last and Liddle's brow cleared in recognition.

'I've heard of Picasso,' he declared.

'Exactly. Who hasn't? And yet this Lambert expects me to pay two million quid for a picture by an unknown artist, someone nobody's ever heard of.'

'Has Ginny heard of him?'

'Ginny said he was a great Renaissance artist. Now I'm landed with it . . . and illegally. I'm not even going to have the pleasure of showing it off with my bride. It has to be tucked away because it's illegally exported. As if *I* get any pleasure from that!'

Suddenly Liddle realized why Varga was so angry. It was because of the marriage. Ever since his interview with Carlo he had been a different man. The chicanery seemed to have bitten into his soul. It had deprived him of the respectability and glamour he so coveted: to have an 'honourable' for a wife; a lord for a father-in-law. It was the first real reverse Varga had suffered since his upward climb began.

It was a very bad time to bring in anything controversial, but Liddle felt he couldn't postpone it indefinitely. He sat down opposite Varga and produced a file from an envelope marked VERY SECRET AND CONFIDENTIAL. This he placed in front of Varga.

'What's this?' Varga barked, opening it to find a single sheet of paper with some rather inexpert typing on it.

'It's a report from our surveillance expert. You *are* being followed.'

'By whom?' Varga seized the paper and scrutinized it.

'He doesn't know.'

'You mean he doesn't follow the person who's following me?'

'His job is to follow you.' Liddle pointed at him. 'He's waiting outside now.'

'What for?'

'His money. Do you want to keep him on?'

'How much?'

'£75 a day.'

'Christ!' Varga leaned back and gave a loud, humourless laugh. 'What a fortune! What kind of hack is he?'

'Plus expenses.'

'No wonder he doesn't find anything.'

'He's young and quite eager to please. He uses a motor-bike. I thought it quite a novelty.'

Varga's humour seemed to return and, as he relaxed, he smiled.

'Have him come up,' he said. 'I'd like to meet this enterprising "secret agent".' He put a mocking emphasis on the words.

Liddle lifted the phone to speak to the receptionist and after a few moments there was a timid knock on the door and Damian, dressed like a Colorado beetle, sidled in. It was very odd to see someone who you didn't know, yet who knew you. The black and yellow outfit certainly struck a chord, weaving in and out of the traffic, eye-catching.

Under Varga's cool appraisal Damian stood nervously on the rug in front of his desk twisting his large space-age helmet in his hands.

'So you don't know who's following me?' Varga barked without preliminaries.

'It's a woman with brown curly hair, sir.'

'A woman?' Varga looked intrigued. 'Attractive?'

Damian screwed up his nose.

'I see, not very attractive.' Varga seemed to find the younger man's expression amusing. He paused for a moment and then leaned across his desk: 'Tell me, young fellow, have you much experience in the surveillance business?'

'Not much,' Damian admitted bashfully, shuffling his feet.

'What did you do before you became a private detective?'

'I was a courier. That's what gave me the idea, using the bike.'

'Very clever.' Varga nodded his head approvingly. 'I call that very enterprising, don't you, Liddle? A young man with a future?'

Liddle couldn't tell from Varga's voice whether he was serious or not. Varga was playing and would probably explode wrathfully after the young man had gone.

'You strike me,' Varga pointed to a seat and waited as Damian, booted and clad from top to toe in shiny leather, clumsily sat down, 'you strike me as a young man full of initiative.'

'Well, that's very kind of you . . .'

'To use a bike for detective work? Excellent. Tell me, Mr . . .'

'Gus, sir, Gus Damian.'

'Tell me, Gus,' Varga spoke in so low a voice that it was scarcely audible, 'have you ever used a gun?'

Gus, momentarily, looked taken aback.

'I'm merely asking,' Varga went on smoothly, 'because you look like the kind of go-ahead guy I could well do with in my organization. I need someone who can give me all-round protection and, of course, you'd have to carry a gun although, hopefully, never use it. Could you do that?'

Damian, obviously torn between greed and fear, nervously licked his lips.

'Think about it.' Varga got up and, rounding his desk,

extended his hand to the younger man. 'There will be a generous salary, full benefits, perks and so on. We have an excellent pension fund and, incidentally, the chance to travel. Might it appeal to you?'

'Very much.' Damian suddenly found his tongue and began to babble. 'Very much *indeed*, Mr Varga. It's the sort of thing I'd love. Of course I don't carry a gun, but I could find out . . .'

'Oh, there are ways of acquiring guns and learning how to use them.' Varga gave him an avuncular pat on the shoulder. 'I assure you, there is no need to have any fears on that score. Everything will be taken care of.'

'Well then, thanks very much, sir . . . when would I start?'

'If you've made up your mind so quickly – and I like that – how about today?' Varga turned to Liddle with a smile. 'It could be arranged, could it not, Tony?'

To Varga's amusement his deputy was practically frothing with suppressed rage, but dared not show it. Without a word he went towards the door, merely gesturing to Damian that he should follow him. Damian, uncertain what to do, looked from one to the other and, as Varga nodded encouragingly, followed Liddle. No further words were spoken.

Varga went over to the french windows and stood there for some time gazing at the fountain bubbling in the courtyard, the fish darting energetically about at its base.

For the first time for days, weeks even, he felt calm; the restlessness, anxiety and fury had strangely disappeared because of a plan he had begun to formulate in his mind.

The only way Varga knew how to find peace was through revenge.

After a quarter of an hour or so Liddle returned to find Varga, apparently in a good mood, sitting at his desk studying a sheaf of documents relating to the many facets of his growing conglomerate.

'Sell cement,' he said to Liddle without looking up.

'But you've only just acquired it.'

'Nevertheless sell it. Jenson should pay a good price for it. It's the sort of thing he's interested in. I have taken your advice Tony, and Ginny's.' Varga sat back with the expression of a cat who has swallowed the cream. 'I shall consolidate. I have too many loose ends, bits and pieces. I'd sell off Oriole if Ginny hadn't become so hooked on it.'

'She's doing a good job there, radical restructuring.'

'Oh, my future wife has talent, no doubt,' Varga smiled proudly. 'She will become increasingly useful to me.' Suddenly his face clouded as one of his mercurial changes of mood swept over him. 'But I want that now, dammit. I don't want to wait two years to be able to make use of Ginny and her valuable family connections. I've waited long enough. I want it *now*.' He banged the desk furiously while Liddle, never sure of which way to react with Varga, stood watching him.

'Don't you think you make use of Ginny enough as it is? She loves you unreservedly; your name is openly linked with hers. She's devoted to you, the organization. She has not yet seen through you, Simeon. Why I don't know. What do you think will happen when she does? Is that why you're in such a hurry to marry?'

Liddle had never been physically assaulted by Varga, but he came close to it now. Varga almost vaulted over his desk and, seizing the smaller man by the lapels, shook him until his teeth started to chatter.

'What the fuck do you mean by that? "Seen through me"?'

'You know what I mean,' Liddle replied between clenched teeth, 'but if you don't let me go I shan't tell you.'

For answer Varga flung him against the opposite wall and watched him contemptuously as he staggered to his feet.

327

'Don't do that, Simeon,' Liddle said, collapsing into a nearby chair. 'Don't do that to me again. I have so much information in here,' he tapped his head, 'that I could sink you. You need me.' Despite his grave words his teeth began to chatter again. 'I know all about you. I'm the only one who does. You're involved in so many underhand, illegal activities that it's a wonder your share price still holds.

'And as for acquiring this guard,' Liddle was picking up courage as he started to feel that Varga was faltering, his self-confidence diminishing, 'what the hell do you need him for? We know nothing about him. For all we know he may go straight from here to the police.'

'Well I hope he won't. I hope you took care of that.' Varga's eyes narrowed again.

'I offered him two hundred a week clear. He thought it was a fortune. I said he'd have to get the pistol next time you went to America and he could have firearms training there. He seems to imagine he's some kind of Mickey Spillane creation. Why the hell do you really need him, Simeon?'

'Because I'm being followed, that's why,' Varga said, slamming the table. 'And if people are following me I want to get rid of them.'

'You don't mean by shooting them?' Liddle looked dumbfounded.

'Yes I do mean by shooting them. Dead.'

'But you don't know who, or what . . .'

'I do know who, or what!' Varga sat carefully on his desk. 'I am, as you say, heavily involved in illegal activities. I have no choice but to eliminate my enemies, Liddle, one by one, and that simpleton can pick them off for me. No one will have a clue who he is. Then when he has done his job we can get rid of him.'

Liddle sat for a long time, blinking like a man in a state of deep shock. He *was* in deep shock. Simeon Varga had done many unprincipled things in his life, but he had never yet, so far as he knew, attempted murder.

'Simeon,' he said shakily, after making another attempt to recover his composure, 'I do urge you not to get into this sort of thing too deeply. There is time to back out. Sell the airline. Sell Planz Steel. Stop importing antiques into this country with fake certificates. Finish with the drugs, most dangerous of all. If you stop now you could perhaps cover your tracks. You are a very rich man if you never lift another finger. As for Melissa,' he said, looking up into his eyes, 'get rid of her too. I don't mean eliminate her, but get her out of your life. If you want a happy, respectable life as a wealthy man with Ginny, why try to destroy yourself? Begin again while you can.'

Varga seemed to listen to Liddle, but a ceaseless tapping of his fingers on his desk showed the degree of annoyance his deputy was causing him. Finally, when Liddle stopped speaking, Varga ceased drumming and, after a while, he rose and, coming casually round to Liddle, sat next to him. He gazed at him for a few moments and then put his hand on his arm.

'Tony,' he said, 'I know you're a good friend, loyal to me, and thank you for your advice; but if you think I'm taking it you're not the wise man I took you for. What I make in legal business, with all the tax ramifications, government control and what not, is peanuts compared to what we do through our offshore companies and everything else that goes on here. I can't stop, Tony. You never have enough. As for Melissa, yes, I think she *is* becoming a burden. Sometimes I question her loyalty. She is jealous of Ginny.'

'Understandably.'

'She never thought I'd marry Ginny. She thought when I divorced Claudia that I would marry her! I ask you, marry a heroin addict, a prostitute!' Varga again grew serious, even sentimental. 'My attachment to Melissa, however, is very real, very deep. It goes back a long, long way. I want to close down that side of our operations – the way I started in business. That certainly *is* very

329

dangerous and, with who knows who following me, it has to stop.'

'What will you do with Melissa?'

'Offer her a large sum of money and put her on a plane.' Varga paused again and smiled.

'And don't forget, Tony: you are so close to me, too. You know everything about me, how I tick, my inner secrets, my innermost being. You are as close to me as my skin. I will never let you go. If you ever desert me or try to leave me or betray me, much as I value you, Tony, I will find you, and I will kill you. There will be no rest, no hiding-place for you. You belong, whether you like it or not, heart and soul to me.'

PART IV

Whispers in the City

CHAPTER 18

The factory high up in the hills above Grasse was as old as, if not older than, the Oriole building on the outskirts of Paris. Yet there was charm in its antiquity, and the old-fashioned methods used to secure the absolute, or essence, of the millions of petals needed for L'Esprit du Temps were still in use. An ancient hand press used to crush the petals was still operated manually whereas most other presses in the business were now hydraulic.

But since Ginny had taken over, the laboratory equipment had been modernized. The latest gas chromatography and spectrometry machines had been introduced into a newly equipped and refurbished lab. New technicians had been taken on, some poached from their rivals in the nearby factories that made Grasse the centre of the perfume industry.

On a bench in front of him Pierre, dressed in a white coat, was using one of those machines to analyse the components of the new perfume being manufactured under conditions of the greatest secrecy, guarded night and day by huge alsatian dogs which roamed the building controlled by a hired guard from a firm of security agents in Nice.

It was all becoming very exciting and Ginny peered over his shoulder trying to decipher the meaning of the squiggles he made on the pad beside him.

'Good?' she asked, an enquiring smile on her face.

'Smell!' Pierre commanded, lifting the test tube with its almost opaque contents. Putting her nose to it, her sense buds were assailed by such a strong, heady vapour that she felt the membrane was being peeled from the inside of her nose.

'Oh!' she cried standing well back and holding her nose with her fingers. 'Goodness, it's so terribly strong. It's not *that*, is it, Pierre?'

'Not yet,' Pierre said, delighted by her reaction. 'That is the essence. It *is* very strong. It has to be diluted many times or else even this expensive perfume would be out of the reach of most people. Your investments would never see dividends if we didn't reduce it.'

'Oh!' The membrane of her nose was still tingling, her eyes shining, and Ginny produced a handkerchief and used it vigorously.

'Good for the sinuses, though,' she said.

'Exactly.' Pierre smiled and, with a final glance at his figures, pushed back his stool and stood up.

'Lunch, Ginny?'

'Lunch is fine.' Ginny glanced at her watch and saw, to her surprise, that it was after two. The absorbing morning had seemed to fly by.

It was a Saturday and the laboratory was almost deserted. Ginny had flown to Nice the previous day to be met by Pierre, who had booked her in to a local hotel. He was living in a small cottage with magnificent views on the outskirts of Grasse; this again had apparently been in the family since it was built. In the time they had worked closely together their relationship had remained formal, though friendly, but she had never visited his country home.

However today he said:

'I hoped you'd come back for lunch. I have a woman who looks after me and she has prepared something for us. Would you like that?'

'Very much,' Ginny said, touched. 'How kind of you to think about it, Pierre.'

'Oh, I've often thought about it,' Pierre said with a shy smile, 'but I have never dared.'

'Why not?'

'The boss's wife.'

'The boss's wife-to-be.' She gave a nervous laugh. 'But there's no need for that to scare you.'

'The wedding date fixed yet?' he asked casually as they made their way to a door where they were let out of the building by the security guard, who carefully locked it after them.

'Well we have about eighteen months to go before Simeon can get his divorce. His wife stopped him, you know.' She stooped over to get into the car as he held the door open for her.

'No I didn't. I'm sorry.'

'She's determined to try and stop it altogether; but we'll get there in the end.'

'A woman scorned?' Pierre murmured as he switched on the ignition and headed out of town.

'Exactly.' Ginny put on her dark glasses and looked about her at the miraculous view. 'Oh, it is *heaven* here, isn't it?'

'Heaven,' he agreed, smiling.

'I must tell Simeon to come and have a look at it. He'd love it, too.'

'Look at what?' Pierre turned to her, surprised.

'Well, look at the place. Of course he knows it, I'm sure. But to have a villa here would be lovely.'

Pierre made no reply, his attention on the road, and after a few moments had passed she looked at him.

'Would that disturb you?'

'It might.'

'You don't *like* Simeon, do you, Pierre?' she enquired in a low voice.

'There's no reason why I should.'

'But he has put a lot of money into the business. He's turned it round.'

'But only for you.'

'Well, that's a good enough reason isn't it?'

'I've never been able to forget how condescending he was to us. How he humiliated my family, my father . . .'

Now Ginny was silent, thoughtful. People often did forget the effects of their behaviour on others; the festering wounds that snubs and humiliations could bring.

'He didn't do it consciously. It was business.'

'It's the same. It's people, isn't it? Or does someone like Mr Varga forget that?'

'I think he does, to be truthful.' She grimaced. 'I'm always trying to remind him of the human factor in everything. He buys companies and forgets they're run by people. He strips them and sells the assets. Inevitably people suffer, but I like to think that, because of me, Simeon is as generous in redundancy terms as he can be.'

'Have you ever visited an "asset" after he had "stripped" it, and seen its effects?' Pierre enquired dryly.

'No.'

'Maybe you should.'

He ran the car on to a grass verge at the side of the narrow road that wound down the mountainside and Ginny could see beneath them the tiled roof of a Provençal house, its terracotta tiles shimmering in the afternoon sun, though it was winter and the nights were bitterly cold, the peaks of the surrounding Alpes Maritimes snow-capped.

Pierre politely helped her out, though his expression was now strained, and she wished they had kept their relationship formal, that she hadn't come. But to have refused would have been rude when obviously he had had lunch prepared for her and, after what he had to say about Simeon, she would not like to have let him down.

Pierre opened a wooden gate and they went down a short path flanked with cypresses, so that, for a moment, she had a vision of a painting by Matisse or Van Gogh, to a small stone-built house, the white shutters closed, surrounded by a balcony. Through the double doors she could see a table laid for two.

'The entrance is round the side,' Pierre said, leading her to the side of the house that faced the mountain. 'Whoever built the house thought the view was the all-important thing.'

'And it *is*, my goodness.' She stood for a moment shielding her eyes, gazing towards the shimmering silver of the Mediterranean on the far horizon.

Inside the house was cool – after all it was February – but not cold. She wore a dress of a very light wool mixture, almost summery, and a cashmere coat. They were both white and she had red accessories. As she removed her coat and glanced at herself in the mirror to make sure that her hair was tidy, Pierre could not conceal his admiration and, fleetingly, their eyes met. He seemed embarrassed by the encounter and led the way into the front room where she had seen the table in front of the open French windows.

'Not *quite* warm enough to eat outside,' he said, looking at the table. 'All I can offer is a cold collation. I hope you don't mind.'

'Just what I wanted,' she assured him, going to the windows and gazing once more at the spectacular scene. 'I'm never much of a person for lunch.'

'Nor am I.' Pierre was opening a bottle of wine and, aware of the exchange of glances in the mirror, she was glad to observe that he had regained his composure and was smiling as he drew the cork.

'At least a glass of wine,' he said, handing her one.

'Oh, at least.' She smiled again and held out her glass. 'To you, Pierre.'

'To Silk,' he said and then, drawing back a chair, held it for her as she sat down.

'I thought you'd like to face the view.'

'You're very thoughtful. I'm dumbstruck, spellbound. I wonder you don't come and live here all the year round.' She flicked open her white linen napkin and laid it across her lap. There was already cold vichysoisse in front of them and on the sideboard a collection of sliced meats and salads and an enticing-looking board of cheeses. She realized that she was hungry and took up her spoon.

'I'm starving after all.'

'It's the air,' he suggested and, passing her a basket full of pieces of *petit pain*, he then took one for himself and began to eat his soup. 'As for living here all the year round,' he leaned back gazing reflectively at her, 'I have to think of my father.'

'Of course. How is he?' she asked after a tiny pause.

'Getting frailer, but glad that the fortunes of the company are reviving. Very grateful to you.'

'And *I'm* grateful to the company. You know, Pierre,' she too broke into her bread, savouring the delicious soup, and looked into his eyes. 'I don't just want to be the wife of a rich man. I have always worked. I'm very lucky that Simeon has given me this chance because now I am a person with my own company, my own identity.'

'And you're still going to marry him?' Pierre came out with the question rather jerkily, as though he'd been bottling it up.

'Of course I'm going to marry him.' She looked surprised.

Pierre fussed a bit more with his bread, his spoon, and when they'd finished took the soup dishes and put them on the sideboard. Then he took a plate and turned to her:

'Shall I serve you?'

'Please do.'

'A little of everything?'

'Fine.' She sat back, feeling awkward, and some moments passed as he filled first her plate then his, then helped them both to more wine and sat down. 'Cheers!' He lifted his glass again.

'Cheers!' she replied.

'You think I'm very rude.'

'No. Why?'

'Because of what I said.'

'About marrying Simeon? Well,' she leaned back and put her napkin to her mouth, 'I already said I knew you didn't like him. Perhaps,' she lowered her voice as if in an effort to make her tone more gentle, 'we should eschew personal matters and stick to business. Now, when do you think the trials of the perfume will be ready?'

Pierre threw back his head and studied the ceiling. He had a handsome, though rather austere, profile: ascetic, a man who, as well as a great parfumier, could perhaps have been a monk.

'Three to six months from now.'

'As long as that?' Her face fell.

'Why do you want to hurry it?'

'We want to launch it at the wedding the following year.'

'Oh, it will be ready for that.'

'We have to think of the bottle design, publicity.'

'Then you had better start to think of it now. In my opinion the name says all.' He held out his hand: '"*Soie*". You have a publicist's gift.'

'That's why we want to keep it so secret.'

'You have a good publicist?'

'I thought myself.' She attempted an expression of modesty but, instead, started to laugh. 'As you say I'm quite good.'

'And your French is good, too.' Once more Pierre saluted her. 'Tell me . . .' he carefully put down his glass and looked at her. 'At the risk of destroying our new-found friendship, do you think Varga *is* the sort of man you ought to marry?'

'Oh Pierre, *please*,' she threw her napkin on the table in irritation. 'That is a very naughty thing to say.'

'I know,' he replied with no apparent sign of contrition, 'but I am serious because . . . I like you so much, Ginny, not only as a person, a woman, a friend; but you are a good human being. You are kind and you care. I can't think how you got involved with him.'

'You have the same kind of snobbish approach as my family,' she said with an air of disdain, looking at her watch. 'Lunch was very nice, Pierre. I should really be going.'

'I've offended you.' He attempted now to look contrite.

'Of course you've offended me.' Refusing his offer of cheese she folded her napkin, placing it carefully by her plate. 'What else did you expect?'

'It is just that I know Varga,' Pierre said meaningfully.

'What do you mean you "know" him? You only met him once.'

'Yes, but I know his type, the sort of man he is. It is nothing to do with his background, of which I am completely ignorant. It is the sort of person he undoubtedly is. He is ruthless, opportunistic . . .'

'He's a businessman. There are plenty of others like him. *I* happen to love him.' Ginny stood up and, looking at Pierre, said in her coldest, most detached voice, 'Would you be kind enough to drive me back to the hotel? I have some packing to do.'

'But I thought you were staying until Monday?'

'I was, but not now.'

'Oh please, Ginny.' Pierre folded his napkin and put it to his mouth. 'I should never have spoken.'

'It would have been far better if you hadn't,' she agreed. 'But, as you have, I think I will confine our meetings in future strictly to business.'

'Of course.' He bent his head. 'I'm sorry.'

'Strictly business,' she said, 'and mostly by fax.'

In the basement was the 'entertainment room', so called because in certain circumstances special guests were allowed to see what went on there. Some clients wanted to watch because they could only get sexual satisfaction through voyeurism. But, whatever the circumstances, a fat fee was charged every time.

340

Varga, of course, could use the entertainment room for nothing. Whenever he liked, he could sit behind the one-way mirror laughing at the antics of his fellow human beings at their worst; wondering how men could so degrade themselves, or allow themselves to be degraded.

There was not only the rack — by far the favourite — there were the whips, the irons, the mechanical horse and a number of other gadgets and implements of torture that, at some time or other, had been brought in from the Continent.

Varga, on his various journeys abroad, had amused himself by brief sorties to various recommended places of assignation where he was offered some instrument of bondage at an exorbitant price. He had become something of a connoisseur, a discerning collector, and, now that he flew in his own aeroplane, importing such things was no trouble at all.

Having enjoyed his own afternoon of illicit pleasure with a new girl called Xanandra — an oriental who had done her apprenticeship in the brothels of New Orleans — Varga, showered, shaved, and now with a gin and tonic in his hand, went down the stairs from the private suite to a room which was covered in drapes. Along one wall was a low sofa and a console with switches. This could operate a television with pornographic videos, films, a hi-fi which had the sounds of torture on it — often more arousing than the real thing — or a switch which operated the curtain on the other side of the room. There were several pornographic magazines lying around and, after sitting on the sofa and glancing at one or two of them, Varga put his drink on the ebony table in front of the black leather sofa and flicked the switches that operated the curtain, which very slowly, tantalizingly, drew back.

As usual the bondage room was in semi-darkness but enough could be seen to provide enjoyment to the voyeur on the other side. The events were usually filmed

341

and could be viewed again at leisure on the TV screen later on.

Varga sat back, drink in one hand, the other resting on the back of the sofa.

Melissa stood there stripped to the waist, her body gleaming with the oil she loved to apply before any form of sexual congress. She wore a black belt with long suspenders and black stockings, no knickers; black shoes with high pointed stiletto heels. On each arm was a broad leather bracelet and in one hand she held a long, thin stick with a fine point, in the other a whip. On the wheel in front of her lay a man, strapped by his hands and feet, facing away. He was entirely naked and in a state of tumescence which was the subject of Melissa's attentions. She would bend over it, run her hands up and down it, pretend to embrace it and then back away and give him a sharp stab in his buttock, breast, thigh or calf. He reacted sharply with cries of pain, either real or pretended, while slowly the wheel revolved and Melissa, like a lioness stalking its prey, walked round with it, the whip, which she alternated with the stick, darting out like a serpent's tongue.

Varga enjoyed watching Melissa, his long-time mistress. She had been working as a stewardess on the ship on which he escaped, to pay her own passage from Cairo, and they became attracted to each other. It was not only physical but also emotional and cerebral. They had been in harmony then and remained in harmony to this day – that is, until the advent of Ginny.

Melissa resented Ginny more than she had resented Claudia. She feared her power and knew that Varga had changed; but there was little she could do about it. She was a heroin addict who had been hooked since she was a girl. Her mother had been African, her father Egyptian, and she had the most beautiful smooth brown skin, a face apparently unravaged by the excesses of her vice, all-knowing.

When she got to London, Varga set her up in her own

establishment and she made a fortune on the side from drugs. She was ten years older than Varga and could easily have retired, lived a life of ease; but she enjoyed her work: vice, risk, and a way of life.

Sometimes Varga feared for Ginny because of Melissa's jealousy, her possessiveness. He thought she might try and blackmail him or inform on him, but she never had. She liked risks and he liked risks and this was a risk he had to take. Besides, he thought she really loved him in a way that was part physical, part maternal.

Melissa knew by now that he was watching and as she passed him she made an obscene gesture with her behind towards him and he felt a twitch in his thighs. Usually voyeurism didn't stimulate him, and he had had a very fulfilling, satisfying afternoon with the new girl who had suited his mood. Melissa was never jealous of the girls he played about with in the house, because no emotion was involved.

He was about to finish his drink and close the curtain when the man turned towards him and he could see the agonized features clearly. His lips were set in a grimace and, clearly, he was enjoying his pain. With an exclamation Varga put down his glass and rose in his seat, going to the window to peer closely at him just to make sure.

He was sure.

'How long has Carlo Bernini been a patron?' Varga asked Melissa when, later, she came upstairs and threw herself on the bed still dressed or, rather undressed, in her flagellation gear. She removed the belt and stockings and lay there with nothing on at all. Taking a cigarette from the bedside she lit it, blowing away the smoke from his direction as he sat on the bed beside her.

He never tried to stop her because he knew she needed it for her work.

'Who?' She glanced at him, a frown on her face.

'Your recent client. What's his name?'

343

'Giacomo, he calls himself.'

'Just that?'

'Yes.'

'How does he pay?'

'Cash, always cash.'

'He's my brother-in-law.'

She turned to the table to flick her ash into a tray and faced him again.

'Get away.'

'How often does he come?'

'Oh not often. Once or twice a month.'

'Always for the "entertainment"?'

'No.' She shook her head and flicked her ash again. There was a thin film of sweat on her brow. 'But he's not straight. He always likes something different.'

'How long has he been coming?'

'Oh, a long time. You mean you never saw him here before?'

'Never.'

'Well it's chance that you recognized him. He's a regular. He usually telephones an hour in advance. I think he works somewhere near here.'

'He does.'

'That's it, then.'

Melissa stubbed out her cigarette, jumped off the bed and went into the bathroom. Varga could hear the sound of water running, and completed the dressing which he had begun before she came in. He felt excited, elated, and curiously stimulated, but not by lust or, rather, it *was* lust of a kind: lust for power, for domination, for revenge on his brother-in-law.

He went into the bathroom and sat on the side of the bath where Melissa was soaping herself. In the bright lights of the bathroom she looked drawn and old and he could see signs of strain now, as well of age, in her face.

'I tell you, you could pack it all up and go away,' he said, bending over her and stroking her brow tenderly. 'You're a very rich woman.'

344

'What would I do? Where would I go?'

It was a question, because she was after all middle-aged. If only she would marry.

'Look, if you became thoroughly respectable,' he got up and began to walk back and forth across the bathroom floor, 'you'd marry.'

'You mean settle down?'

'Yes. Why not?'

'Like you?'

'Why not like me?'

'Because I don't want to be like you, Simeon.' She had a curiously strange and cutting edge to her voice.

Melissa was moody, not surprising in view of her occupation and her habit. But of late her moods had grown stronger and he wondered if her dependency had deepened. Sometimes it could kill people at a relatively young age. It was partly the reason that she didn't enjoy sex; hadn't had an orgasm since her teens. But she was wonderful at making love, a consummate actress playing a well-rehearsed part.

She got out of the bath, suds dripping on the floor. Varga handed her a heavy fleecy bath towel and she wrapped herself in it and, returning to the bedroom, sat on the side of the bed and lit another cigarette, her hands shaking slightly.

Varga finished tying his tie and shrugged on his jacket, glancing at his watch.

'Must go,' he said. 'We'll be in touch.' He went up to her and, stretching out his hand, ran it tenderly through her hair.

'Think about what I said. You want to give it up, get away. You know I'll look after you, always, for the rest of your life.'

'I shan't need you,' she said, raising her head proudly.

He looked deeply into her eyes for a few moments, holding her face firmly between the palms of his strong, powerful hands.

'Remember,' he said, 'you are my oldest, greatest love . . . the best.'

Melissa returned his gaze, her expression unfathomable, but in her manner, her sagging shoulders and limp inert body, there was an air of despair, rejection.

'Ha!' She suddenly threw back her head and gave a loud, mirthless laugh and Varga, as if angered by her response, abruptly let go of her face. Her scorn seemed to echo hollowly in his ears as he hurried out of the room, and ran down the stairs into the viewing room. The video had stopped, as it automatically did when a client left. He took it from the machine and put it in his pocket.

He would very much enjoy playing it back.

Carlo looked at the video that Varga had put on his desk as though it mesmerized him.

'You can play it back if you like,' Varga said.

Carlo got up and went to the window where he stood looking down into Albemarle Street. The one-way traffic whizzed by towards the turning that led into Dover Street and from thence to Berkeley Square.

All the money he'd paid, and no one had ever told him. He'd had Varga followed, but he was never told he went to a brothel. A deep rage welled up inside him and he felt like murder. Instead he turned, clenching and unclenching his hands.

'I suppose this isn't "extortion" is it, Simeon? I mean, you're here for another purpose?'

'I merely want my divorce, that's all. You can then have the video. Very cheap at the price.'

'You could have copies made.'

'I wouldn't go to the trouble,' Varga said with a sneer. 'All I want is my freedom.'

'My mother will never allow it.'

'Then your mother will see the video . . . all of it!'

'You know I can't permit that!'

'I can,' Varga smiled. 'I would love to sit there watch-

346

ing it with your mother. Mama mia,' he shook his hand up and down, Italian style, 'what would she say?'

'I'll do what I can,' Carlo said thickly. 'But even then I don't have any proof you won't use it against me.'

'I am not interested in your perversions, Carlo. Your sexual inadequacies, though pathetic, are entirely your own affair. I only want justice for me, and my freedom.'

Varga went to the desk and pocketed the video. 'I will give you a week and no longer. Ciaou, Carlo.'

He felt light-hearted as he shut the door behind him and took the lift to the ground floor.

Kelly always woke at about six and lay for some time listening to the sounds of the house, the seemingly perpetual flow of traffic in the street outside. The cat slept on her bed, the dog in a basket in the kitchen. At about six both animals began to stir and this sense of movement woke her up.

She lay awake for some time acclimatizing herself to a new day and then, gently shifting the cat, she got out of bed into her slippers and padded to the kitchen where she was greeted with customary rapture by the dog, who was immediately let out into the tiny back garden.

Kelly then made tea and sometimes she took it back to bed and lay watching the early news on breakfast TV. Two cups of tea revived her, made her ready to face the day, and she then accomplished the rest of her morning tasks, including ablutions, dressing, snatching breakfast and briefly walking the dog in about an hour, enabling her to leave the house at around seven-thirty. She was a disciplined creature; ruled by the clock, by habits of a lifetime.

She also liked to be first in the office and, if possible, to read through the faxes that had come in overnight and open the mail herself.

Kelly had known Edward Thomas in the Metropolitan Police Force. Their relationship had always been professional, always close, based on mutual respect. They never mixed socially and in all the years she had known him she had never met his wife or children. He had never been to her house.

This anonymity suited them both and provided for a close working relationship. Kelly guessed that she would remain with Thomas until he pensioned her off and she found that thatch-covered, dream retirement cottage in the country.

Kelly's car was black or dark coloured and her clothes always sober, usually suits in black or navy, low-heeled shoes. Anyone would have taken her for a civil servant leading just the sort of life she did lead, with a flat or a small house in the suburbs, a dog and a cat and not many friends. She had two close women friends, one with whom she had been to school and another she had met in the police college. One was married and one wasn't. She was closer to the one who, like her, was unmarried and occasionally they went on holiday together. Usually, though, Kelly chose a package holiday from a brochure and went for a fortnight to Greece or Sardinia or North Africa, putting the dog and the cat in kennels and the cattery respectively.

She was just like any unattached middle-aged woman – pleasant, agreeable, independent and enjoying her vacation. No one would have ever guessed she was a surveillance expert, one acquainted with violence and the darker side of human nature.

This morning Kelly got to the office just before eight and, as she'd hoped, she was first there. She unlocked the door, turned off the alarm and put on the lights. She inspected the faxes, opened the post and was making her first cup of coffee and lighting her second cigarette of the day when Edward arrived, followed by two of the operatives who had come to get instructions for the day. Their secretary, Mavis, usually arrived at about nine and got straight down to work.

So far it was just like any other day of the week and,

as usual, at nine-thirty Kelly went into Edward's office for a briefing.

'How was your weekend?' he asked.

'Fine.' She smiled. 'How was yours?'

'Fine.'

That was usually the extent of their personal chat. Sometimes he would say he'd played golf or held a barbecue or something like that; but she hardly ever filled in what she'd done. She knew in any case that he wouldn't be very interested.

Kelly had a pad in her hand and they went over some of the routine chores; the reports that had come in, continuing work, new projects, and then Edward suddenly looked at her and said:

'Bernini wants us to discontinue the surveillance.'

'Oh?' She drew a line and wrote a note on the pad. 'That's interesting, because I was about to suggest it.' She looked at Edward with her clear, honest brown eyes. 'Did he say why?'

'They're not opposing the divorce.'

'That's interesting, too.'

'Why?'

'They seemed so determined to screw him.'

'Maybe they have and we don't know about it. I didn't trust him all that much.'

'Anyway, it's a relief,' Kelly said. 'I hate people throwing their money away, even people like him.'

'You really had nothing on Varga did you?' Edward shuffled some papers as though already he were turning to something else.

'No.' Kelly paused and put her chin in her hands. 'Yet I was always sure that there was something more to Varga than we know; more than normal surveillance would reveal.'

'Bernini never wanted to spend money on investigation of the offshore companies.' Edward shrugged. 'And I agree with you, I don't think it was worth it either. Now . . .'

'There *was* one thing about Varga that really surprised me.'

'Oh?' Edward looked at her as though he were just a little impatient at the time she was spending on this unimportant subject.

'He visited a Mayfair brothel.'

Thomas appeared unsurprised by this news.

'Well that's not so extraordinary. Did we tell Bernini this?'

'No.'

Edward leaned forward and frowned. 'Surely that should have figured in the report, Kelly?'

Kelly scratched her head and lit another cigarette.

'Varga is a real shit, but I liked the girl,' she said. 'Ginny, the one he's going to marry. She appealed to me. We were asked to discover something about Varga that would discredit him business-wise. This had nothing to do with business.'

'Perhaps you're right.' Edward looked doubtful but drew a line under the paper in front of him, tossed it into a file and put it on one side.

'File closed,' he said. 'Next?'

Kelly had enjoyed those days when she could get out into the field. She liked sitting in her car playing tapes. She was keen on the classics, Mozart, Schubert and Bach in particular. The operatives changed cars quite a lot, and many of them worked on foot and took taxis for convenience.

That day was a routine one; she had no outside jobs and she didn't leave the office until nearly six, when she joined the rush hour traffic going over Westway, looking forward to getting home to the cat and the dog, the routine of domestic life.

In her mirror she could see a motor-cyclist in black and yellow weaving in and out of the traffic and, suddenly, something clicked in her mind and she wondered why it had never done so before. Maybe she was ceasing to be a good surveillance expert, becoming careless, and she shouldn't spend so much time in the office doing routine work. It was little things that good operatives noticed and this one she'd ignored until now.

She took out her pad to make a note of the courier's name as he flashed past her, aware that she had seen him, or one dressed in the same outfit, several times in the past few weeks.

She usually went south over Putney Bridge, another sure-fire spot for a traffic jam, so she positioned herself in the near-side lane to exit at the turn to Shepherd's Bush. She saw the motor-cyclist approaching and she held her pencil ready to note down the name on his despatch box.

As he drew alongside she looked up into his face and he looked into hers.

He leaned right through the window until his face was a few inches away from hers. His eyes, hidden by the glare on his space helmet, momentarily beamed out at her. She had no chance to see the gun, to panic or take any evasive action before she was dead, the bullet entering her throat and slicing her trachea in two.

Her car rolled down the incline towards the Shepherd's Bush roundabout and crashed into another, slightly injuring the driver.

Soon after that there was the wail of police sirens, but no sign of the motor-cyclist in his Colorado beetle outfit, who had got clean away, charging onwards towards Ealing.

CHAPTER 19

It was a lovely day for a wedding: a July day, not too hot and not too cold. A marquee had been put up on the lawn in case of rain and a covered passageway made from there to the house where the more elderly guests – and there were dozens of ancient Silklanders and assorted relations – could sit in comfort and be served by attentive waiters.

Most people chose to stroll on the lawn and sit at the many tables scattered there, white tables with white chairs under colourful umbrellas, while the catering staff wove skilfully in and out with their laden trays dispensing drink to those who had helped themselves to food from the buffet inside the marquee.

Ginny and Varga made a striking pair. She was dressed in white but not in a traditional bride's dress. She wore a white suit, the jacket with a round neck, and no blouse. She wore, too, the family pearls which had been her mother's, grandmother's and, before that, her great-grandmother's. One day, she hoped, she would pass them on to her daughter on her wedding day.

Simeon was slightly shorter than Ginny, a stocky yet attractive man, his thick black hair brushed back. He looked upright and confident, yet his deeply recessed brown eyes had an expression that was at once sensual and rather sad. His expensive suit had been made for the wedding in Savile Row, blue barathea with a fine white stripe. He wore a blue shirt with a soft, button-down collar and a club tie. He didn't look English. He wasn't English; but, now, he didn't care.

He had fulfilled an ambition: to marry into the English aristocracy, to capture the love of one of its finest off-shoots, and he was a very, very happy man. They looked rapturous together, tightly holding hands. Both wore wedding rings exchanged in the registry office in Gloucester which had been followed by a brief service of blessing at the local parish church.

Only family came to the ceremony. Lambert was best man and Pru assisted her sister. Lady Silklander cried all the way through, even though Ginny was the fourth of her children to marry.

The little Silklanders scampered about watched over, in the case of the most junior members, by nannies. The older Silklanders sauntered about with an aristocratic air, perfectly at home in the grounds of a large country house.

The previous night they had been given 'the tour' and approved everything they saw without ill-bred comment but, perhaps, with a little envy.

The Georgian completion had been remarkable, the pastel colours – yellow, rose, aquamarine, duck-egg blue – toned perfectly. The white plasterwork, friezes, cornices and coronals of leaves looked as though they'd been there for years and had merely been freshened up. Not all the furniture was in place yet, and the walls were almost bare: but the essentials were there and, as the wedding had after all taken place a year before everyone expected it to be, a remarkable amount had been accomplished in time.

Large, light, gracious and airy – the house was perfection, Ginny's life-style as a wealthy woman assured.

But, oh, they *did* so wish it had been someone else. Ever since that business with Angus, how the Silklanders had hoped that, somehow, Ginny would get out of the marriage, end up with someone like Robert, someone more her age, someone just like them.

Still, Varga was undoubtedly wealthy and there was even less doubt that he loved her; it shone from his eyes, his expression of tenderness when he looked at her, was heard in his voice; seen in his manner, the possessiveness with which he touched her.

Oh well, perhaps they'd get used to him in time.

Philip di Suiza, despite his name, was a Scot, a banker and, of course a friend of the Silklanders, the families having been associated for generations, if not centuries. The Scottish connection had been interrupted only briefly when his great-grandmother, a McNeil and a relation of Moira Silklander, had married a Spanish nobleman. That had upset the applecart some time at the beginning of the nineteenth century, except that he was awfully wealthy, very handsome and, unlike Varga, about whom no one knew a thing, possessed of a pedigree stretching back to Philip II of Spain. He was also most happy to come and live on his bride's vast estates in Scotland and turn himself into an Scottish gentleman, and of course his sons and daughters, and he had quite a few, were the genuine thing. Only the name remained.

Di Suiza, although a banker by profession, was an art lover by inclination. He had inherited one of the finest collections in Scotland and kept adding to it. His wife Elizabeth was a sculptor and they were just about as cultured and rich as it was possible to be, knowing everybody who was anybody in almost every walk of life.

They quite liked Simeon, but then they were more cosmopolitan than Gerald and Moira, who still regarded a trip beyond the Channel as an adventure. To the di Suizas the Silklanders were rather homespun and cosy, Ginny a delightful exception.

Elizabeth was very sociable and chatty. She was a lovely girl, tall and fair, and she wore a large picture hat which showed off the highlights in her striking blond hair. Ginny was hatless, the sheen of her own coiffeur like a mane which curled lightly to her shoulders, beautifully offset by the classical lines of her white suit. Elizabeth thought Simeon very attractive and, even on his wedding day, flirted a little with him. The upper classes were like that.

Philip was less gregarious, a solitary man who didn't like parties as much as his wife, but had to go to them just the same. If he could he liked to slink off, preferably to a library, where he could bury himself in a book, a large glass of something by his elbow, until it was time to leave.

Some of the Silklanders were staying at the house, but half the bedrooms were not yet finished despite the efforts of Maggie, and so the main body of people were staying in the Purborough Arms nearby, including Elizabeth and himself.

He drank some champagne, had a plate of salmon and asparagus, and then with a glass in his hand wandered into the house to find some shade, a little peace and, perhaps, a book to read until it was time to go.

Across the entrance hall, huge and beautiful, he made his way towards the main staircase, knowing that the library was on the first floor although, of course, there were hardly any books in it yet. Doubtless Simeon would have them imported, bound in fine vellum, by the case as soon as he could. Doubtless too he would never read a word of any of them.

The hall was practically deserted and he lingered for a while inspecting the paintings on the wall, large, solid paintings, not very valuable, of English country scenes.

It was really a magnificent house, skilfully refurbished – thanks, undoubtedly, to that taste of the Silklanders which could only be inherited, never acquired. He looked round with approval as he mounted the stairs, stopping every now and then to glance back and survey the scene of grandeur, splendour and opulence.

Ginny was a lucky girl.

He wandered along the corridor of the first floor,

which was completely deserted, occasionally glancing out of the window at the scene on the lawn below, the large striped marquee, the tables and chairs dotted about, the elegantly dressed crowd, the beautiful bride and distinguished-looking groom. Yes Ginny *was* lucky; she was a lovely, talented girl with good taste, lucky enough to find a man who could afford to indulge her. What did it matter if his origins were obscure, his manners sometimes a little strange, and that he was years older than she was? Some women liked older men, needed them. Philip smiled to himself, took a sip of champagne and opened a door, peering round.

This was the library. No, he paused for a moment. It was not the library. It was a room he had not seen during the official tour the previous evening. It was a small, rather intimate room with a desk, several chairs and some packing cases on the floor, one or two pictures on the walls, which were covered in pale green silk. A splendid room in the making, no doubt of that.

Ah, he had it. Varga's study. This was why it had not been included in the itinerary. It was not finished. An electrician had temporarily abandoned his task of putting sockets in the wall for faxes and telephones; flexes lay on the carpet and there was even an abandoned screwdriver.

Feeling a little like an interloper, Philip was about to back out when in the corner, almost concealed by the open door of a cupboard, he spied a painting on the wall. His eyes opened very wide even as his heart beat more quickly and he gently shut the door again: like a prowler fearing to be caught out, he stole softly over the carpet towards it.

Surely a reproduction? But was Varga, advised by an expert like Lambert, likely to have such a bourgeois possession as a *reproduction*? But . . . Philip, his hands trembling with excitement, took his reading glasses out of their case and fumblingly put them on his nose, peering at the picture.

Mantegna. Undoubtedly: a fine example of his grisaille method – painting like sculpture. A Sybil and the Prophet . . . but the figures were facing the wrong way. And yet . . . he tried to visualize the painting he had seen, as it happened, not so many months before, at the Cincinnati Art Museum when he and Elizabeth had been on a trip to the States, she on the track of a commission, he on business connected with his bank. As usual they had spent half their time in museums and art galleries, or in the homes of wealthy private collectors like themselves.

Tentatively he put out a finger and, almost not daring to, touched it. But no, it was real. He could feel the varnish, patchy, as it was on the painting in Cincinnati. Gold on gold. The picture had never been intended to be varnished.

Suddenly he realized that he was trembling all over and he sat down abruptly and slowly finished his champagne.

But what could he do with his knowledge? He was a lifelong friend of the Silklanders, Lambert was godfather to one of his children.

Yet he knew, without any doubt, that the picture had in all probability been stolen and that few people – certainly not he, an expert – were meant to have seen it.

Now almost all the guests had gone and they were alone, or rather they were alone in their bedroom because the rooms that were furnished were still full of relations; her parents, Angus and Betty, Pru and Douglas and the children. The rest had gone off, very late, to the hotel and in a breeze that had sprung up, a soft, summery breeze, the fairy lights among the trees seemed to flicker gently, like fireflies.

Ginny and Varga stood by the window naked, his arms round her. He stood behind her, her body pressed against his, and she felt his strength and his power, a feeling, awesome in its profundity, that they were one.

In their union it seemed to her that they owned the

whole world, not just this beautiful house and park.
Material things meant nothing.

'I love you,' he whispered gently, pushing her hair
back from her ear.

'And I love you,' she said and turned to him. Their
lips touched, her arms stole round his neck, his arms
embraced her waist, his breasts brushed hers. The whole
world simmered with a marvellous, incandescent light.

The Vargas didn't go on honeymoon. There was no time.
Simeon was about to complete a deal – to acquire one
of the largest manufacturers of paper in the country,
whose management and workforce were putting up a
strong protest because of his reputation as tough, ruthless, an asset stripper.

The day after his wedding he was back in his office
where he sat at his desk, a telephone in each hand, his
eyes anxiously scanning the share prices on the VDU.

Liddle had not been invited to the wedding. He was not
surprised, not angry. He would have been embarrassed,
because neither he nor his wife would have fitted in.
They had sent a small gift, just a token, because what
could you possibly give a couple who had everything?

However he was quite surprised to see Varga back and
went into his office, a sheepish smile on his face.

'Couldn't you sleep?' he asked, indicating the
announcement in *The Times* which he carried in his hand.

*Mr S.G. Varga and the Hon Virginia Silklander, younger
daughter of . . .*

Varga affably waved a hand at him, smiled and indicated that he should take a seat.

He finished giving instructions down one phone to his
broker, spoke briefly to his solicitor on the other and
then put down both receivers simultaneously. Then he
leaned across his desk and took Liddle's proffered hand.

'Congratulations,' Liddle said.

'Thanks.' Varga gave a brief nod.

'Did it go off well?'

'Very well.' Varga's eyes were still on the screen. 'A perfect day. Loved every minute. Have you noticed the movement in the price of Baltic crude?'

Work, work, work. Varga would never think of anything but work.

They spent half an hour talking business; the new acquisitions planned in England, continental Europe and America.

The share price was still rising, but not as fast as he'd hoped.

'Anything wrong?' he asked Tony, his eyes never leaving the columns of figures. 'I would have thought we would have been over fifteen hundred by now.'

'The City isn't happy about Consolidated Paper.'

'Why on earth not?'

'The workforce are opposing it.'

'To hell with them.'

'It has to be handled properly, Simeon. You'd better get Ginny back to chat up the papers.'

'Look,' Varga leaned over the desk and tapped his finger sharply on it, 'from yesterday Ginny is *Mrs Varga*. She is no longer *Miss Silklander*. No longer anything to do with this business. Except for the perfume,' he added as an afterthought. 'We have agreed about that. For the time being it will keep her happy.'

'How's it coming on, by the way?' Liddle examined his nails.

'I've no idea.' Varga consulted his memo pad and reached for the telephone again. 'Oh well I think, we . . . as long as she's happy. She planned a big launch for the new perfume for the wedding. Of course it wasn't ready, thanks to Claudia giving in, but, maybe for the first wedding anniversary, or the birth of our first child,' he beamed, 'I'm not sure which will be first.'

'Oh, it's to be as soon as that?'

'Oh yes,' Varga nodded emphatically. 'We want a family as soon as we can. Incidentally, Tony,' Varga got up and, crossing to the door, opened it, looked outside and then shutting it again, locked it. He then returned to his desk and, lifting the phone, spoke briefly and rapidly into it. 'Dorothy, no calls until I give you the word. Right? Thanks.' He smiled into the mouthpiece. The loyal Dorothy of so many years' standing had not been invited to the wedding either.

Ginny had demurred but Varga had been insistent. It was an occasion for family and friends only. Staff were not strictly speaking friends. Staff were, therefore, not to be invited.

They compromised on an agreement that there would be a party for them later in London.

'Now, Tony, I want to talk to you very seriously.' Varga, instead of returning to his desk, drew up a chair next to Tony so that their knees almost touched. Tony put his files on Varga's desk and turned attentively towards him.

'Yes, Simeon?'

'I want to change my life, Tony. I am serious about this. I am a married man, very happily married. I not only admire and love my wife, but she is a member of the British aristocracy. Do you know we had at least five lords at the wedding and I don't know how many "sirs".'

'Is that a fact?' Liddle looked impressed.

'At least, and an ambassador. No, two ambassadors I think.'

Liddle could see why he hadn't been asked. He and his humble wife would have made a very poor showing.

'Now, Tony,' Varga placed a hand on his desk and his fingers began their characteristically impatient tap, 'I made a very important decision yesterday as I made my vows. I became a new man, determined to break with the past. I may at one time have appeared to you cynical in my pursuit of Ginny. My motivations *may* not always have been pure. I may have sought to gain something: position, prestige as the son-in-law of a peer of the realm.'

Varga leaned back like a man who has, perhaps, caught sight of the Holy Grail. 'All that has gone, changed. It is no longer important who my father-in-law is. I am deeply and passionately in love with my wife. I have fallen in love, and fallen hard.'

His fingers recommenced their nervous tapping.

'I want to wipe the slate clean. To be true to Ginny and her family. Now, as you know, in the past I have not always dealt straight. I have done some rather foolish, crooked things and I want all this to go. I want the slate cleaned *completely*, do you understand, Tony?'

'I think I understand,' Liddle said, scratching the side of his nose. 'But I don't think it will be so easy, Simeon.'

'Christ, I *know* it won't be easy, but I want it *done*.' He banged the desk firmly.

'I advised you to do this before, Simeon.'

'Just sell the lot, for God's sake. Sell Planz, sell Acapulco. For God's sake, plug up *that* hole immediately. My God, they were having me *followed*. By the way,' he looked sideways at his deputy, 'anything in the paper . . . about the woman?'

'Well it wasn't in the headlines. It made a column in the *Evening Standard*. Death a mystery. Murder on the motorway. It didn't say she was an enquiry agent. Seems to have died down.'

'I see.' Varga appeared able to dismiss murder from his mind with the same ease with which he could forget about an unhappy or discontented workforce. 'Anyway, you got rid of that damned motor-cyclist?'

'He was a creep,' Liddle agreed with obvious distaste. 'I gave him fifty thousand, as you said, with orders to disappear and not reappear again. I said there was nothing to link us with the, er, accident, nor him. If he kept quiet we'd keep quiet.'

'Good.' However, Varga now showed a trace of unease. 'I'm sorry it had to be done like that. It should have appeared more of an accident. It was clumsy . . . maybe we didn't think it through properly.'

'Well, it's done.' Liddle started to doodle on his pad. 'Can't bring back the dead.'

'Yes, clean everything up.' Varga picked up the phone and said: 'Any calls, Dorothy? Well, get him on the line and then get Sir Monty Fenton again.'

Liddle still marvelled at the way his boss was able to compartmentalize his life. For himself, the night after the woman was killed he was unable to sleep, and for many other nights after that. Murder took some getting used to.

'You saw a what?' François Betoine leaned over the lunch table at the Garrick, holding his knife poised in mid-air.

Nervously, Philip di Suiza looked round at the room full of chattering members.

'A Mantegna,' he whispered, leaning as close to François as he could. 'You know *The Sybil and the Prophet*? Gold on gold.'

'Yes, yes, one of his finest grisaille paintings incidentally – go on, where?'

'I can't tell you, but I swear it's the missing half. I'm almost sure of it.'

'Where, here in England?' The Frenchman excitedly resumed his meal.

'In England.'

'At a private house?'

'Yes.'

'Then it is stolen.' Bentoine neatly put his knife and fork together and mopped up the tasty gravy on his plate with a morsel of bread.

'Exactly. That's what I thought.'

'I would absolutely love to see it, Philip.' The Frenchman looked grave. 'It belongs to a friend of yours?'

'A friend of the family, shall we say,' Philip replied cautiously.

'You should warn them to keep it well out of sight. The governments of all the major countries are tightening up on art thefts. In England alone, do you know that *two billion pounds'* worth are stolen every year and hardly ever recovered? Now I know where they go. To the homes of unscrupulous art collectors.'

'This man is not a collector,' Philip said slowly. 'He is not cultured. He would have acquired it for its rarity, as a cachet, not because he values it. He knows nothing about art.' Philip paused and gazed at his plate. 'But his wife . . . his wife is another matter. I wonder what *she* thinks about the Mantegna?'

The expression on Pierre Jacquet's face was rather strained, but his eyes gleamed with excitement. Ginny, dressed in the white suit she'd worn at her wedding, was calm and controlled. The meeting was at the Oriole factory outside Paris and Roger Bennet was present too, together with a handful of technicians.

Ginny stretched out her hand and he shook it.

'Mrs Varga, may I wish you *every* happiness on your marriage.'

'Thank you, Pierre.' Her smile was warm and genuine and, as their hands touched, she felt a response.

'I think at last I pulled it off.' Pierre turned to the bench behind him on which there were various liquids in a series of test tubes. 'I think I have made a wonderful blend. Truly wonderful,' he said with enthusiasm. 'And then, if you agree, we are to meet the marketing people.'

'How exciting.' As Pierre held out the phial Ginny put it gingerly to her nose. It was indeed a wonderfully subtle blend of aromas, the chief of which was rose, a deep, heady rose.

They had already established their first rose garden at Purborough, although it would not mature properly until the following year. Ginny already had visions of the wonderful launching party they would have there to celebrate their first wedding anniversary, and she knew that Simeon hoped also the birth of their child.

'This *is* gorgeous,' she enthused.

'But wait until you smell this.' Pierre held another small phial under her nose.

'Yes . . . even better, a little more positive, perhaps. I don't know,' she frowned, 'may I smell the first one again please?'

'But there are four others for you, madame, and from that will come the final blend.'

It was a heady, even thrilling morning, each new fragrance, it was true, different in a subtle way from the rest. First she preferred this, then that, then another would send her senses reeling.

Whichever they chose she knew that Silk would be sensational. A feeling of happiness overwhelmed her which seemed a combination of her excitement about the perfume with her love for Simeon, the change in her fortunes in the last six months. Everyone in the room responded to her mood and, after a morning spent in the laboratory, they went to the boardroom where lunch had been prepared.

Already the change in the premises was remarkable. Rebuilding and restoration were almost complete. Half of it had been redecorated, with new layouts and the most up-to-date instruments. Above all, she detected a note of genuine optimism among the staff that had been absent before. Roger was particularly cheerful and even Pierre Jacquet, whom she sat next to at lunch, looked happy and relaxed, a little guarded, but friendly.

'How's your dear little house?' she enquired, leaning towards him as they tackled the first course of pâté maison.

'I haven't seen it for some time, madame. At a certain stage I have to do all my work here because of the scientific instruments that are now an important part of our art. Incidentally, Madame Varga,' he paused and looked round.

'Yes?' she said encouragingly.

'I do wish to apologize for my remarks when we last met. About . . .'

'Oh, I quite understand.' She smiled reassuringly at him. 'That is completely forgotten.'

'I can see you're very happy. Besides, they were completely uncalled-for.'

'Consider them unsaid,' she assured him gaily. 'I hope one day you'll come and visit our house. It's very beautiful and tomorrow in Paris I have an appointment to see some treasures which I hope we'll be able to buy.'

'Are you meeting Mr Varga there?'

'Oh no. He's very busy in England. Now, when do you think you'll have the final brew, as it were, and we can begin the launch?'

'In a matter of weeks. The launch we can start thinking about today.'

As lunch was coming to an end, Roger stood up and, tapping his glass, called for silence. The five other people around the table looked expectantly at him.

'I just wanted to use this opportunity to welcome Madame Varga once again and to thank her for all she has done to restore the fortunes of Oriole since she has been chief executive. I would also like to wish madame and her husband the greatest happiness on the part of the staff of this organization and I therefore . . .' he produced a small box from his pocket which he handed to Ginny who, totally unprepared for such an event, was not quite sure what to do. Should she for instance stand up, or remain sitting?

Compromising in a half-rise she took the box from his hand and then she sat down again to open it.

'Oh!' she exclaimed. 'Why, it's absolutely *beautiful*.' It was a miniature perfume bottle apparently made of diamonds which was intended as a lapel brooch. The tiny stopper had a ruby at the top and the whole thing was of precise and expert workmanship. 'It's the most exquisite thing I ever saw,' she said, taking it from its case and holding it against her suit.

'Madame, it is *not* from the profits of the firm,' Roger said earnestly. 'Each member of staff contributed from his or her own pocket, and gave most generously, from the heart.'

'I can see that,' Ginny exclaimed and, with fingers which trembled slightly, she undid the safety chain and fastened it to her bosom just above the left breast.

Everyone exclaimed in admiration.

'It matches your beauty, Madame Varga,' Pierre said with a light in his eyes. 'Yes, I think it is a triumph.'

'Words cannot express my gratitude, or how I feel,' Ginny said, getting to her feet and looking from one eager face to the other. 'Believe me, my greatest satisfaction over the past years is to have assisted in restoring the fortunes of Oriole, that is after my marriage to the chairman of AP International, without whom none of us could have done anything. I assure you the firm has a very special place in my husband's heart. I can tell you now that he has given me a very generous budget for the establishment of Silk. As you know it was the intention to launch Silk on the occasion of our marriage but, happily, we were able to bring forward the date. Now it is our earnest hope that the launch will take place at our country home, Purborough Park, on the occasion of our first wedding anniversary, that is approximately in nine months' time.'

Everyone clapped.

'Thank you again, gentlemen, and please thank all the staff for me. I will write to each one individually.' She fingered the brooch at her breast. 'I can assure you that this precious gift from you is, and will remain, very close to my heart.'

Everyone clapped again and as Ginny, slightly flushed, sat down the door opened and a secretary popped her head round. 'Monsieur Debrès is here from Paris, Monsieur Bennet.'

'Ah, the publicity people have arrived.' Roger stood up and gestured towards Ginny. 'I think you will be very pleased with the work they have already done.'

*

Varga sat in a chair, Ginny squatted on the floor, the preliminary designs in front of her.

'This one I like particularly.' She held up a mock-up of a perfume bottle of elegant and unusual proportions which rested in a bed of silk. The whole effect was of tones of golds cleverly and subtly blended into one flowing harmonious montage, with the simple words: *Soie: l'essence suprême* underneath.

'That is lovely,' Varga nodded, holding it at arm's length. 'Yes I think I agree. The fluidity . . . very expressive.' He handed it back to her, smiling at the childish excitement on her face. He leaned towards her until their faces almost touched. 'Really, my darling, I think you are more excited about this than about us.'

'Oh *no*,' she protested, putting the design to one side and bringing his hand to her lips. 'I am much more excited about *us*, Simeon.'

'I wish you would take off your clothes and sit in front of me naked,' he murmured.

'Would it give you inspiration for the launch?' She looked teasingly up at him.

'It would give me an erection,' he said, leaving his chair and squatting beside her.

It was a Sunday and Ginny had returned from her successful trip to France the day before. He had met her at Heathrow and they had driven straight to Purborough, one of their rare chances to spend some time together: a whole day to themselves. They had dined quietly together the night before and been in no hurry to rise this morning.

She felt satiated with love; loving and being loved. She took his hand as he sat beside her and put his arm round her waist raising her T-shirt so that he could feel her bare flesh.

'I love you,' he said, kissing her neck.

How many times a day did he say it? Her mind was fast losing its concentration on the project at the prospect of making love on the carpet as they had at the office.

Only, in this huge room, who could be sure that one of the staff would not come in, that someone would not peer through the windows? An amorous, erotic situation would descend into farce. Sex, after all, was comical in the eye of the beholder. She looked nervously around as his intentions became obvious.

'Not *here*, darling,' she said.

'Wouldn't you like it?'

'Yes; but I would dislike being seen by someone else, besides,' she glanced at the thin gold band of her watch, 'I have to send all this artwork back by tonight so that they can get started on it first thing tomorrow.'

'But, darling, it's not for ages.' He withdrew his hand and, practical now, seized another design and, legs crossed, chin in hand, examined it.

'I like this, too.'

'I like that *very* much,' she said, taking it from him.

This was a completely different concept with no bottle, just yards and yards of sumptuous material arranged on a plinth. 'It's more subtle.'

'But I do think we should use the perfume bottle. After all it will establish the style. The bottle will be like this, won't it?'

'Yes.'

'Then we have to use it.'

'I think you're right.' She leaned out and touched his cheek, letting her fingers linger on it. 'It's so lovely to work with you like this, Simeon, in the intimacy of our own home.' She put the designs to one side and folded her hands around her knees. She wore jeans and a T-shirt and squatted there barefoot. Varga had on a white shirt and twill trousers, his feet in slippers. They had breakfasted late and it was now mid-afternoon.

He put his arm around her waist again and she felt the craving for him that was like a drug. They kissed. He touched her breast and she felt her nipple hardening. She made a conscious effort to fight off the drowning effect that his caresses had on her.

Suddenly he straightened up, his arm remaining firmly around her waist, and she saw him looking at her still with love, but there was a gravity, almost an anxiety, in his expression she had not seen before.

'Ginny, there is something I want to tell you. I want to get it off my mind.'

Almost at once the happiness left her, to be followed by foreboding. She seized his hand.

'No, no, don't be frightened.' He touched her cheek. 'It's not meant to alarm you. It's meant to reassure you.'

'Then what is it, darling?'

For a moment he did not seem to know what to say, and then he started to speak very rapidly, as though driven.

'Ginny, I have not always been a very good man. I have done things I regret, things I am ashamed of . . .'

'Simeon, there's no need . . .'

'There is a need.' His clasp on her hand tightened. 'I feel a need to get it off my chest, like a confession. I have never told you about my life because I could never find the words.

'The "born in England" on our marriage certificate was a lie. You suspected as much, I know. I was born in the Carpathian mountains in a little village near the town of Uzhok on the border with Poland. My parents were peasants and I grew up without any learning. When I was ten or so they moved to the city; my father died and my mother moved, with my brothers and sisters – I had two of each – to the city of Mukachev where she had a sister who was a little better off than she was.

'I did not like my new home and when I was twelve I ran away. I spent the next few years travelling through Hungary and Romania until, finally, I arrived in Bulgaria. I was about sixteen. It was a very, very poor country, desperately poor and backward, and in the grip of the Communist tyranny. I worked first in Sofia and then in Plovdiv.'

'What did you do?'

'I was always some sort of merchant. I began as a runner for a merchant, but by the time I was sixteen I knew a lot about trading, except that it was the last thing you were supposed to do in the Communist state. So, eventually, I escaped into Turkey and then finally in Istanbul I jumped on a ship and stowed away. I got to Alexandria and, finally, I made my way to England. I had great difficulty getting permission to stay here and was nearly deported, but I managed to convince the authorities that I was a refugee from communism, that I would be killed if I went back, and they allowed me to stay.

'I worked very hard. I studied English very hard. I wanted to speak it without accent. I wanted to be successful.'

'And you were, very,' she said, aware that there were tears in her own eyes.

'Yes I was successful, but I had to claw my way to the top. On the way I did things I regret.' He swallowed and paused as if uncertain as to whether or not to go on. 'When I met you, Ginny, I was impressed because you were an aristocrat. I wanted to marry into the English aristocracy and I courted you deliberately.' Seeing the sudden hurt in her eyes he stopped but then, tightly pressing her hand, he continued in the same hurried tone. 'I very soon knew, Ginny, that whatever you were didn't matter to me. I loved you for yourself. I loved you and I wanted you, and I can't believe my good fortune that I have got you . . . so much so,' he gently released her hand and leaned back against the armchair in which he had been sitting, 'that I am terrified of losing you. But I knew that if I did not tell you and make this confession I would not deserve you. I want you to know me as I am, and for what I am.'

For a moment there was silence as, still sitting cross-legged on the floor, her hands hanging loosely between her knees, she gazed at him. She saw a sad, weary man, suddenly much older. She saw the defeats he had suffered; they were all there, etched on his face: the loneliness and insecurity of his peripatetic youth.

'I had to learn everything,' he said quietly. 'I never went to school. I had to learn to read and write, but in the process I acquired many languages and a mastery of business. But also I was ruthless. I did many things I regret . . .'

'Darling, we all do. It's over now.' She reached out and took his hand.

'Aero Acapulco, Planz Steel, things like that. You were right. I should not have got into dubious enterprises and I have given Liddle instructions to sell them, to clean the slate. Even if I become a little less wealthy it is worth it to have my mind at peace. But I can tell you one thing, Ginny, everything I have is for you. You will never want, never starve . . .'

She leaned over and they kissed. He lay down beside her and she realized that desire had been succeeded by a sense of intimacy such as she never remembered feeling in her life before. They were silent for quite a long time and she was aware from his deep, regular breathing, almost as though he were asleep, of the effort it had cost him, a man so devoted to secrecy that it was part of him, to speak as he had.

'Why didn't you tell me all this before?' she said. 'It would have helped, not me but you.'

'I couldn't tell you before. I didn't even know if I could tell you today. But I have and it's out and now you know.'

'But nothing . . . criminal, Simeon?' She looked doubtfully at him.

'Oh, nothing criminal,' he assured her. 'You can rest your mind on that.'

'But how did you manage . . . your birth certificate? It said you were born in Tunbridge Wells.' She started to laugh. 'Why Tunbridge Wells?'

Her laughter increased and, as the tears ran down her cheeks, she rolled helplessly on the floor.

'Tunbridge Wells!' she cried, almost choking.

'I rather liked Tunbridge Wells. It seemed *so* respectable.' Simeon also had tears of mirth in his eyes. 'You know, dowagers and members of the English middle class.'

'Simeon,' she looked sternly at him. 'Did you *forge* it?'

'Darling, *I* didn't "forge" it.' He looked at her with astonishment. 'I had it done. In the same way that the export certificate of the Mantegna was arranged. It is expert . . .'

'Simeon,' suddenly she felt real fear. 'Simeon, you didn't illegally import the Mantegna? It's simply not worth it.'

'Darling!' His hand closed over hers again, his eyes gazed appealingly at her. 'Lambert convinced me I had to have it. I felt with Lambert's insistence and, incidentally, approval, it couldn't seriously be wrong.'

He glanced at her swiftly, shrewdly. 'After all, surely your brother is a man of honour, isn't he?'

CHAPTER 20

It was four in the morning and Melissa, as usual, couldn't sleep. Her fix wore off at about four and it was usually necessary to have another one before she could sleep; but tonight she lay on the bed smoking cigarettes, one light burning low, the distant roar of traffic on Piccadilly a block away increasing. There were some times when one became aware of it more than others, like in the silence of the night.

Five girls slept in the house apart from her but, by four, almost all activity had ceased and would not begin again until around noon. The girls liked a lazy morning in bed drinking tea, slopping around. They took great care with their make-up and toilet and the most elaborate hygienic precautions possible. There was never any sex without a condom in these days of HIV; but a lot of the men liked oral sex and that came at a very high price because of its inherent danger.

Melissa's fiftieth birthday had long come and gone. She had known Varga since she was thirty and, in so far as she was capable of love, she supposed that all that time she had been in love with him. She remembered seeing him on board ship, an unhappy, tormented youth, yet even then there was the aura of the success which he would ultimately achieve and which, ultimately in its turn, would exclude her.

Varga was her mentor. It had not always been like

that. In the early years they had lived together as lovers until the drug habit got a firm hold on her and Varga, beginning to look for legitimate business, had met Claudia Bernini.

A business arrangement, he'd said. But one never knew with Varga: part of his attraction was that he had always been a consummate liar. During the years of his marriage to Claudia he had set Melissa up in a town house in Mayfair. He had arranged for the delivery of the drugs that not only satisfied her habit, but enabled her to supply other users. As an addict herself, he knew he could rely on her. For himself, he had never indulged. Drugs, smoking, artificial stimulation of any kind was anathema to him. Occasionally he drank wine or whisky, but that was all. Through the drugs racket Varga was wealthy enough to have spent the rest of his life on some pleasure beach, had he so fancied it, but of course he never would.

It made him work harder. The harder he worked, the richer he became, the more he craved respectability . . . and power. To the son of a peasant from the Carpathian mountains, that was important. The racket had made Melissa rich, too, but increasingly she had felt that Varga was trying to rid himself of her. She had become an embarrassment, an anachronism. After he'd met Ginny the change in his attitude had been even more pronounced.

Sometimes Melissa felt she wanted to get her own back on the man who, despite everything, obsessed her, like her drugs. Like them she knew he was bad for her, but there would always be the last time. It never came. As you got hooked on drugs, you got hooked on people. She was the obsessive type.

Melissa stirred restlessly, unsure whether to have a fix or try and get to sleep without it. One of the holds Varga had on her was the drugs. She could not supply herself; they all came through him. They had helped finance his empire and make him independent of his shareholders, his wife, or any person or thing in the world. Yet despite this there were all the things that he craved: public approval, honours (Sir Simeon Varga) and a wife with aristocratic connections.

There was a ring at the front door and Melissa jumped. Her room was on the first floor and she rose and ran swiftly down to the ground floor to look at the video screen above the door. A man stood there whom she vaguely recognized as a client. She believed he was a user. Maybe he had run out of his supply. Still, four in the morning . . . She spoke into the intercom.

'Yes?'

'May I come in?' The man raised his head and looked intently at the door. He was wearing a raincoat and had his hands in his pockets. He was bald-headed. Yes, she was sure she'd seen him before.

'What is it you want?' she said. 'The place is shut up.'

'Please open the door,' he said, 'I'm desperate.'

'I'm sorry, transactions are impossible outside business hours,' she told him coldly.

'You had better open or we shoot out the lock.' The tone of the voice was completely different, and then she saw a gun in his hand pointing through the door at her navel. 'You'll have to do this quietly, Melissa, or you'll wake the whole of Mayfair. Police.'

Melissa pressed the button that would alert the girls upstairs. She stood for some moments looking at the face on the screen and then she decided to let him in. Security was such in the house that he would find nothing.

She opened the door and suddenly the man pushed against it, flinging it open. At the same time a searchlight from a car parked opposite was trained on the house and about six men in plain clothes, appearing from nowhere, crashed in and began to fan out through the house. The man for whom she had opened the door put his pistol back in an inside pocket and looked at her.

'This is a raid, Melissa. We have reason to believe you are supplying drugs to clients.'

'I've seen you here before,' she said, looking at him closely. She was too vain to wear spectacles as she ought, even contacts.

'Yes, for several weeks. Strictly in the line of business.'

'I hope we gave you a good time.'

His answering smile was without humour. 'You told me all I want to know. The drugs, Melissa.'

'There are no drugs,' she said, giving him a myopic stare. 'I keep a clean house. We've more sense. Okay, arrest me for keeping a brothel, but no drugs. Strictly not. That's not my business.'

The man suddenly pushed her against the wall and, in a few swift movements, brutally tore off her gown. Underneath she was naked and he stared at her for a moment as though he had lust in his heart. But he was looking at her arms, her thighs, for the tell-tale pinpricks: the marks of an addict.

He had no difficulty in finding them.

Twenty-four hours later Melissa was in a cell in Paddington Green police station, shaking. She had not been so long without heroin for many years, and she had never felt so ill. She pulled the blanket more tightly around her; she was freezing and yet the sweat poured from her.

Cold turkey. It was horrible.

The door opened and the young, rather attractive uniformed policewoman stood looking at her. Melissa even imagined it was possible to discern some sympathy on her face.

'Inspector Howe wants to see you again.'

'I can't make it,' Melissa said. 'I can't walk.'

She tried to get up from the bed, but staggered back. She tried again and fell on the floor. Finally the prison doctor was called and she was sedated.

Inspector Howe said, 'Melissa, you are heroin dependent. The only way to save yourself from going barmy is to tell us everything. Where did the drugs come from?'

376

'I can't tell you,' she said, eyeing him defiantly.

'Can't, or won't?'

'Can't. Won't,' she shrugged. 'It's the same sort of thing.'

'It's not the same at all, Melissa.' With the tape running Howe had to be careful. Gone were the days when even a little gently applied physical abuse would have worked wonders. Now there was a tape recording and soon there might be video.

One day the prisons would be empty because everyone would be getting off scot free. Howe was a traditional policeman to whom a villain was a villain. He cleared his throat.

'Melissa, it's in everyone's interests to clear this matter up. When we do we can put you under proper medical supervision. You'll get help.' He leaned urgently towards her. 'You're still a beautiful woman. Now,' he leaned back and studied the notes in front of him. Sometimes the softly-softly approach really did work because these girls, especially the ones on drugs, were lonely, hopeless, longing for a protector. He raised his head and gave her a warm, human smile. He had not been to bed with her but with the other girls, several of them. It had been an agreeable experience and one which didn't come regularly in the course of duty. She'd greeted him in the foyer, given him a drink, introduced him to his companion. She'd been a good madame.

'Melissa,' he said, 'does the name Simeon Varga mean anything to you?'

'Nothing,' she said.

'Varga. *Quite* sure?'

'Absolutely nothing.'

'Medium height, dark . . . you must have heard his name. He was married quite recently to a society girl. It was in all the papers.'

'I never read the papers,' she said. She didn't even blink.

*

They lay in bed in the quiet of the morning. He had got up early and drawn the curtains, standing there for some time as the dawn broke through the mist, the silhouettes of the patient deer grazing in the park reminding him of his boyhood.

It was all so timeless, unhurried. As life had been then.

He turned back and looked at his sleeping wife and he knew one of those moments of pure happiness, of thankfulness and then, suddenly, there was the guilt, the fear of the past; the shadow that would keep creeping over him, to threaten his new-found happiness.

In the past few weeks of his life Simeon Varga had been visited by a sea-change. He had become a new man; in love for the first time in his life. He had felt re-born and, like all those experiencing re-birth, he had an earnest desire to expunge the past. He desired that the rest of his life should be free of that dark, bad side – a product of his deprived youth – that not only haunted him but made him afraid for the future.

To comfort himself he crept in beside her and lay listening to the sound of her breathing. Turning his head to gaze at her, he felt overwhelmed by her tranquil beauty, the black lashes lying on white cheeks, the curve of her slightly parted lips.

He leaned over, his hand on her breast, and kissed her very gently. Without opening her eyes she murmured, held out her arms for him and they melted into each other without speaking; fusing harmoniously as they always did: two in one flesh.

They lay quietly, sharing in the communion of love. He had never been in love with a woman as he was with Ginny. She had shown him truth, beauty, had given him hope. He trembled as he touched her.

'What's wrong?' She looked concerned.

'It's chilly.'

'I think you must be getting the 'flu.'

'I hope not.' He trembled again.

She put her arm around him and he stopped shaking,

soothed like a baby at its mother's breast. The child in him father to the man.

'Better now,' he said smiling, and kissed her.

'What time do you have to go?' she asked, looking at the clock.

'I should leave here about nine.'

'Are you worrying about the threat of a strike up north?'

'Yes, it's worrying.' Like a man banishing a nightmare he threw back the bedclothes and sat on the side of the bed. 'I've never had an experience like this. Randolph is up there dealing with it.' Randolph Jones was the newly appointed manager of personnel. 'But I have to go myself. You see, the worrying thing is that already it's affecting shares. We have had our first drop for over two years. Only slight, but enough to worry me a little – not much, darling.' Oh, if only a strike in the north, a slight dip in share price, were all he had to worry about, he would not have had a care in the world.

He leaned over and ran his hand along her brow. 'I do love you so much, Ginny. I want nothing to disturb the harmony of our love.'

'Nothing will.' She looked surprised. 'What could?'

'Who knows, in a busy world?'

'Simeon!' Ginny sat upright and folded her arms around her knees. 'Darling,' she went on, 'one thing only mars my happiness.'

'What is that, precious?' He rose from the bed and put on his gown, tying the cord tightly round his waist.

'It's about your children.'

'What about them?' His tone changed.

'Don't you think it's *heartless* not to see them?'

'No.'

'But supposing they want to see you?'

'I'm quite sure they don't. Ginny,' Varga sat on the bed again, 'Claudia's family always made it their business to distance themselves from me. They influenced Claudia and the children. They were Italian children, speaking

379

their mother's tongue. Of course their English is perfect, without accent, but essentially they are Italian. They were never really mine. I don't think they ever had much love for me at all. But if it makes you happier . . .'

'It would make me happier if you were quite sure. You see I think,' she smiled, feeling oddly shy, 'well, I'm seeing the doctor on Wednesday.'

'*Ginny*!'

'And I think if I am . . . I wouldn't like to think it was at the expense of your other children. I'm so happy, Simeon. So really happy. I want everyone in the world to feel as I do, too.'

He clasped her in his arms and crushed her.

'Ginny's pregnant,' Varga said excitedly, bursting through the door into Tony Liddle's office. When he saw the blank stare he got from his deputy he added, 'Well we think, we hope. She is seeing the doctor on Wednesday.'

'I'm very glad for you, Simeon,' Tony said, but his voice was still subdued, his manner restrained.

'What's the matter, Tony?'

Without another word Tony passed him a copy of the morning's paper.

MAYFAIR DRUGS BUST

Police raided the premises of a suspected brothel in Mayfair two days ago and are holding a number of people for questioning. It is thought that the question of drugs is also involved.

As Varga stared at the paper he felt slightly giddy, a little sick. When he looked up, Liddle saw a haunted face, the face of a man who sensed that, at last, his past was catching up on him.

'Do we know for sure?' Varga asked, slumping into a seat.

'I passed by this morning, on purpose, of course. The place is deserted. The telephone rings but no one answers.'

'Melissa?'

'She's obviously one of those being held for questioning. What will you do, Simeon?'

'Do? What can I do?'

'Aren't you worried?'

'Worried? Of *course* I'm worried. Very worried. And this day of days when I've so much to be happy about. But if Melissa had split on me we would have had a visit from the police already.'

'She's going to need help.'

'What do you mean, help?'

'Money for her defence.'

'She has plenty of money. She's a very wealthy woman. Probably a millionairess. She's been pushing that stuff like crazy for almost ten years. Mind you, she's been taking a lot too. It's an expensive habit.'

'Well anyway, I've stopped all further transactions.'

'Just as well. Christ!' Varga put his head in his hands. 'Just when things seemed so perfect. Anyway it's the last link in the chain. And Melissa I know will be loyal to me.'

'You seem to be expecting a lot of her, Simeon.'

'How do you mean?'

'She needs support.'

'She knows I can't give that!' Varga sprang to his feet, hands clawing the air. 'If I went anywhere near her it would be the end of both of us. Surely you see that?'

Liddle only saw a man he was beginning to despise. However he kept his features carefully under control.

'You've nothing at all that links you to the place?'

'Nothing. Nothing at all. The house is in her name. Anyway I've hardly been there for . . . ages.' He was going to say since his marriage, but thought better of it.

'Then if Melissa keeps silent you're all right?'

'I'm all right,' he nodded, but he was sweating. Melissa seldom showed her feelings, but when he had married

381

Ginny he'd felt that, with the final eclipse of her expectations, the iron had entered her soul.

'Will Melissa really keep silent?'

'I think so. I'm banking on it. But if she gets bail we'll have to be sure she gets out of the country. I'm relying on you totally, Tony.'

As Liddle remained silent, Varga's eyes narrowed.

'You're up to the neck in it too, you know, Tony?'

'I know.'

'And,' Varga appeared more composed now that his agile brain seemed to have started to function again, 'and if she won't go voluntarily we shall have to persuade her. You do know what I mean?'

'I thought you had forsworn the past, Simeon?'

'I had. I have. Once this is over I swear, never again. A clean, clean sheet.'

If only that were possible. Restlessly Varga rose and went over to the window, where he stood for some time watching the play of the fountain in the courtyard. Already the leaves were falling quite thickly and soon, with the onset of winter, the water would be switched off until, with the spring, it leapt into life again.

By the spring their baby would be nearly full term. Silk would be on the verge of being launched. He closed his eyes with horror at the thought of the abyss that threatened to open before him. He broke out in a sweat again. His head pounded. He wondered if he was having a brain seizure, a heart attack. He stood for a few moments trying to steady himself. It was nerves.

The heat gradually subsided, the pain left his temple, the throbbing stopped, and then there was a curious sensation. It seemed as though the blood in his veins had frozen and that, instead of an inferno, his body had become a block of ice.

He had never felt such fear, never known such panic in his life.

And that was only the beginning.

*

Varga spent a restless morning in his office. The share price had fallen again, and one of the broadsheets had a piece about the trouble with Consolidated Paper, together with a slightly unflattering reference to Varga.

HAS THE GOLDEN TOUCH DESERTED HIM?

the headline ran, though it was only a small paragraph, well towards the bottom of the financial page.

> Simeon Varga has seldom put a foot wrong in his successful climb up the corporate ladder with AP International, the company he bought off the peg thirteen years ago. However, his hostile raid on the northern paper group Consolidated Paper was unwelcome by the board, who emphatically recommended shareholders to reject it. Varga issued a press release claiming that the group was stagnant and he claims he has the management know-how to revive it. So far the City are not pleased by his behaviour; some call it an error of judgement by their golden boy and the share price fell by 5p on the day, continuing a slow decline from its heyday of 1275p.

Later that day, Varga and Liddle travelled to Newcastle in the private plane, and for the next three days he was locked in negotiations with the management of Consolidated Paper and the unions concerned. At the end the board recommended acceptance of a new offer to their shareholders, the unions unwillingly climbed down and Varga emerged triumphant.

But, somehow, this time the victory seemed a hollow one and, despite a new bullish press release, the share price continued to fall, not a lot but enough to continue to worry him – one or two pence a day.

He spent the weekend in Newcastle and late on the day

following the successful outcome of his bid he returned home, driving straight to Purborough from Luton Airport. And there, like a dream, like a good fairy to banish the bad, Ginny was waiting for him at the door.

He bounded out of the car and ran up the steps to be enveloped in her arms.

'Well?' She smiled at him.

'You first,' he said, taking her arm tightly and walking with her into the brightly-lit hall.

'Welcome home, Mr Varga,' the butler said, taking his coat.

'You haven't eaten yet?' He looked at Ginny with concern.

'No, darling, I was waiting for you.'

'Oh, my pet.' He leaned towards her and kissed her cheek. 'We'll go straight into the dining-room, Jones. I'm very hungry.'

'Yes, Mr Varga.'

Unlike the Silklanders, Ginny and Simeon usually ate in the dining-room. They had a small living-in staff and were waited on by their butler, Jones, who was a young man but had been well trained, and a maid.

They sat next to each other, two places laid on a vast circular walnut table around which they could easily have seated twenty.

Ginny had felt rather queasy and had ordered a light meal: smoked salmon mousse and grilled chops. Varga took a whisky to the table and she could feel his scarcely suppressed excitement as the maid put the first course in front of them.

'You can leave us,' he said to her and then looked up at Jones. 'We'll ring when we're ready.'

'Very well, Mr Varga.' Jones held the door open for the maid and followed her. As soon as the door was closed Varga hissed: 'Well?'

'Yes. The result came through today.'

'I love you. I worship you.' He took her in his arms and hugged her. 'Oh darling, when is it due?'

'I'm about two months, which is what I thought. So, all going well, in seven months we'll be parents.'

'Dearest darling,' he crushed her hand to his mouth, 'if you only knew how happy this makes me.'

'I do know, darling.' She put an arm round his neck and gazed into his eyes. 'And I'm just as excited, just as happy as you.'

'What will we have, a boy or girl?' He picked up his fork and began to eat ravenously.

'What would you like, darling?'

'A daughter like you. A son to inherit . . .'

'What about . . .'

'Please, not *again*, Ginny.' He held up a hand, talking between mouthfuls. 'I already spoke to Claudia. I spoke to her myself, breaking a rule, and she was very polite, didn't scream at me for once, and said the children were very happy, but she would ask them and if they wanted to see me, she would not object.'

'Oh, that's *fine*.' Ginny realized how unexpectedly relieved she was. 'Oh, darling, I'm *really* happy about that. Now it's up to them. They will always be welcome here.'

'I know, Ginny, and I love you for your generosity, as well as everything else. And tell me, what exactly did the doctor say?'

'He said everything is fine for someone as old as me.'

'As "old" as you?' Varga looked at her in surprise.

'Medically I'm considered quite old to have children.'

'Rubbish, we'll have four more.'

'Oh, I'm not sure about that.' She put down her fork, realizing that perhaps salmon mousse had not been such a good idea. 'You know, darling, Oriole is taking up a lot of my time. I have to go to France at the end of the week.'

'Oh, *Ginny.*'

'Just for a few days, darling.'

'Well,' he shrugged, 'I have to go back north.'

'Now let's talk about that. How did it really go?'

Varga waved his hands. 'Let's admit they are not one hundred per cent happy, not even fifty. They accept the inevitable. Liddle thinks it is only a pause and the unions will start making trouble again.'

'Then get rid of it, darling. Is it worth it?'

'You know I hate to lose a battle. It's not really the paper I'm after. It's the other things. They have a large office in the centre of Newcastle. It's valuable property which we could get a lot of money for. The head office we shall incorporate in our own. Incidentally, we are going to have bigger headquarters. I'm sorry but the Mayfair house will have to go.'

'Oh, no!'

'Rationalizing makes so much sense, you see. Of course, I'll stay in Central London, or maybe the City where so much building is going on. Some place in Docklands. Anyway it won't happen for a while. Consolidated Paper also has a paint offshoot. I don't want that so I'll sell it, and various other bits and pieces that can go. I'm sitting on a small fortune in hidden assets there and I don't want to give it up. This is a mere blip in the market. However,' he took his fork and began to draw patterns on his plate, 'I did think it might be a good idea, darling, if you could reactivate one or two of your special City contacts. Why not invite them here for lunch? Impress them, you know. And just get them to put in the odd word for me. Do you think you could do that?'

'Do you think they'll listen as I'm your wife?'

'Try, darling. Try. You're brilliant at the job.' He gave her a brief kiss and then rang the bell. The door was immediately opened to admit Jones with the portable phone.

'A call for you, Mrs Varga.'

'Oh, who is it? Can't you say we are at dinner?'

'I did, madam, but it is urgent. Mr Jacquet telephoning from France.'

Ginny looked guiltily towards Simeon and then got up from her chair.

'I'll take it in the other room, Jones. It's a business matter. You may serve the cutlets.'

'Yes, madam.'

And, taking the phone with her, Ginny made a hurried exit, conscious of the expression on Simeon's face as she left.

When she returned to the dining-room he was leaning back in his chair, the food in front of him untouched. The servants had been dismissed again and she slipped gingerly into the seat beside him.

'Well?' he said, staring at her.

'Well?'

'I did hear the name Jacquet, didn't I?'

'Yes, dear.' She bit into a piece of meat and knew that, again, she was not hungry. She had so hoped that she would remain unaffected by her pregnancy, but this aversion to food had lasted for several days. The doctor had advised her to eat anything she fancied, when she fancied it, and not bother about a strict routine according to mealtimes. But, with Simeon to think of too, it wasn't easy.

'You don't mean to tell me that you are dealing with these people, do you, Ginny? Please tell me I'm wrong.'

'I am dealing with Pierre Jacquet,' she said, staring straight in front of her.

'But he was sacked.'

'I know. I re-engaged him.'

'Why didn't you tell me?'

'I knew you wouldn't approve.'

'You're quite right.'

Varga threw his napkin on the floor and, getting up from his seat, stamped his foot petulantly. She was suddenly frightened by his anger, frightened as she knew she was of him. Just below the surface there had always been that fear of a man whose emotions could so easily go out of control. She had been very foolish not to tell him about Pierre.

'Simeon, he is the best "nose" in France. He has produced a wonderful fragrance.'

'Get rid of him.'

'I can't and I won't.' She stood up and faced him, feeling less fearful now.

'I order it, Ginny.'

'But why? Simeon, *please*, sit down.' She tried to drag him back to his seat, but he resisted her. 'See sense. I tried to do without him, but I couldn't. He is the best. Everyone says so. I know it. He is not re-engaged as a director, but he has created a beautiful perfume which will be an international winner.'

She could see that he was stiff with rage and she seized him by both arms. She was reminded of his mood when their wedding plans had first gone awry. Like a spoilt child, he demanded his own way.

'Simeon, what *is* it? Surely it's not just that I've disobeyed you, that you've been thwarted?'

'It is that, Ginny. It is all of these things. I trusted you. I gave you complete control. I poured millions into the blasted firm just to please *you*, never dreaming that you would re-employ that nincompoop under my very nose. I regard it as a serious breach of trust.'

'Simeon he is *not* a nincompoop and it is *not* a breach of trust. Please believe it, darling. Calm down. Why lose your temper on a night that is so happy for us? Please, please don't spoil it for us.'

'But it is you, Ginny,' he said, firmly pushing his chair back under the table, 'who has spoiled it for me.'

And with that he walked out of the room.

Paolo Bernini sat in his office above the opulent showroom in the Via Veneto reading the paper over a cup of black coffee and a cigarette. He followed the world stock markets, the movements of shares, the art prices being fetched and, naturally, gold and precious stones. He was an affable, leisured man who liked to begin his day without that sense of urgency that dogged his brother Carlo.

The two men were very different but they were close and Paolo had been as much affected by the treatment of his sister by Simeon Varga as any member of the close-knit family. Like them he felt she had been dishonoured.

He was about to turn the page when a small paragraph caught his eye:

WILL OF ALBERTO CARACOLI

The will of Alberto Caracoli, who died a few months ago, was published today and caused some surprises. Signor Caracoli's death occurred in Florence at the beautiful Villa Caracoli high up in the hills above Fiesole. He was a widower and his last years are understood to have been stressful, due to the fortune he is alleged to have lost.

He inherited the villa full of beautiful treasures, as well as what was then regarded as a substantial fortune, from his father Enrico who married Isabella Pelligrino of the steel family.

Signor Caracoli was thought to have dissipated most of his fortune in unwise investments and the villa was in grave need of repair. He leaves a son, Antonio, who practises as a doctor in Rome. Dr Caracoli has already lodged with the police information which would indicate that several pieces of value are believed to be missing from his father's fabulous collection, including a bust by Donatello and a valuable painting by Mantegna.

Mantegna. The name seemed to burn itself into Paolo's mind, and for several moments he sat there, the paper in his lap, deep in contemplation.

At last he rose, put the paper on one side and went to the telephone directory where he looked up the name Caracoli. His finger ran down the appropriate column until he came to Caracoli, Dott. Antonio, and he was about to tap in the number when, suddenly, he stopped. After making a note of the first number he tapped in another which he found in his personal telephone book.

'*Pronto*!'

'*Pronto, Leonardo*.' He spoke cheerfully into the phone. '*Come sta*?'

Leonardo was very well. Yes, of course it was good to hear from Paolo but, unfortunately, he had nothing for him.

'Did you ever hear more about that Mantegna?' Paolo said, aware that his voice was shaking.

'Ah . . .' Leonardo sounded curious. 'No, not a word.'

'Your client picked it up?'

'Oh yes.'

'Perhaps I could drop in on my way home, Leonardo. There's something I'd like to talk to you about.'

Of course Paolo was always welcome. Bernini had the distinct feeling that the art restorer had read the item in the newspaper too. Despite his excitement he managed to get through the busy working day of a man who ran the Rome side of a successful business. The brothers were contemplating opening in New York. But all day long the death of Alberto Caracoli and the fate of the missing Mantegna was at the back of his mind.

It was about a year ago; no, more. Maybe eighteen months. For some days his mind had lingered on the curious case of the Mantegna which was uncatalogued, apparently in private hands, yet taken for restoration by a dealer. Then he had forgotten about it. The matter had left his mind completely.

He reached Leonardo's studio at about five o'clock and parked his car in a street nearby. He hurried across the road and rang the bell, in his excitement keeping his finger on it for perhaps longer than he should: the door was flung open and Leonardo peered angrily out.

'All right, all right. I'm not deaf.'

'I'm sorry,' Paolo said, giving him his hand.

'No, no, it doesn't matter. Come in, Paolo.'

The studio was its usual clutter with canvases on easels, on the floor, some on tables, all in various stages of restoration. Leonardo was wiping his hands on a piece of rag as though he had finished work for the day. He then shook hands with Bernini, inviting him to sit down, but the jeweller, feeling restless, began to walk about the studio, inspecting first one canvas then another.

'You looking for something in particular?' The restorer put a cigarette in his mouth.

Paolo turned and handed him a copy of the paper which he had folded in half.

'Have you seen this?'

Leonardo took his time about lighting his cigarette, blew out the match, made sure it was drawing properly and then, adjusting his glasses, took the paper from Paolo's hand.

He read the paragraph carefully and then he sat down and read it again. It appeared that, after all, he had not seen it.

'It doesn't mean to say it's *that* Mantegna, does it?' He handed the paper back.

'But it's curious, isn't it?'

'Well,' Leonardo shrugged, 'I suppose you could say it was.'

'You said that the work had come from a dealer?'

'Yes, I did.' The picture restorer paused and rubbed his hand over his face. 'To tell you the truth, my friend, that matter has always been on my conscience.'

'Oh, really?' Bernini felt a little breathless.

'I knew there was something funny about it.'

'Why?'

'The circumstances were so odd. I was asked to authenticate it as *not* by Mantegna, but I refused. It was unsigned, true, but I recognized the master. Anyway that was it. Then it was taken away.'

'But the dealer, the name of the dealer?'

'I can't tell you, I'm afraid.'

'Why not, Leonardo? Do you want priceless pictures,

part of our heritage, to be *stolen* from Italy?'

'No, certainly not.'

'It's information you should give to the police.'

'Oh, I couldn't do that.'

'The dealer is a good friend of yours?'

'In a way.' Leonardo looked haggard. 'No, Paolo, I couldn't believe he'd do something like that.'

'And you can't give me his name?'

'Sorry.'

'Well . . .' Bernini got up and held out his hand.

'*You* wouldn't go to the police, Paolo?' Leonardo looked anxious.

'I shall have to think what to do.' Bernini scratched his head.

'It might land me in terrible trouble.'

'Then let me help you. You tell me the name of the dealer and you won't be involved any more. I promise.'

'You would never tell the police about me?'

'Of course not. But I am on a committee that stops works of art being exported. It is a duty I take very seriously.'

'See here,' Leonardo looked as though he had an inspiration, 'I won't *tell* you his name but I'll *write* it down for you.'

'Excellent: if that salves your conscience,' Bernini smiled, 'you do that.'

Leonardo went over to the table that served as a make-shift desk and, scribbling a name on a piece of paper, folded it several times like a lottery ticket before pressing it into the hand of his visitor. 'Open it when you get out,' he said. 'I hope that is the last I hear of this, Paolo.'

'Well, if you hear about it you will not be involved. Let us hope that the missing masterpiece can be restored to our country, where it belongs . . . and don't forget, Leonardo. I'm always on the lookout for something special . . . as long as it isn't stolen!'

'All right, Paolo, all right. Enough said about all that. *Arrivederci*!'

'Goodbye, Leonardo.'

The jeweller went out to his car and Forsci watched him drive away. Then, with a heavy heart, he produced a bottle from a cupboard and poured himself a large brandy.

Carlo Bernini kept his eye on the papers, but there was no more news about the raid on the brothel. It was vexing, irritating, maddening. Every day he hoped to see the name VARGA splashed across the headlines and every day he was disappointed.

A secret tip-off had been given to the police. He was the source of the tip-off; but he had named Varga and there was no mention of him in the papers which, as so often happens, soon seemed to drop the story altogether.

His ignorance irked him. He walked past the house several times, but it was impossible to tell anything from the outside. He telephoned, but there was never any answer. His desire for revenge on Varga bordered on frenzy: the humiliation of being exposed as a deviant by the hated man, followed by the realization that he himself was involved. Then the scheme; the sudden idea to make an anonymous call to the police. Simple.

He hated Varga. If anything, he hated him more than his mother or sister hated him. Claudia had gone abroad at the time of the marriage, had missed the pictures of his new house in the papers; of Varga with his happy, beautiful, aristocratic bride. He had been humiliated and pilloried by Varga as a fetishist, laughed at, derided, scorned, ridiculed.

He hated him with a fierce hatred.

The telephone rang and he raised the receiver.

'Hello.'

'*Ciaou, Carlo.*'

'*Ciaou, Paolo. Come sta?*'

Paolo was well. How were Carlo and Matteo, Mama and Claudia, the children? Lengthy reports on each

393

member of the family were given, and finally, Paolo said:

'I have some very interesting news for you.'

'Oh?'

'I think it will make you very happy.'

'How is that, Paolo?' Carlo was courteous but offhand.

'I think that, finally, we may be able to get our revenge on the man who dishonoured our sister. I may be wrong, but it would not surprise me if Varga doesn't have a very valuable stolen painting in his house. The cuttings you sent me about the wedding said it was full of beautiful objects and valuable works of art.'

And he told him about the Mantegna and the part played in its disappearance by Varga's brother-in-law, Lambert Silklander.

CHAPTER 21

The excitement illuminating Pierre Jacquet's normally immobile, even expressionless face resembled that of a small child on Christmas morning. He presented the phial to her as though it were a love token and she suddenly felt excited too, though a little apprehensive, and took it hesitantly.

It was a compound of all the essences he had created in the past six months, and its all-pervasive subtlety stole up on her, infinitely mysterious and alluring. As she removed the phial from her nose the after-effect lingered like an addiction and she was tempted to hold the phial under her nostrils and inhale the perfume again.

Pierre could see by her face how pleased she was, and his own expression of anxiety was transformed to one of satisfaction.

'You like it,' he said, as a statement rather than a question.

'Words can't express . . .' she began. 'It's magnificent, Pierre.'

The white-coated staff gathered round the parfumier breathed a collective sigh of relief.

Madame liked the fragrance. All was well.

'And it *is* Silk,' Ginny exclaimed. 'So subtle, so luxurious. We will make it the finest perfume to be launched next year, or any year. The best since L'Esprit du Temps.'

'And the plan is, Madame Varga,' the PR man moved

deftly forward, taking his cue from the success of her reaction, 'to enlarge upon the legend of its predecessor. To keep it "in house" as it were.'

'Exactly,' Ginny nodded. '"From the creators of L'Esprit".'

'Yes, and "from the grandson of the original creator of L'Esprit".'

'Yes, I see.' Ginny, suddenly recalling her conversation with her husband, turned aside to hide her face from Pierre.

However, her move was not lost on him and, with a slight frown, he replaced the phials on the bench and took off his white coat, joining Ginny after a few moments at the far end of the laboratory.

'So,' she saw the anxious look in his eyes, and smiled reassuringly at him, 'what happens now?'

'The presentation of the advertising campaign, Madame Varga. It is all set up in the boardroom.'

'Excellent. By the way, I thought we were on christian name terms?'

He shrugged and she recalled the awkwardness of their meeting in France.

'As you wish,' he said diplomatically.

Roger Bennet made no attempt to conceal his enthusiasm. 'I hope you'll like our ideas, Ginny.'

'I'm quite sure I shall.' She smiled and then, suddenly, she was overcome by an acute feeling of nausea and leaned against the lab bench for support while several executives rushed up to take her arm.

She fought with the sensation until it passed and, although she felt well again, her feeling of weakness was such that she needed to sit down. Next to her Pierre Jacquet looked at her in alarm.

'Are you all right, madame?'

'Perfectly all right,' Ginny reassured him. 'You might as well know, it's no secret, that I'm expecting a baby. This has not happened before, so I expect that's the reason.'

Everyone looked embarrassed. Someone brought her a glass of water. She sipped, recovered. They coughed.

'Congratulations,' Roger said at last.

There was a murmur in the room and Ginny smiled her thanks.

'Mr Varga must be very pleased.'

'Oh, very.'

'I hope it won't interfere with your interest in the business.' Roger momentarily looked anxious. 'It's entirely owing to you that we have a second lease of life.'

'You need have no worries on that score,' she reassured them. 'I don't intend to be a full-time wife and mother. I shall be frequently hopping over to France, I can assure you.'

'That's very good news.' Pierre had remained at the back of the group, looking reflectively, perhaps a little sadly, at her. 'It would have been quite devastating for us . . .'

'We hope we will launch Silk to coincide with the birth of our baby. It's due early summer.'

'Excellent.' Everyone relaxed. There were renewed murmurs of agreement and Ginny, feeling perfectly recovered, rose to her feet.

'I can't wait to see what you've done for us,' she said, looking at Martin Hamet, the head of the agency, and together they moved out of the lab.

As she entered the boardroom she was greeted by a spectacular sight. One spotlight, in an otherwise darkened room, was centred on an outsize bottle of perfume whose elegant, elongated neck was crowned by what seemed like a huge emerald from which emerged a kaleidoscope of brilliant, winking lights. Beneath and around the display were sumptuous layers of silk, their rich sheen opalescent in the single beam. Timed with her entry the kaleidoscope began to revolve, shooting brilliant colours across the material which appeared to flow like pearly lava down the side of a volcano. Then the perfume bottle started to revolve, very slowly, as the phantasmagoria of lights continued to play upon it but decreasing in intensity until the colours faded completely and only the single spot gleaming on the emerald remained.

There was spontaneous applause from everyone in the room, led by Ginny. When the lights went on and the magic faded it was seen that her face was flushed and her eyes sparkled.

'Absolutely breathtaking,' she murmured.

'Of course there will be an orchestral accompaniment,' Hamet explained. 'We thought Debussy or Ravel.'

'Or we may have something composed especially for the TV,' a henchman of Hamet's said. 'There is a very good woman composer who does a lot of music for the movies.'

'Yes, by all means. Do as you think fit.' Ginny moved across to a table where a number of visuals were on display, some complete, some in initial stages of development.

The meeting went on all afternoon with only a brief pause for tea, and finally Ginny had divided the material into what was to be accepted, what discarded and, of the ones she approved, which were her favourites.

By five everyone was tired and Martin Hamet looked at his watch.

'Thank you for giving us so much of your time, Madame Varga. I hope you feel better now?'

'Oh, I'm fully restored,' she assured him, 'and feeling all the better for your presentation.'

'Would, er, Mr Varga's approval be necessary?' he enquired.

'Well, I think he'd like to *see* them, eventually, but his approval is not necessary at this stage,' Ginny said. 'Naturally the campaign has to be costed and he'll probably want to come in on it then, but I'm sure he'll approve.'

'Excellent. Thank you, madame.'

The staff who had accompanied Hamet began to dismantle the stand and remove the lights; eventually they all departed with the visuals and show material. Finally only Roger and Pierre were left in the room with Ginny, and Roger, glancing nervously at his watch, said:

'Ginny, I wonder if you'd think me very rude if I rushed off?'

'Not at all,' she said, looking at Pierre. 'And you, Pierre, do you have an engagement?'

'I have no engagement,' Pierre said stiffly.

'I'm terribly sorry, Ginny. I thought you might be returning to London.' Roger looked downcast.

'No, I'm here for a day or two. Don't worry, I'll be glad of an early night at the hotel. See you tomorrow, Roger? I'd like to look at our development plans and the latest from the architect about Grasse.'

'Of course. I'll be here first thing. You're sure you'll be all right?'

'I'm sure. Pierre will see me to the hotel. There's absolutely no need for you to hang about.'

'You run along, Roger.' Pierre waved dismissingly. 'You can be sure I will take good care of Madame Varga.'

They both walked with him to the lobby where the commissionaire was in the act of locking the door. When he saw them he unlocked it again.

'Have you anything else to do, madame?' Pierre, still formal, looked at Ginny as Roger hurried away.

'Here? No. It can be done tomorrow.'

'Then I'll take you to your hotel.'

'That would be very nice. Come in and have a drink with me?'

'I . . .' he paused for a moment and then said: 'Thank you. I'd like that.'

His car was at the door and, after they were in, she said: 'Would you like to have dinner with me? I owe you some hospitality.'

'I'm afraid I can't. My father hasn't been too well. I've

got to see him every night. It curtails my time a little.'

'Oh, I am sorry.'

'Well, that's the way it is.' He shook his head, intent on the road in front of him.

'I thought the display was terrific.'

'It is very good.' But he didn't smile or take his eyes from the road, and when they stopped in front of the hotel she said:

'Is there anything wrong, Pierre? You don't seem very happy.'

'I wondered if there was something wrong with you, madame?' He looked gravely at her.

'But I told you I was pregnant. The first weeks are always the worst, so they say.'

'I don't mean that; that is a happy, natural event. But I wondered if you had told your husband about me?'

'Why, shouldn't I have done?'

'I thought you looked disconcerted when his name was mentioned, intent on avoiding my eyes. Does he now know you are employing me?'

'He knows.' Ginny was aware of the leaden feeling in the pit of her stomach which she knew was not solely on account of the baby.

'And he's displeased?'

'I think you can say that.' She turned and looked at him.

'He would like me dismissed again, perhaps?'

'It's out of the question. I told him I was in charge.'

'But still it can't be very pleasant, newly married, expecting a child.'

'No, it's not very pleasant.' She gazed at her diamond and sapphire engagement ring, the thin gold band beside it. 'It is the only thing that has happened to mar my happiness.'

'I'm not surprised.' Pierre sat back, his expression at last relaxed, even philosophical. 'Monsieur Varga is a man who likes his own way.'

'He is.'

'Maybe you would have been wise to give in to him?'

'No!' The vigour in her voice surprised even her. '*I* say whom we employ and whom we don't.'

'However the circumstances were, perhaps, exceptional. He had personally fired me and you took me back.'

'There is no question of your being fired again.'

'How do you know?'

'Because he loves me.' Feeling more confident now, she turned to him and smiled. 'He was angry and annoyed; but it will pass.'

'I'm sure Monsieur Varga loves you,' Pierre murmured. 'He is a most fortunate man. And I hope he will grant your wish?'

He looked at her and he too smiled, a rather sad smile.

'There is absolutely no question of your going, Pierre. You have created a marvellous perfume. I would tell Simeon, anyway, that if you went the fragrance goes too.'

'Oh, I wouldn't be so petty, Madame Varga.' Pierre, still addressing her formally – perhaps a sign of his hurt? – raised his eyebrows as though he found the suggestion in poor taste. 'You have paid me. I work for the company. I'm happy to have been given the chance to do what I do well.'

'I'm sure you are. But that isn't enough. Silk *is* your creation . . .'

'Would you fight your husband for me?' His lips curled a little, perhaps ironically.

'If need be; but I don't think it will happen.' She frowned. 'I think I know your opinion of Simeon, Pierre, and of course I don't share it. Just at the moment my husband is oppressed by business worries. There's something wrong with him. Normally he's confident, buoyant, but lately he is erratic and moody. He loses his temper quickly and immediately he's contrite. He's thrilled about the baby . . . oh, I shouldn't be talking to you like this.'

'But please go on, Madame Varga.' Pierre put one of his long, tapered, artistic hands lightly on her arm. 'I think you need a friend and you have one in me.'

'If you are to be a true friend you must call me Ginny. Anyway, I thought we'd agreed?'

'I'm sorry. I'm rather formal by nature.'

'I know, but I'd like it. Believe me, if ever I needed a friend I would come to you; but I have a friend in Simeon. We sincerely love and understand each other. Only at times he perplexes me. It is the nature of his genius. I'm sure of that.'

Pierre said nothing, appearing to listen politely. A few minutes later he escorted her from the car into the lobby of the hotel where, excusing himself from her offer of a drink, he punctiliously took her hand and kissed it.

'Until tomorrow, Mada . . . Ginny.'

'I'll be there about nine. Do give my best wishes to your father.'

'Thank you. I will.'

'They are sincerely meant.'

'I'm sure they are. Thank you, madame.'

Then he turned and walked slowly back through the hotel lobby to his car. She stood for a few moments watching him as, without looking back, he drove off.

There was a man, she thought, who was as unlike Simeon Varga as it was possible to be, yet one for whom she felt a deep and increasing respect and friendship.

The paragraphs had started in a very small way, a line or two at the bottom of the pages of local papers in the north and confined to the north of England. After all, a strike at a paper mill was not an event of national importance. But strikes were no longer as commonplace as they had once been, and this was in opposition to the new owner, the already legendary Simeon Varga, who was supposed to have such a sure touch. Gradually the story spread from the financial pages of the broadsheets to the tabloids, and everywhere the message was the same.

A crack had been revealed in Varga's armour; it was growing wider; was his magic beginning to desert him? The price of his shares on the Stock Exchange began to accelerate downwards, more steeply every day; not one pence or two, but five or ten.

Because what he had to say was private, Varga needed a large restaurant with well spaced tables, and thus he had eschewed his preferred haunts in favour of Claridges, where people could talk without every word of their conversation being overheard.

Robert was already in the lobby when he arrived and he hurried up to him, apologizing for the delay.

'I'm so sorry, Robert. I had a call . . .'

'That's okay.' Robert had risen politely to greet Varga, who took him by the arm.

'Shall we go straight in? Or would you like a drink?'

Robert pointed to an empty glass.

'Oh dear, I'm much later than I thought.'

'No, I was early, honestly.' Robert's smile seemed particularly warm and Varga felt encouraged. He had had a bad morning on the telephone with his bankers and he felt a glimmer of hope.

They settled down in a corner of the restaurant, fussed over by the *maître d'*, who greeted Varga like a long-lost friend.

'You desert us in favour of Le Gavroche, Mr Varga,' he said soulfully.

'Only sometimes.' Varga waved a finger at him. 'And it *is* just round the corner.'

'Mr Varga,' the *maître d'* looked pained, '*we* are only just around the corner.'

'Anyway, here we are.'

'Will you have something to drink, Mr Varga?'

'I think champagne. It's the only thing I can drink at lunchtime. Robert?'

'Suits me,' Robert said with a smile.

'A bottle of the usual.'

'At once, Mr Varga.'

The *maître d'* hurried off to summon the sommelier while the two men looked at each other, the menu unread before them.

'Well, Robert, this *is* good.' Varga lightly put a hand on his wrist. 'Really good to see you again.'

'And you, Simeon.'

'And I hear you're a father.'

'Yes, we've a son, Jeremy.'

'Congratulations.'

'He's eight months.'

'Ginny's expecting, too.'

Simeon thought that momentarily Robert had an expression of dismay which he tried to conceal.

'That's terrific. When?'

'Late spring, early summer. We hope to celebrate the birth with the launch of a new perfume.'

'Oh? Oriole still in one piece then?'

'Of course.' A spasm of irritation passed across Varga's face. 'Ginny has taken personal control; and it's thriving. She's over there now.'

'I'm delighted to hear it.' Robert took up the menu and began to study it in earnest.

'Yes, what do you fancy?' Varga did the same.

They both settled for asparagus and roast beef, and by that time the champagne had arrived. Varga raised a glass towards his guest.

'To the health of you, your wife and baby, Robert.'

'Thank you. And to you and Ginny and *your* baby, Simeon. Every happiness.'

They both drank and then when they put down their glasses there was a sudden awkward pause which was broken at last by Robert.

'So, how are things in general, Simeon?'

'Well . . . you've read the papers.'

'Yes, I must say I can't help noticing some rather preju-diced comments. People are so spiteful about success, aren't they? Your share price was, perhaps, too high anyway, or the P/E ratio.'

'Exactly. Now it falls a little, but we're still higher than ICI.'

'Yes, it's quite remarkable. I daresay it's a hiccup.'

'People do resent success, you're right.' A note of bitterness entered Varga's voice.

'You see, the trouble is that when you have been so successful any little blip is bound to affect the share price. Frankly, Simeon, can't you settle the dispute with the paper mill? It's only a tiny piece of your empire, isn't it? Is it worth the bad press?'

'Do you think I haven't tried?' Varga paused as the waiter placed the asparagus in front of him and another fussed with the finger-bowls. 'I would settle with the paper mill tomorrow; but it's part of a much larger group. I don't *want* the paper mill, but I can't get rid of it as long as the workforce is striking, and they're striking because of the other parts of the group I want to keep. It's a matter of principle.' Varga looked sternly at his asparagus as he popped a succulent piece in his mouth.

Robert too ate silently, enjoying the thick spears washed down with vintage champagne in an atmosphere that he found congenial; but Varga, he could see, was a worried man. Not quite the Simeon of a few years before.

'Principles sometimes have to be forgone, Simeon.'

'Not by me,' Varga snapped, taking a sip from his glass.

'I understand.' Robert nodded politely. 'Well, I'm sure you'll weather the storm.'

'Robert,' Varga finished his asparagus and dipped his fingers in the bowl of warm water; 'it's a question of confidence. I have to bolster up my share price.'

'Bolster?' Robert immediately looked alarmed.

'Oh, I'm not talking about anything illegal; no share support scheme, nothing like that. However, what is there to prevent you, for instance, placing an order for shares through your broker?'

'You mean personally?' Robert began to look embarrassed.

'Or through the bank. I don't mind which.'

'I'm afraid not, Simeon.' There was a note of firmness in Robert's voice, almost as though he had been expecting the question. 'It's not the sort of thing we do. We'd avoid that kind of involvement, especially if things are starting to go wrong. Look at Guinness . . .'

'I am *not* Guinness,' Varga snapped. 'And nothing is "going wrong".'

'Anyway, we wouldn't. We're not in the risk business.'

'I thought you were.' Varga's tone was icy.

Robert was about to reply, but paused while their plates were cleared and an array of waiters approached with the main course. By the time it was laid before him Varga felt he had little appetite, but Robert's remained unaffected.

'I may need, in that case, to up my facility with your bank,' Simeon said. 'Another hundred million or so, should we say?'

Robert finished his mouthful and then leaned across the table, lowering his voice.

'That too is out of the question, Simeon.'

'But why? I really don't understand.'

'Because when you invited me for lunch I asked for your portfolio and what I saw did not make very encouraging reading. I think you should retrench, not borrow.'

'But a minor strike . . . it's preposterous.' Varga threw down his napkin on the table, occasioning a glance from one or two other diners nearby.

'It isn't that, Simeon,' Robert's voice was even more subdued. 'You're over-extended. You have been for some time. I warned you a long time ago not to be too ambitious, but you thought I was jealous because of Ginny. It had nothing to do with Ginny. It was purely and simply a matter of good banking business. You bought too much, too quickly, and in some cases you paid too high a price. You have too many offshore, private companies which are too secretive. How do you finance them? What surplus funds have you, and where do they come from? Now, when a relatively small blip occurs, everything collapses like a house of cards . . . it's the law of the jungle.'

'It is *not* collapsing, it is *not* a house of cards.' Varga thumped the table again. 'It is people like you who undermine confidence. The market is a matter of confidence, Robert.'

'Oh, I couldn't agree more,' Robert said suavely, 'and, for some reason, at the moment people have lost confidence in you. It shows in the share price and, believe me, it will go on falling until you do something about it.'

'What can I do?' Varga hissed.

'Restore that confidence. Get rid of that blasted paper mill, and all that goes with it if you have to. Settle the strike. Sell the lot. Cut your losses. Realize a few more assets round the world. Don't try to borrow your way out of this crisis but sell. You are rich in assets.' Robert paused and finished with evident relish what was on his plate. 'Some people wonder where all the profits have gone. Perhaps they go to your offshore companies in Panama?'

'They most certainly do not.'

'The City is always nervous about an entrepreneur, Simeon.' Robert's manner became sympathetic. 'You must know that.'

'You mean if one's not Eton and the Guards with a seat in, shall we say, Northumberland?'

'Well, it helps to have known a bloke at school, or for his father to have known your father; but that's just a fraction of the matter. It's important when things begin to go wrong. You are on your own, and I don't suppose Ginny's family are of much help?'

'How can they be? They haven't a penny.'

'But they have a lot of connections. A member of the Board of Governors of the Bank of England is a relation.

Now I don't suppose you knew that did you?'

'No.'

'And I don't suppose they would tell you, because you humiliated them over that business with Angus.'

'How did I humiliate them?' Varga asked indignantly.

'I don't imagine you were even aware of it.'

'I wanted to help them.'

'Yes, but by making yourself seem superior. You wanted to buy not only the farm but the entire estate.'

'You seem to know a lot about it.'

'Things get around.' Robert studied his plate. 'You know how it is.'

'I did not want the castle.'

'No, but everything else. Five thousand acres of land at a knock-down price; telling Angus how to run his farm; Gerald, an expert forester, what to do with his precious trees. Now they both know a lot about farming and the care of timber. They were insulted.'

'They seemed perfectly all right at the wedding.'

'They would be. They have their pride.'

'Well, they kept their precious pride; they got a big mortgage and probably lost a lot of money,' Varga sneered.

'The point is, Silklanders won't forget such a thing and when the chips are down, Simeon, you need friends. You should have tried to get on with your wife's family. After all, some people thought that was really why you married her.'

Before Varga could react, Robert shot out his arm and looked at his watch.

'If you'll forgive me, I must skip pudding and fly. I have a meeting at three and, after all, you were over half an hour late.'

When Varga returned to the office he was in an eminently bad humour, which was not improved by Dorothy who greeted him with an unsmiling face.

'I'm afraid Sir Monty Fenton can't meet you for lunch,

Mr Varga,' she said consulting a pad. 'He could let you have ten minutes in his office on Thursday week at seven AM.'

'Tell him to go and get stuffed,' Varga shouted, going into his office and violently shutting the door after him.

He sat at his desk and realized he was trembling. He was actually afraid, and for someone to whom self-confidence was paramount, it was a new experience. It was as though the fabric of his life, so carefully and painstakingly built up, was beginning to fall apart. He spoke through the intercom to Liddle.

'Come in here for a moment, would you, Tony?'

Nervously Dorothy knocked at the door and put her head round.

'There were some other messages, Mr Varga.'

'Come in, Dorothy.' Varga gave her a strained smile and pointed to a chair. As she sat down he leaned across his desk, joining his hands, and managed a contrived smile.

'Forgive me, Dorothy. I was rude to you just now and you know it's not in my nature to be rude.'

'I quite understand, Mr Varga.'

'I have a lot on my mind. You, who know all my secrets, or almost all, know that.'

'Oh I do, sir, and I understand.' Still there was no forgiving smile.

'I had a meeting with the fickle Robert Ward, who was of no help at all but took lavishly of my hospitality, and then Sir Monty Fenton, who was leaning over backwards to lend me money a couple of years ago has the nerve . . .'

'Oh I know, Mr Varga. I was shocked.' At last Dorothy looked sympathetic.

'My nerves are on edge. I need a holiday. Ginny is always pressing me to take one and I believe once I have cleared up a few things I will.'

'Mr Varga, you never even took a *honeymoon*.' His standing with the faithful secretary was fully restored.

'Nor I did. Well, Mrs Varga and I will have a long, relaxed, extended holiday over Christmas. We'll get in the plane and tell the pilot to fly us somewhere hot.'

'I'm sure it will do you both good, Mr Varga.'

'That's exactly what we'll do, Dorothy.' Varga leapt out of his chair and went over to her, clasping her shoulder. 'And thank you for suggesting it. Everyone needs a holiday . . .'

'There *were* some more messages, Mr Varga.' Dorothy had the hesitant tone of one bringing further bad news. 'Mr Eric Lumpey of the Bankers' Trust can't see you until next week and Mr George Cartwright of Lomax would like to see you immediately. Oh and Miss Kalourie called again.'

'I know no one of that name,' Varga said stiffly.

'That's what I told her, Mr Varga. It's the fifth time she's called.'

'Tell her . . .'

Varga stopped as the door opened again, this time to admit Liddle who was carrying an armful of files.

'Oh, Tony,' Varga pointed to a chair. 'Thank you, Dorothy. I'll deal with this matter and others later. And no calls, please. I want to talk to Tony undisturbed.'

'Oh, and Mr Lambert Silklander called. It sounded quite urgent.'

'In time, Dorothy, in time.' Varga made a soothing motion with his hands.

'Yes, Mr Varga.'

Dorothy gave them both a tremulous smile and made her way to the door.

Tony Liddle remained by Varga's desk, on which he had put the files.

'That damned Melissa.' Varga returned from locking the door. 'What the hell am I to do with her? She keeps on ringing me. Doesn't she know that this place might be bugged? The phones tapped?'

'Well, in my opinion,' Liddle undid his jacket at leisure and sat down, 'you're remarkably lucky you haven't had

410

a visit from the police already. She obviously hasn't implicated you.'

'Yet,' Varga said wearily. 'She's going to blackmail me, make me pay for her silence.'

'Did you ever think that Melissa really loved you?' Liddle asked quietly.

'Pah!' Varga said between clenched teeth.

'It seems to me she does.' Liddle crossed his legs and then, with an air of complete detachment, raised his head. 'Otherwise I agree with you. The place was raided six weeks ago. I would have expected her to have spilled the beans by now, and she hasn't. Maybe she just wants to get away and needs help.'

'Tony,' Varga said suddenly, reverting to his normal, controlled, businesslike manner, 'you must see her. You must tell her that I can't possibly be *seen* to have anything to do with her. You must promise any help she wants. I'll tell Dorothy next time she rings to put her through to you.'

'*If* there's a next time,' Liddle said meaningfully, but Varga, his manner preoccupied, seemed not to hear him. He returned to his chair behind his desk and sat down, running his hand over his smooth cheeks.

'Tony, we must sell Consolidated Paper. We must get rid of it at once.'

'Ward couldn't help?' Liddle looked interested.

'Couldn't and wouldn't. *And* I have been snubbed by Monty Fenton, who was so keen to lend me all the money in the world a while ago. People like that shit have such short memories. He can't have lunch and can only fit me in at seven in the morning! Now he has to insult me. Just wait . . .' Varga clenched his fist and shook it at the ceiling.

'Yes, I've had calls from Barclays *and* Hill Samuel.' Liddle frowned. 'I'm afraid the packs are moving in.'

'Christ, at 1051p a share we are worth *five hundred million pounds*. I don't want to see all that go down the drain.'

'It's the other things they don't like. You're getting talked about; your private companies are speculated about. They don't like that. You haven't got the background they like. You're an interloper, not one of them.

'I think you married Ginny a bit too late, Simeon. You shouldn't have tried patronizing her family. You'll have your work cut out now to stem the advancing tide.'

'But I *will* stem the tide.' Varga sat back, palms on his desk. 'This is my first setback, and don't think I'm going to let it get me down. Now, you go through every one of our companies and see what we can sell and how quickly we can release the cash. Stop that damaging strike up north even if you have to do it yourself. Call in as much as you can . . . and if it takes you all night and all tomorrow, Tony, and the next day, and the day after that . . . *do* it!'

CHAPTER 22

Varga stood in a corner of the airfield, his fur collar turned up against the cold, as the plane taxied towards him. He had watched it come in, swooping down between aircraft of all shapes and sizes – the very large and the very small – as they completed their journeys from all parts of the globe. He eyed it anxiously, watching its graceful descent. What it bore was so precious to him that the muscles of his stomach seemed to contract at the thought of an accident marring its safe arrival. Never a nervous traveller, he was now – on behalf of Ginny.

The door opened, the steps were lowered and, after a few seconds, Ginny stood at the entrance looking around in the dark blustery night. He began to run towards her and she saw the white of his raincoat and waved, beginning to descend gingerly, clutching the rail. As she reached the bottom he swept her into his arms and clung to her, pressing his face into her shoulder.

'Ginny, darling,' he murmured, 'it's so *good* to have you back.' They stood there for a moment battered by the rain, unaware that the car had driven up alongside them, that Peter was holding open the door while Geoffrey, the pilot, was clearing customs formalities.

'Your passport, Mrs Varga?' he asked and she and Varga broke away while she produced it from her pocket. 'The officer would like to inspect your luggage.'

'By all means let him,' she said.

'Just what is this . . .' Varga began, but she put a finger on his mouth.

'Don't antagonize them, darling. It only makes them worse.'

'Come on, let's get into the car. I hate all this officialdom.'

They got into the back; Peter tucked the rug around them and then climbed into the driving seat. They waited.

It seemed an interminable time.

'They're turning the plane inside out,' Ginny said with a rueful smile. 'Do they think I'm smuggling drugs?'

'Darling, shh,' Varga's heart skipped a beat as he put an arm round her. 'Don't even give them the idea.'

At last Geoffrey appeared with Ginny's bags which he and Peter stowed in the boot, and then the customs officer put his head through the window.

'Everything seems perfectly in order, Mrs Varga. Sorry to have kept you.'

Varga nodded and Peter dowsed the lights in the rear. The car moved smoothly forward, leaving the customs officer and the pilot still in conversation on the tarmac.

'I suppose they have to be awfully careful with private aircraft,' Ginny said thoughtfully, glancing out of the back window. 'But they've never done that to us before, have they?'

'I suppose we have to take our turn. Now, darling,' Varga placed his hand over hers, 'how was the trip? Successful?'

'Oh, very.' She leaned back against the seat. 'The perfume is divine. I've brought a tiny drop for you to smell, and the TV commercial . . . they're sending the video of that in a few days. It's spectacular. They love the name, they love everything . . .'

'And how are *you*, my darling?' He pressed his lips against her cheek.

'I've been fine, a touch of nausea but nothing much.'

414

'Nausea?' He immediately looked concerned. 'When was that?'

'Oh, don't worry.' She squeezed his hand. 'I was completely all right and it didn't recur.'

'Darling, you must take it easy,' Varga, still clasping her hand, also leaned back against the leather upholstery, 'and so must I. Dorothy reminded me today that we didn't have a proper honeymoon.'

'We still had a very nice time.' She gave him a glance full of meaning.

'Oh, I agree, and Purborough Park was the best place for it . . . but still, we haven't been away. I thought we'd take a long break at Christmas. How do you fancy Mustique or the Virgin Islands?'

'Either. Sounds marvellous. Yes, what a good idea; but,' she looked at him anxiously, 'is it okay for you? I saw the *Financial Times* last Friday. That was unkind.'

'It does me no good at all, that kind of thing; but Liddle is sorting it all out. I had lunch with Robert yesterday and he advised me to realize some of my assets to restore the markets' confidence in me. I think he's right.'

'But not Oriole.'

'No, we shan't sell Oriole; and, darling,' his hand tightened over hers, 'do forgive me. I could have bitten off my tongue after I said what I said about Jacquet. I know I upset you.'

'And I know I should have told you,' she said contritely. 'Only I knew you would be angry and you were. I knew, and Roger agreed, that he was the very best person to get. If I'd discussed it with you, you wouldn't have listened.'

'Right,' he nodded.

'You might have ordered me to get rid of Pierre before he had created the perfume, and he is a genius. He really is.'

'Yes, I was angry and I was wrong. I don't like being crossed. I'm not used to it and it has made me intolerant.

415

Well, I've learned a few things, Ginny. Above all I've learned how precious you are to me. Also who to trust and who not to trust, who one's real friends are.'

'Was Robert helpful?'

'He was helpful; but I still think he's getting his own back on me because I took you from him.'

'Oh, but they've got a baby. They're very happy.'

'I still think he loves you best. He says I upset your family.'

She didn't reply.

'Did I?' he urged.

'I'm sure they've forgotten it. They were fine at the wedding, weren't they?'

'I thought they were exceptionally nice.'

'Well then – they've put it out of their minds.'

'He said you had a relation who was a governor of the Bank of England.'

'Oh, he's terribly remote. A tenth cousin or something, twice removed. Please don't let's discuss this, darling. I'm home, now, with you.'

Varga continued to press her hand, but he sensed her irritation that he'd involved her family.

'Look,' she leaned over to him, her mouth very close to his, 'I'm yours now, and you're mine. No one else matters but us and our baby.'

Oh, how he wished it were true.

An hour later they swept up the drive of the house, cheered by the lights that blazed from the windows, the welcome from the staff as the door was flung open to greet them. They had acquired a couple of labradors, bred at Silklands, who bounded down to greet them and there was an air of happiness, even festivity, as they entered their home.

Varga, who'd stayed in London while Ginny was away, gave a deep sigh as they stood in the hall taking off their coats, while the dogs, still puppies, frisked about them and the butler solicitously enquired after their welfare.

He told them that the cook had prepared something delicious for dinner and asked when they would like it to be served.

How precious were the comforts of home, of a well-trained staff to cosset and comfort them. And now it all seemed to be in danger of slipping away. In the midst of all this happiness there lurked a nightmare.

Ginny told Jones they would eat at eight-thirty, and they went straight upstairs where, in the privacy of their room, they embraced for a long time, but did not make love.

That would come later.

As Ginny bathed, Varga sat on the edge of the tub passing her the soap, a flannel, a brush with which he scrubbed her back. She lay in the bath, her dark hair held back by a towelling bandeau, her face glistening with moisture. She stretched her long arms to soap herself and her breasts appeared above the water, covered in suds.

He knew this was a moment that would be forever impressed on his memory. As she stepped out of the bath he held out for her the huge bath towel and tenderly wrapped it round her, hugging her. They walked together into the bedroom and he helped to dry her, then they lay for some moments on the bed caressing each other, conscious of desire but, again, not making love.

'This is the most perfect homecoming I've ever had,' she murmured. 'Can they all go on being as good as this?'

'Yes. Always.'

'I feel it can't last.'

'It can. It will.'

'Oh, Simeon, I'm *so* happy.'

After dinner they lay on the floor in front of the drawing-room fire listening to Mozart. Varga was leaning against the sofa, Ginny's head resting on his lap, and he ran his fingers through her hair watching the effects on it of the firelight.

'Ginny.'

'Yes, darling?'

'Happy?'

'Terribly; but . . .' she raised her head and looked anxiously at his face. 'I sense a tension in you, Simeon. You seem preoccupied.'

'It's been a worrying week, darling. It seems so unimportant now that you're back. You're my only reality.'

'But tell me, please. *Is* something wrong?'

'Just the usual business worries.'

'But what specifically? Normally you don't have business worries – you're on top. Is it the share price? The FT article?'

'Basically it's that damn paper mill and the striking workers. It's given me a very bad press, not only in the FT. Robert said it was a chink in the armour, and he's right. I've got to get rid of it. I've told Liddle to sell the damn thing and also look at our assets in general. He has to work non-stop until he comes up with a plan. Now, darling, with your talent for chatting up the press, I wondered if you've thought of this suggestion to host a couple of lunches, say, with well-chosen journalists, people you liked and were close to. Show them the house?'

'Mmm,' she seemed to ponder the idea. 'I was quite close to Gloria Keane.'

'Excellent. Invite her here to see round the house. She hasn't seen it, has she?'

'No.'

'You know, as woman to woman. She'd love it.'

'Okay. Leave it to me.'

He felt weary and closed his eyes, aware of Ginny groping for his hand and kissing the palm, the back, the fingers one by one.

*

'You're sure it's all right?'

'Of course it's all right. I'm not ill.'

'But what about the nausea?'

'Don't be silly.'

'I'll be very careful.'

Very careful, very, very careful. She was so precious. He wished he could lose himself in her for ever, like the baby who nestled in her womb, snug and secure against the ravages, the hostility, the harsh demands of the world outside.

Varga woke very early, before dawn. He felt as though he had only just fallen asleep, but he looked at the clock and it was six. He often woke at six in London and was ready to begin the day, in his office by seven, bathed and shaved, having scanned the morning papers over his breakfast of black coffee and toast.

He generally felt on holiday in the country; relaxed and expansive, luxuriating in the beauty of his wife and his home in equal proportions. Though a lot still remained to be done, it was a real home, a place of his own.

Usually when Varga woke beside his sleeping wife he was overcome by a feeling of peace and contentment, but today was different. Despite their reunion, the passion of their lovemaking, he woke feeling tense, apprehensive, almost afraid.

He knew it was a combination of worries rather than one in particular. It was not just the business, not just Melissa, not just criticism in the press, or a fear of failure, or of his past catching up with him. It was a fear, a real fear, of losing Ginny.

To have sought something for so long, to have found it, and now to have to face the terrible prospect of losing it.

He was juggling with life, gambling.

Restlessly he got out of bed and went and stood by the window, drawing back the curtains and looking out into the dark. Nothing stirred except the branches of the trees, dusted with a fine layer of snow which had fallen during the night. Now, on the horizon, there was a suggestion of dawn breaking above the clouds in the inky sky.

It was cold. It seemed to him abnormally cold. He couldn't stop his teeth chattering. He touched the pipes; the central heating was just coming on. He crept back into bed and Ginny, perhaps woken by the cold body beside her, murmured sleepily:

'What time is it, darling?'

'Six. Go to sleep again.' He bent over her, his lips touching her cheek, and wrapped the bedclothes securely around her shoulders. But Ginny turned to him, her hands touching his cold body.

'Simeon, you're freezing! What were you doing?'

'Just looking. It's been snowing.'

'Darling, you *are* restless, aren't you?' She switched on the light by the side of the bed. 'You really are worried at the moment, aren't you? You tossed and turned all night.'

'Did I, darling? I'm terribly sorry.' He kissed her shoulder.

'I shouldn't have left you at such a bad time.'

'You were only gone a few days.'

'But I shouldn't. My place is beside you.'

'Ginny? Are you abandoning the women's movement?' She saw a mischievous light in his eyes and smiled.

'Not completely; but even liberated women are allowed to fall in love and help their menfolk, as their menfolk in turn are expected to help them.'

'Of course.' His lips lingered on her shoulder. 'Now that you are back everything will be better; but I need you, Ginny. I need you so much. If only you knew.'

Knew what?

She lay beside him, conscious of the heat returning to his body, the palpable tension ebbing away as he relaxed.

Yes, she was very precious to him. Vital. She knew it now. She imagined that he began to doze, and then she found that his anxiety had transferred itself to her, that she, in turn, grew tense and fearful wondering what it was that had made him react with such untypical distress.

But was it untypical? The Varga she had known in the last few months was not the man she had started to work for three years before. Then he never flapped, never shouted or lost his temper; all the time he was, or appeared to be, level-headed, controlled. It was only really in the last six months, since their marriage in fact, that he had changed. But that, he had said, made him happy. What else was it that had happened that perhaps she didn't know about, that he hadn't confided in her, to make him change?

Now it was she who crept out of bed and, gazing through the still partly drawn curtains, saw that the dawn had arrived revealing the park in a kind of beauty she had never seen before: its pristine whiteness unmarked by anything except the footprints of birds and squirrels, the boughs heavy with snow like icing on a Christmas cake. And soon it would be Christmas. Though this year, the first of their marriage, they would eschew the traditional family party at Silklands in favour of two or more weeks alone together somewhere in the Caribbean.

They kept a kettle and tea things in the room and the night before a maid always brought up a tray laid with cups and saucers, a lidded milk jug. Varga liked coffee, Ginny tea. It was one of the pleasant little domestic intimacies for her to make this first drink of the day for them both.

She switched on the kettle and, waiting for it to boil, stood with her arms folded gazing out of the window, watching the pink sky on the eastern horizon beginning its winter progress low across the sky.

She put two teabags in the pot for her, and some

instant coffee into a cup for Simeon. There were so many excellent brands on the market these days that he didn't mind so long as he had real ground coffee for breakfast. She let her tea brew for a few minutes and then poured the boiling water on the powder in his cup, stirred it and took it over to him.

'Half past seven, darling, and a lovely day.'

Varga jerked awake again and at first she saw an expression of terror on his face, as though he had woken from a bad dream. Sometimes these brief dreams between periods of wakefulness were full of horror, but when he saw her sitting on the bed beside him the fear evaporated and he smiled.

'Already? I must have fallen into a deep sleep.'

'*And* had a nightmare, by the expression on your face.'

He struggled to sit up in bed and, rubbing his eyes, reached for the cup and put it to his lips. Black, unsugared, she didn't know how he could drink it but he did, and appeared to find it reviving. He drained the cup with relish and handed it back to her.

'Seven-thirty, my goodness,' he looked at the clock, 'and I have a meeting at ten.'

'You've plenty of time.'

It took just over an hour to get to central London from their home using the M4 motorway. The Jaguar positively ate up the miles with Peter keeping an eye in the mirror for the police.

'What will you do today, Ginny?'

'I'll probably speak to Pierre again and the marketing men about the perfume. Pierre will be relieved to hear that you've sanctioned his appointment.'

'Surely he wasn't afraid of *me*?'

'I think *everyone* is a little afraid of you, darling.' She bent to kiss the tip of his nose. 'Except me.'

'Ginny,' he paused in the act of getting out of bed into the dressing-gown she held out for him, 'how can you *possibly* say a thing like that?' He had the petulant expression on his face of a spoiled child.

'Darling, you *are* a little frightening sometimes, especially recently with your moods. You weren't like that when I first knew you.'

'I was on the crest of a wave when I first knew you.' He finished getting into his gown and pulled the cord tightly round him. 'My company was small and I was expanding rapidly along the right lines. Somewhere, Ginny, I made a mistake. I think you once warned me about diversification and I let my excitement, my self-confidence, my wish to have a huge powerful empire, get the better of me. I did some unwise things . . . however, we must forget about the past, my darling, and hope that only good times lie ahead. Now that you are back with me I'm sure they do.'

He kissed her again and, as she sat on the side of the bed drinking her tea, she could hear the water running in the bathroom and her husband even singing.

Half an hour later they went downstairs together, Ginny in a housecoat. Once Simeon had gone she would bathe and dress at leisure, look at the post and deal with the many small matters that had accumulated during her absence. She would take a walk round the garden to get some exercise and maybe have a nap in the afternoon. She would make an appointment to see her gynaecologist in London the following week for a check-up, though the nausea had not recurred. She didn't even suffer from morning sickness. Only some days she did feel rather tired, more tired than she was accustomed to feel. The nap in the afternoon was welcome.

They never had a cooked breakfast. She had orange juice and cereal and Simeon some real black coffee and toast with marmalade. Consequently by a quarter to nine he was ready to leave and Peter had the car by the front door. Jones had opened the door and Varga had just bent to kiss Ginny on the lips when another car drew up beside the Jaguar and two men emerged.

They stopped for a moment to say something to Peter, who pointed to the door where Varga now stood looking down at them, Ginny just a step or two behind him.

For a moment Varga's eyes met those of the strangers and he had a feeling of terror so acute that he reached back for Ginny's hand.

'Darling, whatever is the matter?' She clutched his hand and rubbed it vigorously. 'You're frozen again. Who are these men, darling?'

'I've no idea.'

Holding tightly on to her hand he watched them as they came up and Jones went down the steps to speak to them. The group then looked again at Varga and Ginny standing beside him, and then continued their progress up the steps. Both men took off their hats.

'Mr Varga?'

'Yes?' His voice sounded tightly controlled.

'Might we have a few words with you, sir?'

'I'm afraid I'm just on my way to London,' he replied politely, looking at his watch. 'I have an important meeting at ten.'

'This is important too, sir,' one of the men replied equally politely. 'We are from the City of London Police and have come on a matter of some seriousness.'

Ginny felt Simeon's hand stiffen in hers.

'Please come inside,' he said in a matter-of-fact manner, releasing Ginny's hand. He then spoke to the butler who hurried down the stairs to tell Peter that his master would be delayed.

'May I come too?' Ginny asked as Varga conducted the police officers through the hall into the drawing-room.

'If you wish, Mrs Varga.'

'I'd rather, Ginny . . .' Varga began.

'I'd like to be with you, dear,' she said firmly.

He opened the door of the drawing-room and stood aside for the policemen to pass through. They stood for a few seconds looking at the room as though impressed by its size, maybe also by the scale and magnificence of the decoration. They then turned courteously to Varga, who motioned them towards the chairs drawn up in the middle of the room.

'Do sit down.'

'Detective Chief Superintendent Bradley,' the older of the two men produced a pass and turned to the man next to him, 'Inspector Ryan.'

They formally shook hands and, after Ginny was seated, the men also sat down and Inspector Ryan produced a notebook from his pocket.

'I'm extremely sorry to call on you at such an early hour, Mr Varga,' the superintendent said, 'but a matter has arisen which directly concerns you.'

Varga tried to moisten his lips but his mouth was too dry. Ginny noticed that he clung to the arm of his chair as if it supported him. She longed to be beside him, but even as the thought entered her mind the senior policeman turned to her. 'It also concerns you in a sense, Mrs Varga. Now if I can stop talking in riddles, as I can see I am bewildering you – the facts of the matter are these. We are questioning Mr Lambert Silklander about a picture by the artist Andrea Mantegna which appears to be missing from a valuable collection in Italy.'

'The Mantegna,' Varga gasped and Ginny, accustomed to his nuances, thought she detected relief rather than fear.

'Ah, you know it.'

'Please go on, Superintendent.' Varga was by now well in control of himself.

'It belonged to the collection of the late Alberto Caracóli who lived in a villa above Florence which he had inherited from his father. The collection apparently was priceless and went back to the Renaissance. Now it happens that I am attached to a special section of the City of London Police which is concerned with the tracing of missing or stolen works of art, and we were informed by an anonymous telephone caller that the picture found to be missing from the estate of the deceased had been taken by Mr Lambert Silklander – your brother, I believe,

Mrs Varga — to a picture restorer in Rome, who recognized it as one of the pieces missing from the late Signor Caracoli's villa. There is also independent evidence that someone — maybe a guest?' he looked enquiringly from Varga to Ginny, '— saw it here and believed it to be stolen.' His expression remained inscrutable. 'Such information has a habit of finding its way to us.

'Mr Silklander, who has been closely questioned, claims that the picture was legally purchased by him from a contact in Bulgaria and he has shown me what he believes is an authentic export certificate, but I believe it to be a forgery. There is no such ministry to authenticate works of art in a country as poverty-stricken as Bulgaria, as you might well be aware.

'Now the question is, Mr Varga, do you have this picture?'

'Why, certainly I have the picture,' Varga said, rising and looking down at his wife who, with a shocked expression, was staring at the elder of the two policemen. 'But naturally I had no idea it was stolen. If Silklander has done anything illegal, please don't involve me.'

'Simeon!' Ginny said indignantly. 'How *could* you say such a thing?'

Appearing more relaxed and at ease, Varga put his hands deep into his pockets and began to pace the room. 'Your brother and sister-in-law have advised me at every stage in the redecoration and refurbishment of this house, as well as of my offices in Mayfair. I am an ignoramus in these matters,' he smiled deprecatingly at the policeman, 'I'm sorry to say. I'm the sort of person who knows nothing about art, nor, do I much care! I was anxious, however, to begin a collection that would help me to impress and entertain the visitors to this house. I was accordingly advised solely by the Silklanders. I had never heard of this fellow Mantegna. Had you, Inspector?'

'He *is* rather a well-known artist, Mr Varga.' The superintendent coughed and got up. 'Do you think we might take a look at the picture in question?'

'Certainly. Come this way.'

Varga gestured towards the door and the inspector and Ginny followed them out of the room.

Ginny felt frightened, confused, as she climbed the stairs in the wake of the men and, after walking along the corridor, followed them into Varga's study where, in the corner by the window, in a relatively insignificant position, the Mantegna hung on the wall; the Sybil and the Prophet in conversation as they had been for centuries.

The superintendent put on a pair of spectacles and, while he carefully examined the painting, kept up a running commentary mainly for the benefit of his colleague. 'Undoubtedly Mantegna. A superb example of his grisaille style. You see the sculptured effect . . . gold on gold . . . Cincinnati . . . most probably the missing half . . .

'I beg your pardon,' he said at last, his face flushed with the thrill of discovery as he turned to Ginny and Varga. 'Art is a passion of mine. I was extraordinarily lucky to land this job. I can understand your eagerness to acquire such a masterpiece, but why, Mr Varga, did you choose to exhibit it in a place so poorly lit, where few people could see it? I would have thought in your beautiful drawing-room downstairs . . .'

'Look, let me level with you, Chief Superintendent.' Varga, by now thoroughly in control of himself, dug his hands deep into his pockets again. 'As I explained, I am not a connoisseur of art. I know frankly nothing about it. I was in the hands of Silklander to choose suitable works of art for me. I am absolutely astonished to hear he may have been party to a theft, and I'm sure there is some misunderstanding. But please, don't involve *me* in it.' He pointed to the painting. 'For God's sake, take the bloody thing.'

'You don't mind?'

'Of *course* I don't mind. I want to do all I can to co-operate.' Varga was about to take it from the wall when the policeman hurriedly stepped forward.

427

'Allow me, Mr Varga. It would never do . . . after five centuries . . .' With great care he unhooked the picture – it was not very heavy – and lowered it tenderly to the ground where once again he examined it closely.

'How much do you say you paid for it, Mr Varga?'

'Two million pounds,' Varga said, in evident disgust. 'And I don't suppose I'll see a penny of that.'

'It might have to go to law. It depends on whether the late Signor Caracoli sold the painting – which Mr Lambert says he did – or whether it was stolen.'

'I'm quite *sure* my brother wouldn't have been involved in a theft,' Ginny said angrily. 'He is a dealer of the highest repute.'

'That is what we all thought, Mrs Varga. The trouble is, there is no receipt, no record of the transaction, which he said was paid in cash. Your brother also *appears* to have lied, quite seriously.' Bradley looked severe.

'Then how did it get from Italy to Bulgaria?' Ginny asked.

'*That* is where the theft may have occurred. It's *possible* Mr Silklander acted in good faith, and Mr Varga undoubtedly did. But . . .' he picked up the painting which was not very large and tucked it under his arm, 'this will find a good home for the moment, in our vault, while we try and sort the matter out.' The policeman looked at his watch.

'I see it's nine-fifteen, Mr Varga. Doubtless you'll be anxious to be off to your meeting.'

'That's all?' Varga looked incredulous.

'That's all, for the moment.'

Ginny shook hands with the two men, allowed Varga to brush her cheek with a kiss and then stood at the top of the staircase as the three of them hurried down the stairs and, crossing the hall, disappeared through the front door, Chief Superintendent Bradley carefully clasping the precious painting.

She went swiftly to the landing window, from which she could see the men chat briefly in the drive with every sign of amiability; then, after shaking hands, they climbed into their respective cars. But for a long time after the cars had vanished up the drive Ginny remained there, transfixed, seeing and not seeing.

CHAPTER 23

Gloria Keane was more than happy to accept the invitation to view the Vargas' new house and renew her acquaintance with an erstwhile business contact. She drove down to Purborough Park in her Porsche and was busy admiring the view from the window of the car as Ginny ran down the steps to welcome her. Her pregnancy did not show, but caftans suited Ginny and this was blue, made of fine wool with large gold buttons and a mandarin collar. The women embraced as Gloria got out of the car, swathed in artificial fur and with fashionably high-heeled boots.

'I say, what a *place*!' She didn't conceal her admiration as she looked up at the house, seen at its best on this cold but beautifully clear and cloudless day in December. The backdrop to the house was a forest of firs gradually sloping up a hill so that, despite the classical style of the building, the setting was vaguely Austrian or Swiss.

'I didn't think it would be *quite* like this, Ginny dear.'

'It's a lovely home. That's the main thing.' Ginny linked arms with her friend and the two women walked slowly up the steps into the entrance hall, where logs blazed in the huge marble fireplace.

'A wedding present from Simeon, I hear?'

'Yes. He wanted me to have it.'

'Very wise.' Gloria nodded and extracted a cigarette

which she popped into her mouth and lit with a slim gold lighter. 'You don't mind do you?'

'Not at all. How do you mean, "wise"?' Ginny looked at her curiously.

'Well, it's wise to disperse one's assets. You never know do you? Now, please, a tour.'

Jones took her coat and Gloria gave him an approving look.

'A butler, too. I like.'

'Let's start at the top,' Ginny said, leading the way to the stairs, 'and work our way down.'

The tour took about half an hour, Gloria pausing every now and then to express her admiration, even though the house was only half furnished. Most of the top floors were bare and the room next to the Vargas' suite was being turned into a nursery. The yellow walls and blue curtains made Gloria pause and look enquiringly at Ginny.

'You're not – are you? Already?'

'Yes. Simeon is anxious for a family.'

'I thought he already had one,' Gloria murmured.

'*Our* family, and so am I.'

'Oh, don't misunderstand me, darling. That sounded rather bitchy. Only I always think of you as a woman devoted to her career. What about Oriole?'

'I mean to be a businesswoman *and* a mother. I want to tell you all about Oriole and our new perfume.'

'Is this the reason for the invite?'

'No. I wanted to have you to lunch because you sent us a very nice present and you haven't seen the house.'

The present had been a set of crystal glasses, quite valuable.

They walked casually along from the nursery suite, peeped into a guest bedroom – 'this is where you'll sleep when you come to stay' – and down the staircase back to the hall where Jones was waiting.

'Drinks are served in the drawing-room, Mrs Varga.'

'Thanks, Maurice.' She smiled at him before turning

431

back to Gloria. 'Now *this* is our *pièce de resistance*, I think you'll agree.'

Gloria did agree and, as she stood with her gin and tonic, she lavished praise on the colour scheme, the furniture, the heavy silk curtains, the paintings. She seemed to take a particular interest in these and walked around carefully examining each one. They were mostly eighteenth-century French masters, a light, delicate theme, reflected in the antique furniture and the luxurious fabrics of the curtains and upholstery. There was a pastoral scene by Watteau, the head of a child by Greuze and a minor but exquisite Fragonard which had echoes of *The Swing* in the Wallace Collection in London. In addition there were pastels and watercolours by lesser-known artists and a huge gilt mirror over the high marble mantelpiece which was possibly by Clodion.

Gloria had put on a pair of half-moon spectacles to examine the paintings and, arms folded, she nodded her approval as Ginny freshened her drink.

'Aren't you drinking?' Gloria enquired, removing her spectacles and folding them into her case.

'Umm, I don't really feel like it. I'll have a glass of wine, maybe, at lunch.'

'I approve,' Gloria nodded. 'I never wanted to be a mother, but if I had I would have done all the right things to ensure that I had the best baby possible.'

'Exactly!' Ginny sat in a chair facing her while Gloria's eyes restlessly continued their examination of the room.

'It's all *quite* exquisite. Is it true you have a Mantegna?'

'Oh, that's what you were looking for? I wondered about the scrutiny.'

'I didn't expect it here with all the exquisite French paintings. But I couldn't see it anywhere in our trip through the house.'

'The Mantegna's gone.'

'Oh they took it away, did they?'

'I expect you really know *all* about it?' Ginny gave her an ironic smile. 'Come clean, Gloria.'

'Don't forget, Ginny, I'm best friends with Lambert and Maggie. They were terribly indignant at the suggestion it was *stolen*.'

'Simeon wasn't too pleased, either.'

'But what exactly happened?'

'Lambert bought it in all good faith during a visit to Sofia. It had apparently been stolen from a collection in Italy, but no one knew that. Lambert's still not sure he won't be charged with something and Simeon's furious.'

'I can imagine; but weren't you a bit suspicious to have been offered a Mantegna?' She looked closely at Ginny who shook her head.

'No, I don't really know all that much about him. Do you?'

'Well, no.' Gloria also looked doubtful. 'But, I mean, if I were offered a Leonardo or a Rembrandt I would be suspicious, and Mantegna *is* in that category, well nearly.'

'Simeon had never heard of him!' Ginny laughed. 'So that makes him all the more angry. Mantegna meant nothing to him and now he's somehow under suspicion.'

'Strictly speaking, who does the painting now belong to?'

'In British law it remains with the original owner who, we're led to believe, is a doctor in Rome. He inherited his father's estate, which was when the picture, a family heirloom, was discovered to be missing. Gloria, shall we eat? You must be famished.'

'I *could* eat,' Gloria admitted, and Ginny led her into a small dining-room where she and Simeon sometimes ate when they were alone.

It was a delightful room overlooking sloping lawns at the back of the house which were fringed by the forest of pines. To eat there was a light fish terrine with a herb sauce, and a selection of cold meats and salads, followed by cheeses of various kinds and lemon syllabub. To drink there was a Chablis, of which Ginny had a glass and Gloria most of the rest.

'I thought we'd have a cold lunch, then we could chat,' Ginny said as the butler helped them to their seats.

'I approve.' Gloria nodded to the door after Jones had quietly closed it. 'Of course, I suppose you were used to this kind of thing?'

'What kind of thing?' Ginny took up her fork, looking puzzled.

'Servants, grand houses, a butler to push back your chair.'

'On the contrary. The Silklanders live very simply. Even my parents were a bit overawed by it all. They have no live-in servants and eat in the kitchen.' Ginny gave her a frank stare. 'If what you're saying is that Simeon is *nouveau riche*, he is. He is and he's proud of it. He likes fine things, a wife like me, and paintings, even if he knows nothing about them.'

'Don't misunderstand me, Ginny.' Looking distressed, Gloria put out her hand. 'Not for a moment. You know I *adore* Simeon, but . . .'

'But what?' Ginny felt a chill of fear; a resurgence of the fear, rather, that had never left her since the visit of the police; the notion that somehow Simeon and her brother were not being frank about the truth behind the acquisition of the painting.

'There are whispers in the City, you know. People are saying things.'

'*What* things?'

'That the company is in a bad way. It isn't very sound.'

'On the contrary, the company is *very* sound.'

'The share price has bombed on the Exchange.'

'It hasn't "bombed", it's gone lower. It was too high anyway. It's mainly this wretched strike at an insignificant paper mill in the north. Simeon admits he handled it badly. He left it to subordinates when he should have seen to it himself. Tony Liddle is a superb deputy; but he's limited. Simeon has a sure touch with people and they like him. Anyway, he's up there now and,

434

hopefully, it will all be sold and disposed of in the next few months.'

'He's sold a *lot*, hasn't he? That steel works in Germany . . .'

'He found it extraneous to his needs.'

'Some people say it was manufacturing parts for the Iraqi supergun; designed by that man who was murdered in Paris.'

'You're *not* suggesting that had anything to do with Simeon?'

'Oh, of course not. I guess that when he found out what it was doing he wanted to get rid of it.'

'He didn't like the set-up.' Ginny realized the feeling of nausea was returning, and she knew she couldn't touch her fish terrine. 'But as for even *implying* that he had anything to do with murder . . .'

'Ginny, I do *assure* you,' Gloria firmly put down her fork, 'I am simply echoing what they are saying in the City. Of *course* he had nothing to do with *that* – that horrible business; but he showed lack of judgement in getting involved with an operation as suspicious as Planz Steel. The shares were far too cheap.'

'Well, he hasn't got it now.'

'Then he had an airline in Mexico . . .'

'How did you know about that?'

Gloria tapped her nose. 'You can't hide anything in the City. They have a way of winkling out information of the most secret or clandestine nature. Let's just say that I know a bod who knows another who knows . . .'

'It was registered in one of his offshore companies. It had nothing to do with AP. It was simply of no consequence, used for flying fruit from South America. He got rid of that, too.'

'He's been cleaning up his act, hasn't he, Ginny?' Gloria looked at her keenly.

Ginny swallowed, aware that she was doing her job, the job that Simeon had asked her to do, badly, and it would have been better if she had not asked Gloria for lunch at all. 'Simeon realized something I'd told him from the beginning. He was overstretched, departing from the core, which was pharmaceuticals. He will keep a few key industries and dispose of the rest. Don't worry, Simeon won't go down. If you think that, you don't know my husband.'

Gloria broke into her bread and sat looking at Ginny, as though undecided how to proceed. Finally, with a deep sigh, she said: 'There *are* other rumours too, dear, not very nice ones, I'm afraid. The sort of things your best friend won't tell you.'

Ginny swayed very slightly, again momentarily overcome by nausea. She held tightly on to the table, her knuckles out of sight.

'Are you trying to tell me,' she said, her eyes fixed on the woman opposite, 'that Simeon has a mistress?'

There was silence while Gloria pushed away her plate and lit a cigarette.

'I don't honestly know,' she said, blowing smoke over her shoulder. 'I was a fool to mention it. A heel, too, I suppose, to smoke in front of you.' Angrily she stubbed out her cigarette. 'But I *have* been concerned about you and when I got your invitation I was anxious, troubled. I wondered how much you knew. You see the collapse in the share price isn't *just* to do with the performance of Simeon's companies. It's to do with him, as well. He's emerging as a distinctly shady sort of character; people are wondering if there was a reason for his excessive secrecy, after all. A few weeks ago there was a raid on a brothel . . .'

'*What*?'

'Oh, Simeon wasn't there; but the story *is* that his name is in some way linked with it. I can't say how. That's all I know. Something to do with drugs . . . all hearsay I suppose.'

'Or a deliberate attempt to *smear* Simeon!' Ginny rose and angrily hurled her napkin into the centre of the table. 'I'm surprised at you, Gloria, always such a good friend of mine, to bring me all this trash. I'm afraid you're no longer welcome here.'

Gloria rose, face flushed, eyes bright. 'Of course. I suppose you won't accept an apology? Because I really am sorry. I thought in a way you might know something; but obviously you don't. I'm very fond of you, Ginny, believe me. If I'm wrong I'll cut my throat, but if I'm not I'm glad I told you, so that when the blow comes, if it comes, you'll be prepared.'

She went swiftly over to her and pecked her cheek. 'Bless you, Ginny, take care.'

It was the most dreadful end to a private visit Ginny had ever known and she remained sitting statue-like at the table for some time after Gloria had left.

Eventually the door opened gently and Maurice sidled into the room. 'Did Mrs Keane not enjoy her lunch, madam?'

Ginny started from her reverie and attempted a reassuring smile.

'These City people are always in a hurry. Actually I'm going to lie down.'

'Of course, madam.' Maurice gazed disapprovingly at the remnants of a ruined lunch. 'I'll send Alice up.'

When Ginny reached her room her maid had turned down her bed, drawn the curtains and was hovering sympathetically with her gown.

'I didn't think you *looked* very well this morning, Mrs Varga. Now you spend the rest of the day in bed.'

'I'll be okay in a couple of hours.' Ginny slipped thankfully between the sheets. 'Frankly, I could have done without her visit, but I'm expecting my husband home tonight and want to be at my best.'

'Naturally, madam,' Alice said in a motherly way, tucking her in with such concern that Ginny half expected a kiss. 'Would you like one of your sleeping pills?'

'No, thank you.'

'Have a good rest, ma'am.'

'Thank you.' Ginny smiled gratefully at her and

watched as she tiptoed out of the room. For a while, she tossed and turned, unable to sleep. Gloria's words, her bitter, unkind innuendoes, went round and round in her head, while she wondered what on earth it all meant.

Six PM, and the place was deserted. Maybe, thinking he wouldn't come back, everyone had gone home early. Maybe they thought they'd earned it. It had been a hard week.

Varga turned on the lights in Dorothy's office and looked at her neat desk, cleared ready to begin business sharp at eight on Monday morning. He then went into his own, switched on the lights and, after putting down his briefcase, thumbed through the notes she'd made for him: a list of people who had called, a number of queries about various outstanding matters, plus a list of the best hotels in the West Indies so that he and Ginny could make a choice over the weekend for their Christmas vacation, now only two weeks away. 'Do make up your mind if you can this weekend, Mr Varga,' she'd written. 'I'm afraid some of them will be booked up. Kind regards to Mrs Varga. Have a nice weekend.'

Varga went over to his drinks cabinet and poured a small measure of scotch. He was not a drinker and the supply in his office was rarely used. Sometimes it wasn't opened for weeks. No *Dallas* life-style here. He took the tumbler back to his desk and sat down gazing at the list of hotels sprinkled among the Caribbean islands. Two weeks to go, and then two weeks alone with Ginny: a Christmas and a New Year together. Was it possible to believe, to hope, that the past was behind him and they could make a fresh beginning? They had so much to look forward to; especially the baby. Sometimes, now that the paper-mill strike was about to be settled, he thought it was and that his forebodings had been the disorder of a mentally and physically tired and overworked man.

He made a note to send Christmas presents to his children. Although he never saw them he didn't forget them, remembering birthdays and presents at Christmas and Easter. As far as he knew they never made any request to see him.

He linked his hands behind his head and, leaning back, gave a deep sigh. Yes he was tired, very tired, but he had come back from the north with the problem solved. He was willing to sell the entire business as a going concern as long as the strike was called off. They had promised to be back to work on Monday. He'd faxed Morgan, who would already have issued a press release and, hopefully, the share price, which had stabilized, would start to rise. Oh, the newspapers would soon sing a different tune.

He felt a gradual lessening of tension as he thought of his achievements over the year. He had got into and out of some pretty nasty situations. He had married a beautiful woman and they were expecting a child. He had a lovely house and, according to the experts, had acquired some fine masters and old antiques. He was not cultured, but from now on he was going to be. He would have a programme to include visits to art galleries, the opera. One painter he would give a clear miss would be Mantegna but, although that issue was far from settled, he hoped the area of art theft was sufficiently murky not to involve him. He would kiss goodbye to two million pounds – what had happened to it? he wondered – but it was a small price to pay for peace of mind.

There remained Melissa. He frowned. She had not called again, and Liddle hadn't seen her. He would like to make contact because he wanted to be sure she remained silent. He thought again of the man in the black and yellow outfit they'd paid off; but no, killing was no longer for him: the killing of the woman, the Berninis, the scandals were behind him. Hopefully.

He lifted the telephone receiver and tapped in the numbers of his home. It rang for some time and then Ginny answered.

'Darling?'

'Simeon!' He thought she sounded surprised rather than pleased. 'Where are you?'

'I'm at the office. I'm about to leave.'

'Already? That was quick.' Her voice was curiously dead.

'I said a week and it took a week. Sorry I couldn't call last night, darling. You all right? You sound odd.'

'I'm fine,' she said, but in the same detached voice. 'I saw Gloria Keane yesterday.'

'Oh good. Did she like the house?'

'Very much.'

'Was she all right? You *do* sound strange, Ginny.'

'I don't think she's convinced that the share price will pick up.'

'She's dead wrong there,' Varga laughed. 'I'm going to sell the paper business, lock, stock and barrel; yes, giving them back all they thought they'd lost, and the strike is settled. There's to be a press release over the weekend. It's a big weight off my mind.'

'Oh good.' Again she sounded apathetic.

'Darling, are you *sure* you're feeling quite well? The gynaecologist gave you a good report?'

'He said everything's fine.'

'And *you* feel all right?'

'Yes, I do.'

'I'll see you very soon, darling.' He blew kisses into the mouthpiece. 'And I love you.'

'See you soon,' she said and put the telephone down.

She didn't say 'I love you' back. Something was wrong with Ginny. He wondered if she was still brooding over the things he'd said about Lambert.

Well, he would soon sort that out. Tonight he would hold her in his arms and love her as she had never before been loved.

He rose from his desk, put the glass back on top of the drinks cabinet and stuffed the list of hotels in his pocket. They would have the most sumptuous delayed honeymoon anyone had ever had. Maybe he would hire a yacht for cruising round the islands. He put out the lights in his office, scribbled a note which he put on Dorothy's desk.

'Please enquire about yacht hire in the Caribbean. Thanks for the list. See you Monday.'

All he could think of now was Christmas and his holiday.

He ran down the stairs, switching off the lights as he went. He spent some time in the lobby re-setting the burglar alarm which he'd switched off when he entered. It had a complex code which only a few people knew.

Once he set it he had ten seconds to get out and, putting out the lobby lights, he went smartly through the main door and double-locked it behind him. The car stood by the kerb with Peter at the wheel waiting for him. Peter, reading the evening paper, did not see his boss emerge, and Varga stood for a moment or two savouring the cold night air. In London the stars were always obscured by a city haze but in the countryside they would be shining brightly over Purborough Park.

There was a movement to one side and a figure stepped out of the shadows. Varga felt a moment of intense fear and was about to shout for Peter when a voice hissed:

'Simeon.'

'Melissa.'

She came up to him and, in the street light, stared into his eyes. She wore a black coat and a headscarf that almost obscured her face. He put a hand on her arm and repeated her name.

'Melissa.'

'I tried to speak to you, Simeon.'

'Look, not here.' He glanced towards the car and saw Peter looking behind him as though he had just discovered the presence of his boss. He leapt out of the driver's seat and came running round, but Varga had already opened the back rear door and bundled Melissa in. He didn't want to take her back into the office. He was anxious to go home.

'Go take a walk round the block, Peter,' he said.

'Are you sure, sir?' Peter strived to peer into the gloom past his boss.

'Of course I'm sure. Take ten minutes.'

'Very good, Mr Varga.'

Peter went round and closed the driver's door. Then, without looking back, he walked out of the mews and turned the corner into Park Street.

Melissa sat upright, very still and tense, in the corner of the back seat of the car.

'Melissa.' Varga climbed in beside her, his voice tender, and put an arm round her.

'Please *don't*, Simeon!' she exclaimed, her teeth chattering with cold, or fear, and she tried to push him away. 'You behaved very *badly* to me, Simeon.'

'I know, Melissa, I know, but I did not forget you, and I would not forget you. What could I do? I was very vulnerable. I left a message that you were to be put through to Tony, but you never rang again. Look, Melissa, I have made arrangements for Tony to help you. He'll get you out of the country.'

'I never betrayed you, Simeon.' She was still shivering violently and he wondered if she needed a fix. She seemed not to be listening to him. He looked at her anxiously.

'I pro . . . tected you,' she rambled on. 'The police tried to get your name out of me – how did they know by the way? – but I said I'd never heard of you.'

'I know that.' He put out a hand and squeezed hers tightly.

'How did you know?' She looked at him sharply.

'Because they would have arrested me by now. I knew you'd be loyal.'

'I did it because I *loved* you, Simeon, and always have. Years ago you were very good to me and I have never forgotten it.'

'And you were very good to me and I have never forgotten that, Melissa. You gave a young insecure man

442

confidence and restored my self-respect.' He leaned forward and touched her cheek with his lips. 'There will always be that love, a deep love, a bond.'

'And yet you wouldn't help me.'

'Darling Melissa,' he held her hand even more tightly, 'I was terrified that the police would contact me. I relied on your loyalty and love. They appeared at the house a few weeks ago to enquire about a painting they thought was stolen and I nearly died of shock. You've got to understand.' He removed his hand from hers and sat upright, staring in front of him as though he were talking to himself rather than her, reliving those nightmarish days. 'I have been a bad man in my life, Melissa, and done many bad things. Maybe we destroyed a lot of people with drugs, who knows? The money made a big difference to me. I was ambitious to succeed and I have succeeded more than in my wildest dreams. But now I want to begin again.' He looked sharply at her. 'Tony will help you to get away. You must disappear. I don't want any trial, anything that could possibly lead to me. I have too much, much too much, to live for.'

'And what will happen to me?' she asked in a small voice.

'You will assume a new identity with as much money as you want for the rest of your life.'

'And will I ever see you again?'

'I hope so, darling Melissa. I hope so.'

'Can one *ever* make a fresh start, Simeon?' Her voice sounded so sad, so broken, that he turned to console her, his lips pressed against hers, seeking her mouth, her tongue. He felt her suddenly stiffen and the shivering stopped.

Whether he even sensed fear, or felt pain, as the low calibre bullet pierced his heart, will never be known.

'Mrs Varga?'

'Yes?' Ginny looked anxiously at the two police officers who came to the house at about nine-thirty. She had

443

just watched the nine o'clock news and when she heard the doorbell she thought it was Simeon; but Maurice had got there before her to open the door and she stood now in the hall, looking at them.

'Could we talk to you privately, Mrs Varga?'

'Of course. Come in. I hope nothing's wrong?'

Nevertheless she started to tremble.

She led the way into the small sitting-room, switched off the TV set: 'The weather throughout England will be . . .' and motioned for them to sit down. They remained standing and so did she. She could feel the nausea mounting but she desperately fought it off. The policemen were looking at her with concern. They had given her their names and ranks but she immediately forgot them.

'Please sit down, Mrs Varga.' She slumped into a chair and the knot in her stomach tightened. 'I'm sorry to say we have some very bad news for you, Mrs Varga.'

'My husband has had an accident!'

It was a statement rather than a question and the two men looked startled.

'Did you know?'

'I guessed by your faces. He was due home about an hour ago. He telephoned me just before seven. I was already feeling apprehensive when you arrived. There was no reply from the car phone.'

'I'm afraid he has been murdered, madam, shot through the heart.'

Ginny leaned forward in her seat and retched so hard she thought she would vomit. A policeman went to the door and asked Maurice, hovering uneasily in the hall, for water. By the time it arrived Ginny was feeling a little better, but her heart was hammering in her breast so violently that she thought it would stop. In a way she wished it would.

'I can't believe this,' she said faintly.

'I'm terribly sorry to bring you this news, Mrs Varga.'

Maurice stood by, a look of shocked horror on his face.

'Should I get Alice, Mrs Varga? Madam is pregnant,' he explained to the policeman, who looked more concerned than ever.

'You'd better get her doctor,' the senior officer said. Maurice went off to telephone.

'How . . . why?' Ginny said at last.

'It was outside his office, Mrs Varga, at about seven PM. We only know it was a woman.'

'A *woman* . . .'

'You wouldn't know, have any idea . . . ?'

'Of *course* I have no idea.'

'It seemed to be someone he knew. She appeared on the pavement and he invited her to sit with him in the back of the car.'

'But Peter . . .'

'He told the driver to go for a walk. He had no fear, no apprehension, but as he left they were talking earnestly together in the back seat as if they knew each other well. The woman wore black with a headscarf and the chauffeur had no chance to see her face. When he returned after ten minutes Mr Varga was lying in the back . . . he was bleeding profusely from a gunshot wound straight through the heart which would have killed him instantly. He can't have suffered. I am so sorry to give you this terrible news, Mrs Varga.'

What a useless, empty, but above all inadequate little word 'sorry' was, Ginny thought, at a time like this.

The sensational murder of a man on the verge of a City scandal made headlines throughout the world. Immediately any mud that anyone could discover about Varga was raked up and flung at him, and his shares went into free fall until they were suspended on the Stock Exchange. In a single day five hundred million pounds was wiped off their value.

There were pictures of Ginny and of the first Mrs Varga, who appeared almost as shocked as the second and retreated to her mother's home where the press were barred by a burly Italian at the gates.

Edward Thomas, private investigator, sat watching the news as the story unrolled. Pictures of Varga, of his office, of his beautiful home in Gloucestershire. Pictures of his first wedding, none of his second, as it had been a private affair and even the most diligent member of the press couldn't get hold of a picture. The second Mrs Varga was three or four months pregnant. Sad.

Varga emerged as a man of mystery, and, where the facts of his meteoric career were not known, they were speculated upon. Thomas slumped deeper in his chair and his hand went out to pat the dog who sat by his side as if she too had somehow linked the news with the death of her mistress.

Varga was dead and Kelly, who had spied on him, was dead. The police obviously had it in for the first Mrs Varga and the killer was known to be a woman, a woman probably envious and jealous, out for revenge. What woman would want to avenge herself on Varga in such a hideous fashion if not a spurned wife? Mrs Varga was taken in for questioning, but subsequently released because her alibi was unassailable. She had been at a dinner with friends, given by a charitable Italian society in the West End of London. However, the police still didn't seem satisfied because of the Italian connections. The mystery of the stolen Mantegna was brought into the daylight and the fact was that *that* story had originated in Italy. Was there a link? The scandal gathered momentum.

Edward thought of the evening after Kelly had been shot. He could remember it with such clarity as though it were yesterday. He had never visited her house in his life before and knew so little about her, even the fact that she had a cat and a dog who had sat patiently behind the front door waiting, a little anxiously perhaps, for her to return.

He had stroked the dog, fondled the cat — he liked animals, though he had none of his own — and looked round the house, a small terraced house in Wandsworth. It was a conversion and she had had the ground floor. There wasn't a thing out of place; no unwashed dishes, except the bowls for the cat and the dog neatly side by side on the floor. You'd have thought she would have put her cup into the sink before she went to work – she always got there before anyone else – but no, she'd washed it, made her bed. Everything was fresh, ready for her return; but she never would. He'd thought of her body in the morgue looking quite as it usually did except for the shattered windpipe which was hidden by a sheet. Calm, even serene, in death, she was the Kelly he had always known, yet actually known very little about.

In her armchair, beside the television set, in front of her bewildered cat and dog, he'd sat down that night and wept.

The cat and the dog he'd adopted. He didn't know their names, so he called the cat Floss and the dog Bunty. His children were delighted to have animals and they had settled down well. They gave no indication of missing their mistress as much as he did. As long as they had their food and comforts cats were all right. Maybe the dog pined for her a little. But her death had angered Thomas because it had been dirty and messy and wrong, and also because there was no one to care very much, no evidence she had ever really been loved.

The police had no clues, he had no clues. Cases were searched, but nothing came up. As a private investigator she seemed to have less priority than the humblest member of the public because the nature of her work made her vulnerable – drugs, industrial spying, contraband of all kinds. Her file seemed to go to the bottom of the police orders of priority.

But as he watched the news bulletins about the death of Varga, who clearly was at the top of their priorities, Thomas thought about the fact that Kelly had once watched Varga and had also been shot.

And, for some reason that he couldn't fathom, he

thought of the one piece of information Kelly had had which she'd hidden from her client Bernini and, until the last minute, from him. Up to now he had never considered its significance.

Varga patronized a brothel, just around the corner from his office in Mayfair.

Melissa had been dead about a week when the police found her. They'd searched high and low after the visit from Edward Thomas, as she'd jumped bail. In the end they were alerted by the landlady of a bed-sit in Maida Vale, an anonymous room in an anonymous house in one of those long, anonymous streets which are hard to tell apart. It was easy to get lost in Maida Vale: Sutherland Avenue, Elgin Avenue, Warwick Avenue, Lauderdale Road, Castelnau Road, Randolph Crescent, all so like one another with the same tall terraced houses, once the homes of the affluent middle classes, and now largely flatlets or bed-sits for the great amorphous sub-culture of London.

Melissa's death was due to a massive dose of heroin. She lay in bed in her nightclothes as though she'd just got in and fallen asleep. But the smell in the room was terrible and, although there was no gun, no bloodstains, no note, nothing to connect her with Varga's death, few entertained any doubts that she had killed him.

Pru had trained to be a nurse and was on the staff of a large hospital when she'd met Douglas and given it all up to marry him. Ever since then she'd been wife and mother, happy in her role as a farmer's wife. She was older than Ginny and, in truth, she had never understood her younger sister very much or what motivated her, made her so different from the rest.

Sometimes she'd envied Ginny her drive, determination and ability; but now she was glad she'd eschewed life in the fast lane for that of a farmer's wife. It was now, too, at a time when Ginny desperately needed her, that her style of life was shown to be superior to, as well as different from, that of her younger sister. She could give not only succour and support but also the benefits of her rich, deep experience of looking after people and animals and mothering children.

Ginny had miscarried spontaneously on the eve of Varga's funeral. In the opinion of the doctors the foetus had been deformed and she would have aborted anyway: just as well. In a way it was providential because, although the public didn't know then what they were later to know, Ginny knew everything. She knew all about her late husband that the police knew, that Liddle had told them, and that Melissa had always known.

Melissa was cremated quietly in an undenominational ceremony which no one attended except a solitary police officer. There was no one to mourn her or cry for her. Where were her friends? She had no one. The one and best friend she'd had she'd killed. No, no one to remember or mourn Melissa and what money she had, if she had any left, was never found.

Matteo Bernini attended the funeral of his brother-in-law on behalf of his family. Carlo stayed away, perhaps because he may have thought he was responsible for it. Neither Claudia nor his children attended.

Angus represented the Silklanders because he had known his brother-in-law least. There was a sprinkling of business colleagues, Liddle, and Dorothy, who wept quite unashamedly all the way through.

Simeon Varga was cremated and his ashes were scattered in the grounds of the crematorium.

Dust to dust.

Pru moved away from the window where she'd been thinking of those terrible events in the weeks before Christmas. She gazed at her sister's sleeping form and her face softened because she saw there the small girl that Ginny used to be; face a little flushed, dark hair thick and luxurious on the white pillow.

She wished then that her younger sister could return

to that childhood and begin all over again, take another path and never meet a man called Simeon Varga or encounter all the grief that meeting had brought her.

Ginny fluttered her eyelashes and opened her clear blue eyes. She saw her sister and smiled and then at once, as always, the smile was replaced by a stricken look as the memories came flooding back.

Pru sat on the edge of her bed and tenderly stroked her brow.

'How do you feel, darling?'

'I wish I could sleep for ever.'

'It'll take a long time, Ginny. You can't rush this.'

'It's as though he'd never been,' Ginny said suddenly, echoing Pru's thoughts. 'Nothing of him left, not even the baby.'

'Yes.' Pru paused and tentatively drew a piece of paper out of her pocket. 'At least there's *some* good news. No trace of HIV in you . . . or him . . . or her. We thought it best to ask the doctors to be certain, because of his life-style.'

'Yes.' Ginny's eyes glazed over. Extraordinary, no impossible, to think of the relationship between her husband and a drug-addicted prostitute that had continued all the time she'd known him.

She shuddered.

'Just as well it's all over, everything.'

'You're going to get away for a good long rest. Mummy's been persuaded to go on a cruise.'

Ginny thought of the plans she and Simeon had had for Christmas.

'As long as it's not the Caribbean.'

'It can be anywhere you like,' Pru said. 'But it certainly won't be the Caribbean.'

Christmas at Silklands was a restrained affair. There were no guests and no parties. Ginny came down for lunch on Christmas Day but only stayed for half the meal. She was constantly attended by a member of her family in

450

case her despair should make her harm herself; but her long periods of thoughtful silence were never suicidal.

In January she and her mother flew to Australia and then joined the QE2 on a cruise around Borneo and across the South China Sea to Hong Kong.

Ginny recovered, but slowly, and spent many an hour on deck staring into the depths of the sea.

Sometimes she imagined that, reflected in its shining surface, she could see the face of the man she had loved so much and lost gazing up at her with that soft, sad look in his eyes.

Then, and only then, sometimes she thought she forgave him.

EPILOGUE

È finita la commedia

Some thought that the woman – statuesque, elegant, beautifully dressed, had aged prematurely because of her experience. Others thought that maturity had made her even more beautiful. Yet, somehow, there lurked an air of sadness beneath the carefully applied but not over-elaborate make-up.

The smile was gracious, infinitely charming, as she took her seat in the front row looking at those around her. As the lights went down and the single spotlight illuminated the giant crystal bottle, a huge emerald twinkling on top, a roar of appreciation went up from the well-dressed, sophisticated crowd and everyone applauded. In the half-light Ginny could be seen, appreciative, serious, even a little critical. Miss Silklander, as she was now always known, was a perfectionist.

Silk; its essence of voluptuousness, of luxury. It had no memories of the past. Next to her Pierre Jacquet leaned forward in his seat in the room at the Ritz where the perfume was being launched.

It was eighteen months following his death, but a lot had happened since the concept of the campaign had been initiated when Varga was alive, Ginny married to him and expecting a baby.

Silk: it had a touch of the past, a feeling for the present, a hope for the future, and France was now Ginny's home. She had settled in a villa near Grasse, not far from the equally reclusive Jacquet. People were beginning to talk of them as a couple, but no one knew the truth.

Purborough Park had escaped the wholesale seizure of Varga's assets following the scandal after his death as he had, perhaps percipiently, put it in the name of his wife, who sold it as soon as she could. That once happy home, full of high expectations, had become a tomb. It fetched a high price, and with the proceeds she was able to buy Oriole from the receiver and revive its fortunes as she had promised she would.

Silk: it was tactile, clinging, slipping through the fingers, encasing the body in luxury. The perfume's subtle fragrance permeated the room, and when the kaleidoscopic presentation reached its climax there was a renewed roar and, as the lights went up, everyone cheered and turned to clap the perfume's originator and inspiration, who regally acknowledged the ovation.

She was dressed in a suit by Ungaro, a rich blend of tapestries on a grey background which could be worn for day or evening. She was becoming known for her style and her chic.

A widow with a past that no one envied.

She said little but smiled a lot; what words she spoke were carefully chosen. She already had an aura, the stature of a famous film star or the wife of an eminent man.

She was a survivor, a creator, the past firmly behind her. She believed in the future. At the end of the presentation several celebrated couturiers leapt forward to lavish kisses on her hand, maybe hopeful that one day she would create a fragrance for them. But there were no promises; a nod, a smile, a firm handshake. Silk would be hailed as one of the great fragrances of the century, Jacquet one of the greatest perfumers.

People turned to watch her walk out of the salon, Pierre at her elbow, his face turned attentively towards her.

Maybe, they thought, life would be kind to her yet.